Diff
Diagnosis
pocket

Clinical Reference Guide

Börm
Bruckmeier
Publishing

Authors: Christian Sailer, M.D., sailer@media4u.com
Susanne Wasner, M.D., wasner@media4u.com
Cover Illustration: Lucy Mikyna
Production: Sylvia Engel

© 2002–2007, by **Börm Bruckmeier Publishing LLC**
63 16th Street, Hermosa Beach, CA 90254
www.media4u.com
Second Edition

IMPORTANT NOTICE – PLEASE READ!
This book is based on information from sources believed to be reliable, and every effort has been made to make the book as complete and accurate as possible and to describe generally accepted practices based on information available as of the printing date, but its accuracy and completeness cannot be guaranteed. Despite the best efforts of author and publisher, the book may contain errors, and the reader should use the book only as a general guide and not as the ultimate source of information about the subject matter.
This book is not intended to reprint all of the information available to the author or publisher on the subject, but rather to simplify, complement and supplement other available sources. The reader is encouraged to read all available material and to consult other references to learn as much as possible about the subject.
This book is sold without warranties of any kind, expressed or implied, and the publisher and author disclaim any liability, loss or damage caused by the content of this book.
IF YOU DO NOT WISH TO BE BOUND BY THE FOREGOING CAUTIONS AND CONDITIONS , YOU MAY RETURN THIS BOOK TO THE PUBLISHER FOR A FULL REFUND.

Printed in China
ISBN 978-1-59103-216-8

Preface to the First Edition

Differential Diagnosis pocket is intended to help both students and physicians in their everyday clinical and private practice by placing at their disposal the basic materials for working through differential diagnostic questions. Here, for the first time, we have laid the groundwork by including clinical pictures as well as lab values, syndromes, cardinal symptoms, subjective complaints, and clinical signs. This forms the basis for the most comprehensive and broad-based approach possible with a single book.

We have placed special emphasis on manageable presentation. **Differential Diagnosis pocket** is arranged alphabetically, which makes it possible to locate items quickly. Related subjects or further explanations are cross-referenced by page number. The structured layout gives the reader a quick overview of a specific subject, and can then lead further to the details of possible differential diagnoses when required.

Each individual differential diagnosis begins with an introduction that contains important information, such as definitions, basic pathophysiology, incidence rates, or comments to get you off to a quick start. Reference ranges for lab values are also included.

We hope that **Differential Diagnosis pocket** will help you avoid the long, tedious process of searching out and compiling information from the various standard reference works. We would be happy to hear your criticism, ideas, and suggestions for improvement. Please write to us at **sailer@media4u.com**. We hope to hear from you!

Best wishes from

Christian Sailer, M.D.   January 2007
Susanne Wasner, M.D.

Additional titles in this series:
Anatomy pocket
Canadian Drug pocket 2006-2007
Drug pocket 2007
Drug pocket plus 2007
Drug Therapy pocket 2006-2007
ECG pocket
ECG Cases pocket
EMS pocket
Homeopathy pocket
Medical Abbreviations pocket
Medical Classifications pocket
Medical Spanish pocket
Medical Spanish Dictionary pocket
Medical Spanish pocket plus
Medical Translator pocket
Normal Values pocket
Respiratory pocket

Börm Bruckmeier Publishing LLC on the Internet:
www.media4u.com

Abdominal Discomfort

Very common complaint. Pay attention to concomitant symptoms like fever (→ 143), diarrhea (→ 101), nausea, vomiting (→ 252), hemorrhage and peritoneal irritation. See Abdominal Pain, Acute → 7

Diffuse abdominal discomfort
▶ Gastroenteritis (→ 101)
▶ Peritonitis
▶ Pancreatitis
▶ Leukemia
▶ Sickle cell crisis
▶ Appendicitis
▶ Mesenteric adenitis
▶ Abdominal aortic aneurysm
▶ Intussusception
▶ Colitis
▶ Ileus (→ 206)
▶ Inflammatory bowel disease
▶ Metabolic, toxic, bacterial causes

Epigastric and upper quadrants
▶ Gastrointestinal
 • Dyspepsia
 • Gastroesophageal reflux disease
 • Peptic ulcer disease
 • Gastritis
 • Irritable stomach
 • Stomach emptying disorder
 • Gastric tumors
 • Colon cancer
 • Cholecystolithiasis
 • Postcholecystectomy syndrome
 • Tumors of the gall bladder and bile ducts
 • Pancreatitis
 • Pancreatic tumors
 • Ulcerative colitis
▶ Hepatopathy (→ 226)
 • Congested liver
 • Hepatic tumors
 • Parasitosis of the liver
 • Cholecystitis

▶ Miscellaneous
 • Splenic rupture
 • Splenic infarction
 • Spleen tumors
 • Kidney cancer
 • Lymphomas
 • Myocardial ischemia
 • Basal pneumonia
 • Pleuritis
 • Pyelonephritis
 • Pulmonary embolism
 • Chronic infections
 • Lamblia
 • Tuberculosis
 • Aortic aneurysms
 • Diseases of the spine with pain radiating into the abdominal cavity

Left upper quadrant
▶ Splenomegaly
▶ Splenic rupture
▶ Splenic infarction
▶ Spleen tumor
▶ Renal pain
 • Pyelonephritis
 • Kidney cancer
▶ Gastritis
▶ Gastroduodenal ulcers
▶ Pancreatitis
▶ Pericarditis
▶ Empyema
▶ (Basal) pneumonia
▶ Pulmonary infarction
▶ Pleuritis

Right upper quadrant
▶ Cholecystitis
▶ Choledocholithiasis
▶ Pleuritis
▶ Pulmonary infarction
▶ Renal pain
▶ Pancreatitis
▶ Peptic ulcer
▶ Budd–Chiari S./ hepatic vein obstruction
▶ Hepatomegaly
▶ Hepatic abscess
▶ Hepatic tumor

A

▶ Hepatitis

Mesogastrium
- ▶ Mesenteric infarction
- ▶ Ileus (→ 206)
- ▶ Invagination
- ▶ Sigmoid volvulus

Lower quadrants
- ▶ Non-organic
  - • Intestinal motility disorders
  - • Irritable colon
  - • chronic constipation
- ▶ Organic
  - • Gastrointestinal
    - ○ Diverticulosis
    - ○ Inflammatory bowel disease
    - ○ Ischemic colitis
    - ○ Adhesions
    - ○ Neoplastic
  - • Urologic, nephrologic
    - ○ Urolithiasis
    - ○ Pyelonephritis
    - ○ Glomerulonephritis
    - ○ Hydronephrosis
    - ○ Polycystic kidneys
    - ○ Renal artery stenosis
  - • Gynecologic
    - ○ Adnexitis
    - ○ Cystitis
    - ○ Ovarian cysts
    - ○ Endometriosis
  - • Miscellaneous
    - ○ Vertebral problems
    - ○ Hernias
    - ○ Anorectal diseases (hemorrhoids, anal fissures)
    - ○ Lactose intolerance
    - ○ Opiate withdrawal
    - ○ Porphyria
    - ○ Aortic aneurysms
    - ○ Familial Mediterranean fever
    - ○ Lead intoxication
    - ○ Retroperitoneal fibrosis
    - ○ Retroperitoneal hemorrhage
    - ○ Diseases of the spine with pain radiating into the abdominal cavity

Right lower quadrant
- ▶ Appendicitis
- ▶ Inflamed ileal diverticulum
- ▶ Terminal ileitis/Crohn's disease (Inflammatory bowel diease)
- ▶ Adnexitis
- ▶ Ovarian cyst or torsion
- ▶ Ectopic pregnancy
- ▶ Ureteral colic
- ▶ Endometriosis
- ▶ Salpingitis
- ▶ Mittelschmerz
- ▶ Inguinal hernia
- ▶ Psoas abscess
- ▶ Seminal vesiculitis
- ▶ Renal pain
- ▶ Uteral colic
- ▶ Perforated ulcer
- ▶ Colon carcinoma
- ▶ Leaking aortic aneurysm

Left lower quadrant
- ▶ Diverticulitis
- ▶ Intestinal obstruction
- ▶ Appendicitis
- ▶ Gastritis
- ▶ Ureteral colic
- ▶ Psoas abscess
- ▶ Seminal vesiculitis
- ▶ Renal pain
- ▶ Adnexitis
- ▶ Ectopic pregnancy
- ▶ Ovarian cyst or torsion
- ▶ Endometriosis
- ▶ Salpingitis
- ▶ Mittelschmerz
- ▶ Ureteral colic
- ▶ Inguinal hernia
- ▶ Colon carcinoma
- ▶ Leaking aortic aneurysm
- ▶ Inflammatory bowel diease
- ▶ Splenomegaly

Flank pain
Dorsolateral origin with possible inguinal radiation, See Flank Pain → 146.

Abdominal distention, See Ileus → 206

Abdominal Enlargement

Sudden or progressive enlargement of the abdomen. Localized or generalized, intermittent or persistent.

Abdominal mass (localized abdominal enlargement, swelling)
► Hepatomegaly (→ 179)
► Cholecystitis
► Splenomegaly (→ 337)
► Pancreatic abscess
► Pancreatic pseudocyst
► Abdominal aortic aneurysm
► Crohn's disease
► Bowel obstruction
► Diverticulitis
► Volvulus
► Tumor
  • Colon cancer
  • Stomach cancer
  • Kidney cancer
  • Liver cancer
  • Gallbladder tumor
  • Neuroblastoma
  • Uterine leiomyoma (fibroids)
► Bladder distention
► Hydronephrosis
► Ovarian cyst
► Ureteropelvic junction obstruction

Generalized abdominal enlargement
► Ascites (→ 43)
► Ileus (→ 206)
► Large abdominal cyst
► Generalized peritonitis
► Congenital megacolon
► Large retroperitoneal tumor

Abdominal Pain, Acute

Acute abdomen
The acute abdomen is a serious acute intra-abdominal condition with pain, tenderness, and muscular rigidity. Emergency surgery must be considered.

Most common causes
► Acute appendicitis
► Acute gastroenteritis
► Acute cholecystitis
► Acute diverticulitis
► Acute pancreatitis
► Ileus (→ 206)
► Perforated gastric or duodenal ulcer
► Mesenterical infarction
► Gynecologic diseases

Abdominal pain in surgical emergencies
► Twisted ovarian cyst
► Ectopic pregnancy
► Intestinal obstruction
► Appendicitis
► General peritonitis from unknown cause
► Perforated peptic ulcer
► Perforated diverticulitis
► Leaking abdominal aneurysm
► Mesenteric embolism or thrombosis
► Biliary tract disease
► Pancreatitis
► Kidney stone

Abdominal pain in neonates, infants, and children
► Meconium peritonitis
► Intestinal obstruction from
  • Atresia
  • Stenosis
  • Esophageal webs
  • Volvulus
  • Imperforate anus
► Enterocolitis

Abdominal pain in women
► Dysmenorrhea
► Mittelschmerz (middle pain)
► Pelvic inflammatory disease (→ 279)

A
- ▶ Endometriosis
- ▶ Intrauterine contraceptive device (migration)

Intra-abdominal causes
- ▶ Infection and inflammation
  - Acute appendicitis
  - Acute cholecystitis
  - Acute gastroenteritis
  - Acute pancreatitis
    - ○ Necrotic pancreatitis
  - Acute peritonitis
  - Acute diverticulitis (poss. Meckel's diverticulum)
  - Inflammatory bowel disease
    - ○ Crohn's disease
    - ○ Ulcerative colitis
  - Abscess (subphrenic)
  - Pyelonephritis
  - Acute adnexitis
  - Splenic abscess
- ▶ Perforation, hemorrhage or rupture
  - Gastric ulcer
  - Duodenal ulcer
  - Anastomotic ulcer
  - Gastric carcinoma
  - Abdominal aneurysm
  - Acute appendicitis
  - Acute cholecystitis
  - Diverticulum
  - Spleen, liver or kidney rupture
    - ○ After blunt abdominal trauma
  - Tubal pregnancy
- ▶ Obstruction of a hollow organ
  - Ileus (→ 206)
    - ○ Mechanical
      - *- Colon tumor*
      - *- Stenoses*
      - *- Hernias*
      - *- Volvulus*
      - *- Invagination (children)*
    - ○ Paralytic
      - *- Toxic (peritonitis)*
      - *- Reflex (postoperative)*
    - ○ Metabolic
      - *- Hypokalemia*

- ○ Spastic
  - *- Lead intoxication*
  - *- Porphyria*
- Obstruction of the bile ducts
  - ○ Cholelithiasis
  - ○ Choledocholithiasis
  - ○ Stenosis of the bile papilla
- Obstruction of the urinary passages
  - ○ Kidney stones (renal colic)
  - ○ Ureter stones (ureter colic)
  - ○ Ureteral stenosis
- Urinary tract obstruction
  - ○ Misplaced urinary catheter
  - ○ Prostate hypertrophy/hyperplasia
  - ○ Prostatitis
- Testicular torsion
- Twisted ovarian cyst
- Ovarian tumor rotation
- ▶ Vascular
  - Abdominal bleeding
  - Abdominal angina
  - Mesenteric artery infarction
  - Mesenteric vein thrombosis
  - Omental ischemia
  - Portal vein thrombosis
  - Renal artery infarction
  - Aortic aneurysm
  - Splenic infarction
- ▶ Gynecologic
  - PID
  - Acute adnexitis
  - Extrauterine pregnancy
  - Ovulation (intermenstrual pain)
    - ○ Mittelschmerz
  - Dysmenorrhea
  - Ovarian cysts
  - Ovarian torsion
  - Ovarian tumor rotation
- ▶ Cancer
  - Stomach
  - Pancreas
  - Colon
  - Liver
  - Kidney
  - Metastatic tumor

- Peritoneal carcinomatosis
- ▶ Functional disorders
  - Irrritable bowel syndrome
  - Nonulcer dyspepsia
  - Sphincter of Oddi dysfunction
  - Functional constipation
- ▶ Pelvic disorders
  - Inflammation
    - ◦ Pelvic inflammatory disease
    - ◦ Tuboovarian disease
    - ◦ Endometris
    - ◦ Salpingitis
    - ◦ Cystitis
    - ◦ Seminal vesiculitis
    - ◦ Epididymitis
  - Mechanical disorders
    - ◦ Ovarian cyst
    - ◦ Ectopic pregnancy
    - ◦ Omental torsion

Extra-abdominal
- ▶ Metabolic, endocrine
  - Diabetic coma
    - ◦ Ketoacidosis
  - Hyperlipidemia
  - Hyperparathyroidism
  - Hypercalcemia
  - Tetany
  - Thyrotoxic crisis
  - Addisonian crisis
  - Uremia
  - Porphyria (!)
  - Hemochromatosis
- ▶ Hematologic
  - Hemolytic anemia
  - Henoch-Schönlein purpura
  - Sickle cell anemia
  - Leukemia
  - Lymphoma
  - Polycythemia
- ▶ Neurologic
  - Herpes zoster
  - Tabes dorsalis
  - Herniated disc
- ▶ Bones
  - Lumbago

- Vertebral body degeneration
- Intercostal neuralgia
- Diskitis
- Coxitis
- Pelvic osteomyelitis
- ▶ Cardiovascular
  - Angina pectoris
  - Myocardial infarction
  - Perimyocarditis
  - Acute right ventricular failure
    - ◦ E.g. after pulmonary embolism (capsular pain from congested liver)
  - Aortic aneurysm
    - ◦ Dissecting aneurysm
  - Pulmonary embolism
  - Infectious endocarditis with splenic infarction
- ▶ Thoracic
  - Esophagitis
  - Esophageal ruptur (Boerhaave's syndrome
  - Pneumonia
  - Pulmonary embolism
  - Penumothorax
  - Empyema
  - Pleuritis
- ▶ Collagen vascular disease
  - Polyarteritis nodosa of the mesenteric vessels
  - LE
- ▶ Toxins
  - Snake bite
  - Insekt bite
  - Lead poisoning
- ▶ Psychiatric
  - Depression
  - Anxiety disorders
  - Schizophrenia
  - Factitious abdominal pain
- ▶ Miscellaneous
  - Acute abdomen in patients with AIDS
    - ◦ Infectious gastroenteritis (common)
    - ◦ CMV enterocolitis
    - ◦ Atypical mycobacterioses
      - - M. avium

- *M. kansasii*
- *M. fortuitum*
- *M. xenopi*
- Salmonellosis
- Mycobacterium avium infection of the retroperitoneum and spleen
- Acalculic cholecystitis or sclerosing cholangitis due to CMV infection or cryptosporidiosis
- Perforation
- Non-Hodgkin's lymphoma of the gastrointestinal tract
- Kaposi's sarcoma of the gastrointestinal tract
- Narcotic withdrawal
- Heat stroke
- Behçet's syndrome (aphthoid-ulcerative changes of the oral and genital mucosa, iritis, erythema nodosum and arthritis)
- Unexplained intractable abdominal pain

Acanthocytes
See Erythrocyte, Morphology → 132

Achalasia

Failure of the esophagus to relax, inability of the lower esophageal sphincter (LES) to open and let food pass into the stomach. Caused by degeneration of the myenteric plexus, resulting in dysphagia (→ 110), regurgitation and dilation of the esophagus (megaesophagus).

Primary
▶ Idiopathic achalasia (cause unknown)
Secondary
▶ Chagas' disease
▶ Neoplasms
  • Gastric carcinoma
  • Bronchial carcinoma
  • Lymphoma
    ○ Non-Hodgkin's lymphoma
    ○ Hodgkin's lymphoma
  • Prostate cancer
  • Mesothelioma
▶ Chronic idiopathic intestinal pseudo-obstruction
▶ Syrcoidosis
▶ Amyloidosis
▶ Ischemia
▶ Neurotropic viruses
  • Herpes zoster
▶ Drugs, toxins
▶ Radiation therapy
▶ Postvagotomy

Acid Phosphatase (AP)

Group of enzymes that liberate inorganic phosphate from phosphoric esters. The enzyme is localized in the lysosomes of all body cells, with high activity in the liver, bone marrow, prostate, erythrocytes and thrombocytes.

Reference range
0–5.5 U/l
Increased
▶ Prostate disease
  • Prostate cancer
  • Benign prostatic hypertrophy
  • Prostatitis
  • Prostatic manipulation
▶ Bone diseases
  • Osteosarcoma
  • Bone metasteses
  • Paget's disease
  • Osteogenesis imperfecta
▶ Hematologic disease
  • Multiple myeloma
  • Polycythemia
  • Leukemia
  • Megaloblastic anemia
  • Hemolysis
  • Thrombocytosis
  • DIC
▶ Hyperparathyroidism
▶ Breast cancer
▶ Gaucher's disease

▶ Liver disease
▶ Chronic renal failure

Acidosis, Metabolic

A condition of low arterial pH, reduced plasma HCO_3^- concentration, and usually compensatory alveolar hyperventilation resulting in decreased PCO_2. Increased accumulation of acid equivalents through metabolism or impairment of the regulatory ability of liver or kidneys. Compensation is made through the lungs. If the acid load overwhelms respiratory capacity, acidemia (arterial pH < 7.35) will result.

Disorder	H^+	pH	HCO_3^-	pCO_2
Met. Ac.	↑	↓	↓↓*	(↓)
Met. Alk.	↓	↑	↑↑*	(↑)
Resp. Ac.	↑	↓	(↑)	↑↑*
Resp. Alk.	↓	↑	(↓)	↓↓*

* primary change

See Alkalosis, Metabolic → 18
See Acidosis, Respiratory → 12
See Alkalosis, Respiratory → 19

Primary metabolic disorder
▶ pH changes in same direction as bicarbonate, pCO_2
▶ Metabolic acidosis
  • Serum ph decreased
  • Serum bicarbonate and $paCO_2$ decreased
▶ Metabolic alkalosis
  • Serum ph increased
  • Serum bicarbonate and $paCO_2$ increased

Primary respiratory disorder
▶ pH changes in opposite direction as bicarbonate, $paCO_2$
▶ Respiratory acidosis
  • Serum ph decreased
  • Serum bicarbonate and $paCO_2$ increased
▶ Respiratory alkalosis
  • Serum ph increased
  • Serum bicarbonate and $paCO_2$ decreased

Classification I
▶ Addition acidosis
  • Endogenous acid production:
    ○ Ketoacidosis
      - *Diabetic (pre)coma (typical in diabetes)*
      - *Starvation*
      - *Alcoholism*
      - *Thyrotoxicosis*
    ○ Lactic acidosis
      - *Vasomotor ataxia*
      - *Shock*
      - *Hypoxia*
      - *Hyperventilation*
      - *Mesenteric insufficiency*
      - *Sepsis*
      - *Pancreatitis*
      - *Severe burns*
      - *Hepatic failure*
      - *Leukemias, lymphomas*
      - *Congenital metabolic disorders*
      - *Chronic respiratory alkalosis*
      - *Drugs (biguanides, salicylates, sorbitol and xylitol infusion, ethanol intoxication, isoniazide)*
    ○ Fever
    ○ Heavy physical work
    ○ Fetal emergency situation during childbirth
  • Exogenous acid supply
    ○ Intoxication
      - *Barbiturates*
      - *Salicylates*
      - *Carbonic anhydrase inhibitors*
      - *Methyl alcohol*
      - *Glycol*
      - *Methionine*
    ○ Spironolactone intoxication
  • Increased chloride absorption
    ○ Ammonium chloride medication

A

- Infusion of 0.9% NaCl-Solution
  - Potassium substitution with neutral salts
- ▶ Retention acidosis (reduced renal acid elimination)
  - Renal failure
    - Glomerular/tubular retention acidosis
    - Chronic interstitial nephritis
    - Distal tubular acidosis (type I)
    - Acute renal failure
- ▶ Base loss
  - Biliary fistula
  - Small intestine fistula
  - Diarrhea
  - Inflammatory intestinal diseases
  - Ileus (→ 206)
  - Following chronic hyperventilation
- ▶ Renal bicarbonate loss
  - Proximal tubular acidosis (type II)
  - Distal renal tubular acidosis
  - Hyperkalemic renal tubular acidosis
  - Therapy with carbonic anhydrase inhibitor
  - Acetazolamide

Classification II
- ▶ Lactic acidosis without hypoxia
  - Drugs, toxins
    - Alcohol
    - Methyl alcohol
    - Salicylates
    - Acetaminophen
    - Sodium nitroprusside
    - Catecholamines
    - Biguanides
    - Isoniazide
    - Infusions
      - *Fructose*
      - *Sorbitol*
      - *Xylitol*
  - Severe hepatopathy
  - Diabetic regulatory dysfunction
    - Diabetic ketoacidosis
  - End-stage renal failure
  - Tumor

- Leukemia
- ▶ Lactic acidosis with hypoxia
  - Circulatory insufficiency
  - Shock
  - Myocardial infarction
  - Hypovolemia
  - Sepsis
  - Pulmonary embolism
  - Cardiac pump failure
  - respiratory failure
    - COPD
    - Status asthmaticus
    - CO_2 intoxication
- ▶ Physical activity

Classification III
- ▶ Increased anion gap (→ 34)
- ▶ Normal anion gap (→ 34)

Acidosis, Respiratory

A condition of low arterial pH, hypoventilation resulting in an elevated PCO_2, and usually compensatory increase in plasma HCO_3^- concentration. Decrease in blood pH is often caused by retention of carbon dioxide due to inadequate pulmonary ventilation or hypoventilation (→ 319), unless compensated by renal retention of bicarbonate.

Disorder	H$^+$	pH	HCO$_3^-$	pCO$_2$
Met. Ac.	↑	↓	↓↓*	(↓)
Met. Alk.	↓	↑	↑↑*	(↑)
Resp. Ac.	↑	↓	(↑)	↑↑*
Resp. Alk.	↓	↑	(↓)	↓↓*

* primary change

See Respiratory Failure → 319
See Dyspnea → 112
See Acidosis, Metabolic → 11
See Alkalosis, Metabolic → 18
See Alkalosis, Respiratory → 19

Causes
▶ Airway obstruction
- Laryngeal spasm or edema
- Tracheal stenosis or edema
- Sleep apnea
- Mechanical
  ○ Foreign body
  ○ Neoplasm
  ○ Aspirated fluid
- Bronchospasm
▶ Cardiopulmonary, thoracic
- Cardiac failure
- Pneumonia
- Pumonay edema
- Respiratosy distress syndrome
- Restrictive lung disease
- Pulmonary embolism
- Pneumothorax
- Chest trauma
- Smoke inhalation
- Inadequate mechanical ventilation
- Kyphoscoliosis
▶ Neuromuscular
- Drugs, toxins
  ○ Sedatives
  ○ Tranquilizers
  ○ Anticholinesterases
  ○ Anesthetics
- Injury or infarction
  ○ Cerebral
  ○ Brainstem
  ○ High spinal cord injury
- Neuromuscular
  ○ Myasthenia gravis
  ○ Guillain-Barré syndrome/ Polyradiculitis
  ○ Amyotrophic lateral sclerosis
  ○ Poliomyelitis
  ○ Tetanus
  ○ Botulism
- Myopathy involving respiratory muscles
  ○ Hypokalemic myopathy
  ○ Familial periodic paralysis
  ○ Muscular dystrophy

- Primary hypoventilation
- Sleep apnoe syndrome
- Diaphragmatic paralysis

Acrocyanosis

Persistent, painless, symmetric cyanosis of the hands and less commonly the feet caused by vasospasm of the small vessels of the skin.

DDx
▶ Localized peripheral cyanosis
- Raynaud's syndrome
- Vegetative vasomotoric hyperexcitability
- Venous thrombosis
- Peripheral arterial occlusive disease
- Constitutional acrocyanosis
- Cold agglutinin disease
- Paroxysmal cold hemoglobinuria
- Perniosis
- Acrodynia (Feer's disease)
- Waldenström's syndrome
▶ Congenital cardiac defect with right-to-left shunt
- Tetralogy of Fallot
- Patent ductus arteriosus
- Acquired cardiac defects
- Cor pulmonale
- Left ventricular failure
- Mitral stenosis
- Congestive cardiomyopathy
- Mitral valve insufficiency
▶ Pulmonary
- Chronic bronchitis
- COPD
- Pulmonary emphysema
- Pulmonary fibrosis
- Bronchiectases

Acromegaly, See Growth Hormone → 159

ACTH

Adrenocorticotropic hormone

Polypeptide hormone of the anterior lobe of the hypophysis stimulating growth of the adrenal cortex or secretion of its hormones. Indicator in differential diagnosis of hypercortisolism (Cushing's syndrome (→ 91), and adrenocortical insufficiency.

Increased

▶ Central Cushing
- Pituitary ACTH secreting adenoma (usually microadenomas)
- Hypothalamic hyperfunction (increased corticotropin-releasing hormone)

▶ Ectopic ACTH syndrome
- Practically any tumor can cause ectopic ACTH syndrome. In over 50% of cases it is caused by lung cancer, followed by islet cell malignancies and thymomas.

▶ ACTH therapy

▶ Primary adrenal cortical insufficiency (Addison's disease). See Addison's Disease → 14.
- Autoimmune/idiopathic (~80%)
- Congenital
- Hemorrhage/infarction
  ○ Waterhouse-Friderichsen
- Iatrogenic
- Infections
  ○ Tuberculosis
- Drugs
- Infiltrative, neoplasm

Decreased

▶ Adrenal Cushing
- Adrenal adenoma
- Adrenal hyperplasia
- Adrenal carcinoma

▶ Iatrogenic hypercortisolism
- Long-term glucocorticoid therapy (most common cause)

Addison's Disease

Adrenal cortical insufficiency

Chronic insufficiency of the adrenal cortex due to insults to the adrenal including physical trauma, hemorrhage and tuberculosis of the adrenal. Characterized by bronzing of the skin, anemia, weakness, and low blood pressure.

Primary adrenocortical insufficiency (Addison's disease)

▶ Autoimmune/idiopathic (~80%)

▶ Congenital
- Adrenal aplasia/hypoplasia
- Familial glucocorticoid deficiency
- Adrenal leukodystrophy
- Congenital adrenal hyperplasia

▶ Hemorrhage, infarction
- Anticoagulation
- Arteritis
- Coagulopathy
- Embolus
- Hypotension
- Neonatal
- Pregnancy
- Sepsis
  ○ Waterhouse-Friderichsen syndrome
- Surgery
- Thrombosis
- Trauma

▶ Iatrogenic
  ○ Bilateral adrenalectomy
  ○ Radiation (therapy)

▶ Infections
- AIDS
  ○ CMV
  ○ Cryptococcosis
  ○ Kaposi's sarcoma
  ○ Mycobacterium avium
  ○ Toxoplasmosis
- Fungal
  ○ Blastomycosis
  ○ Coccidiomycosis
  ○ Cryptococcosis

- ○ Histoplasmosis
- Syphilis
- Tuberculosis (~20% of all Addison's)
▸ Drugs
  - Aminoglutethimide
  - Barbiturate
  - Etomidate
  - Ketoconazole
  - Metyrapone
  - Mitotane
  - Phenytoin
  - Rifampin
  - Spironolactone
  - Suramin
  - Trilostane
▸ Infiltrative
  - Amyloidosis
  - Hemochromatosis
  - Sarcoidosis
▸ Neoplasm
  - Leukemia
  - Lymphoma
  - Metastases
▸ Coma
▸ Uremia
▸ Volume/electrolyte disorders

Secondary (pituitary) or tertiary (hypothalamic) adrenocortical insufficiency
▸ After surgery of cortisol-secreting tumor
▸ Drug withdrawal
  - ACTH
  - Glucocorticoids
  - Megestrol acetate

Adrenal Tumor

Unilateral
▸ Functional
  - Adrenal adenoma
  - Adrenal carcinoma
  - Pheochromocytoma
  - Primary aldosteronism
▸ Nonfunctional
  - Adrenal adenoma
  - Adrenal carcinoma
  - Ganglioneuroma
  - Myelolipoma
  - Hematoma
  - Adrenolipoma
  - Metastasis

Bilateral
▸ Functional
  - ACTH-dependent Cushing's syndrome
  - Congenital adrenal hyperplasia
  - Pheochromocytoma
  - Conn's syndrome (hyperplastic)
  - Micronodular adrenal disease
  - Idiopathic bilateral adrenal hypertrophy
▸ Nonfunctional
  - Infection
    - ○ Tuberculosis
    - ○ Fungi
  - Infiltration
    - ○ Leukemia
    - ○ Lymphoma
  - Amyloidosis
  - Hemorrhage
  - Bilateral metastases

Adnexitis
See Pelvic Inflammatory Disease → 279

Adrenal cortical insufficiency
See Addison's Disease → 14

Adrenocorticotropic hormone
See ACTH → 14

Adult respiratory distress syndrome
See Pulmonary Edema → 303

Adynamia, See Fatigue → 140

AFP

Alpha-Fetoprotein

AFP is formed by the fetus in the gastrointestinal tract and the liver, as well as embryonic yolk sac. It is thought to protect the fetus from maternal estrogens and immunologic rejection, as well as substituting for the albumin that predominates later. Concentrations > 50 µg/l in adults are pathognomonic for an AFP-producing tumor.

Normal values	
Newborns	< 140,000 µg/l
Non-Pregnant:	< 25 ng/ml
Fetal serum	Peak: 3 mg/ml (13th week)
Amniotic fluid	Peak: 30 ug/ml (13th week)
Maternal serum (MSAFP)	Peak: 100 ng/ml (30th week)

Increased AFP
▶ Hepatocellular carcinoma
▶ Ovarian tumors
▶ Germ cell tumors
▶ Testicular tumor (non-seminoma)

Slightly increased AFP
▶ Pancreatic cancer
▶ Gastric carcinoma
▶ Bronchial carcinoma

Increased maternal AFP
AFP > 100 µg/l in the 16th-20th week of gestation (abnormal maternal serum AFP =MSAFP)
▶ Fetal malformation
  • Anencephaly
  • Spina bifida
  • Abdominal wall defects
▶ Multigravida
▶ Intrauterine malnutrition
▶ Exomphalos
▶ Astroschisis
▶ Placental abnormalities
▶ Threatened abortion
▶ Fetal death in utero
▶ Multiple pregnancy (twin gestation)

Decreased maternal AFP
▶ Chromosomal abnormalities
  • Down's syndrome

Agranulocytosis, See Leukopenia → 223

Alanine aminotransferase
See Aminotransferases → 23

Albumin

Main protein in human blood. Only reduced levels are clinically relevant. About 70% of total body albumin is found in the interstitial space. Also occurs in liquor and muscle. Function: regulation of the oncotic pressure of blood, transport protein for water, salts (calcium), pigments (bilirubin), free fatty acids and drugs. Since many drugs are bound by albumin, a hypoalbuminemia can lead to an increase in pharmacologically available drug with the same dosage.

Reference range	
In serum:	3.5-5.2 g/dl
In urine:	< 10 mg/g (morning urine) < 30 mg/24 h urine

Hypoalbuminemia
▶ Liver diseases (decreased synthesis)
  • Cirrhosis
  • Hepatitis
▶ Nephrotic syndrome
▶ Gastrointestinal
  • Severe malnutrition
  • Malabsorption
  • Protein-loosing enteropathy
▶ Infection/inflammation
  • Inflammatory bowel disease
  • Acute and chronic infectious and inflammatory diseases
▶ Malignancies
▶ Iatrogenic

- After hemodialysis
- Oral contraceptives
- Rapid intravenous hydration
▶ Severe burns
▶ Pregnancy
▶ Pre-eclampsia
▶ Cystic fibrosis
▶ Lymphangiectasia
▶ Prolonged immobility
▶ Miscellaneous
  - Rheumatoid arthritis
  - Lupus erythematosus
  - Rheumatic fever
  - Waldenström's syndrome
  - Idiopathic hyperlipidemia
▶ Rare causes
  - Sarcoidosis
  - Leishmaniasis
  - Leprosy
  - Ménétrier's disease

Hyperalbuminemia
▶ Iatrogenic albumin substitution
▶ Dehydration (pseudohyperalbuminemia)

Albuminuria, See Proteinuria → 298

Aldosterone

Mineralocorticoid hormone produced by the zona glomerulosa of the adrenal cortex. Facilitates potassium exchange for sodium in the distal renal tubule, causing sodium reabsorption and potassium and hydrogen loss. Regulating the balance of salt and water in the body and regulating blood pressure.

Reference range

Plasma	At rest	< 8 ng/dl
	After stimulation	2–6 x increase
24 h urine		5–19 µg

See Hyperaldosteronism → 186
See Hypoaldosteronism → 198

Aldosteronism. See Conn's syndrome, aldosteronism → 186

Alkaline Phosphatase (AP)

Group of enzymes that hydrolyze many orthophosphoric monoesters and are present ubiquitously (liver, kidney, bones, intestine and placenta)

Reference range

55–170 U/l

Increased serum AP
▶ Physiologic
  - During growth (bone AP, up to 700 IU/l)
  - In last trimester of pregnancy (placental AP)
▶ Pathologic
  - osteogenic (increased osteoblast activity)
    ○ Rickets
    ○ Osteomalacia
    ○ Fracture healing
    ○ Osteonecroses
    ○ Osteomyelitis
    ○ Hyperparathyroidism
    ○ Paget's disease
    ○ Bone tumors
    ○ Osteosarcoma
    ○ Metastatic bone tumors
    ○ Multiple myeloma
    ○ Osteoblastic metastases
    ○ Prostate carcinoma
    ○ Breast cancer
    ○ Osteomyelosclerosis
  - Gastrointestinal
    ○ Bowel disease
      - *Ulcerative colitis*
      - *Bowel perforation*
    ○ Hepatic cholestasis
      - *Fatty liver*
      - *Alcoholic hepatitis*
      - *Benign or malignant liver tumor*
      - *Primary biliary cirrhosis*

A

- *Drug induced liver disease*
- *Hepatic granuloma*
- *Hepatic cyst*
  ○ Biliary cholestasis
    - *Cholecystitis*
    - *Cholelithiasis*
    - *Primary biliary cirrhosis*
  ○ Hepatitis (liver AP)
  ○ Cholestasis (bile duct AP)
  ○ Cirrhosis
  ○ Cholangitis
  ○ Liver abscesses
  ○ Hodgkin's lymphoma with and without liver involvement
  ○ Liver metastases
  ○ Hepatotoxic
    - *Drugs*
    - *Intoxications*
- Miscellaneous
  ○ Endocrine
    - *Hyperparathyroidism*
    - *Hyperthyroidism*
    - *Acromegaly*
  ○ Sarcoidosis
  ○ Polyarteritis nodosa
  ○ Diabetes mellitus
  ○ Acute pancreatitis
  ○ Renal failure (renal osteopathy)
  ○ Right ventricular failure (→ congested liver)
  ○ Fanconi's syndrome (hereditary impairment of amino acid metabolism with cystine storage in miscellaneous organs, rachitic microplasia and nephropathy)
  ○ Paraneoplastic
    - *Hodgkin's lymphoma*
    - *Hypernephroma*
    - *Bronchial carcinoma*
  ○ Pregnancy
  ○ Hereditary hyperphosphatasemia

Decreased serum AP
▶ Vitamin D intoxication
▶ Pernicious anemia
▶ Hypothyroidism

▶ Celiac sprue
▶ Malnutrition
▶ Fibrate therapy

Alkalosis, Metabolic

Loss of acids or retention of bicarbonate (HCO3). Respiratory compensation. Through transmineralization: Hypokalemic alkalosis. (pH > 7.45, HCO3 > 29 mmol/l)

Disorder	H$^+$	pH	HCO$_3^-$	pCO$_2$
Met. Ac.	↑	↓	↓↓*	(↓)
Met. Alk.	↓	↑	↑↑*	(↑)
Resp. Ac.	↑	↓	(↑)	↑↑*
Resp. Alk.	↓	↑	(↓)	↓↓*

* primary change

See Acidosis, Metabolic → 11
See Acidosis, Respiratory → 12
See Alkalosis, Respiratory → 19

Base excess
▶ Overcorrection of acidosis with bicarbonates
▶ Hepatic coma
▶ Administration of citrates (banked blood)
▶ Milk alkali syndrome
▶ Alkali therapy for stomach problems

Acid loss
▶ Loss of stomach acid
  • Vomiting
  • Hyperemesis gravidarum
  • Gastric juice drainage
▶ Hypokalemia
  • Saluretic therapy for hypokalemia
  • Renal potassium loss
  • Conn's syndrome
  • Bartter's syndrome
  • Gastrointestinal potassium loss
    ○ Diarrhea
▶ Mineralocorticoid therapy
▶ Cushing's syndrome
▶ Cystic fibrosis

▶ After respiratory acidosis

Alkalosis, Respiratory
Hyperventilation

Disorder	H⁺	pH	HCO₃⁻	pCO₂
Met. Ac.	↑	↓	↓↓*	(↓)
Met. Alk.	↓	↑	↑↑*	(↑)
Resp. Ac.	↑	↓	(↑)	↑↑*
Resp. Alk.	↓	↑	(↓)	↓↓*

* primary change

See Hyperventilation → 197
See Acidosis, Metabolic → 11
See Alkalosis, Metabolic → 18
See Acidosis, Respiratory → 12

Alopecia
Increased loss of hair. Pathologic if
> 100 hairs/day. Hypotrichosis is reduced
hair growth, particularly of secondary hair.
Common causes
▶ Nonscarring alopecia
  • Androgenetic alopecia
  • Telogen effluvium
  • Anagen effluvium
  • Trichotillomania
  • Traction alopecia
  • Alopecia areata
  • Ssecondary syphilis
▶ Scarring alopecia
  • Inflammatory dermatoses
  • Systemic lupus erythematosis
  • Infection
  • Physical or chemical agents
  • Neoplasm
  • Congenital defects
Causes
▶ Genetic causes (90%)
  • Androgenetic alopecia (men and
    women)
▶ Endocrine

• Thyroiditis
• Hypothyroidism
• Hyperthyroidism
• Hypogonadism
• Cushing's syndrome
• Sheehan's syndrome
• Hypoparathyroidism
• Pituitary insufficiency
• Adrenocortical insufficiency
  ○ Primary
  ○ Secondary
▶ Stress
• Psychic trauma
• Operation
• Labor
▶ Folliculitis
▶ Dermatosis
• Seborrhea
• Scleroderma
• Chronic disciform LE
• Mycosis fungoides
• Lichen ruber atrophicans
• Psoriasis
• Neurodermatitis
• Dermatitis exfoliativa generalisata
• Chronic lupus
▶ Scarring
• Chemical or physical trauma
• Lichen planopilaris
• Extensive bacterial or mycotic
  infections
  ○ Trichophytosis
  ○ Favus
  ○ Microsporosis
  ○ Secondary syphilis
  ○ Leptospirosis
  ○ Typhoid fever
• Herpes zoster infection
• Scleroderma
▶ Drugs
• ACE inhibitors
• Allopurinol
• Androgens
• Anticoagulants
• Anticonvulsants

A

- Antimycotic agents
- Arsenic
- Azathioprine
- Beta blockers
- Borates
- Cadmium
- Chemotherapeutics
- Chlorambucil
- Cisplatin
- Clofibrate
- Cyclophosphamide
- Cytarabine
- Estrogens
- Ethyl urethane
- Fluoruracil
- Gentamycin
- Gold compounds
- Heparins
- Indomethacin
- Levodopa
- Linolic acid
- Mercury and derivates
- Methotrexate
- Monoiodoacetic acid
- Niacin
- Oral contraceptives
- Propranolol
- Retinoids
- Salicylates
- Selenium
- Spironolactone
- Squalenes
- Steroids
- Thallium
- Thallium
- Thyroid depressants
- Undecylenic acid
- Vitamin A overdose
- Warfarin
▶ Miscellaneous
- Testicular feminization
- Turner's syndrome
- Cirrhosis
- Autoimmune disease
  ○ Hashimoto's thyroiditis

  ○ Addison's disease
  ○ Diabetes mellitus
  ○ Schmidt's syndrome
- Cachexia
  ○ Malignant tumors
  ○ Anemia
- Postinfectious
  ○ Pneumonia
  ○ Scarlet fever
  ○ Abdominal typhoid fever
▶ Temporary hair loss
- Pregnancy
- Malnutrition
  ○ Malabsorption
  ○ Malresorption
  ○ Protein deficiency
  ○ Tryptophan deficiency
  ○ Nontropical sprue
  ○ Vitamin A deficiency
  ○ Vitamin B deficiency
  ○ Vitamin D deficiency rickets
▶ Mechanical effects
- Traction alopecia
- Pressure alopecia
  ○ Alopecia after extended bed rest
- Trichotillomania (compulsion to pull out one's own hair)

Alpha-1 Antitrypsin

Alpha-1 antitrypsin inhibits or prevents the activity of proteolytic enzymes (trypsin). Alpha-1 antitrypsin deficiency is an inherited disorder leading to damage of various organs, principally the lungs with dyspnea or the liver with jaundice, ascites, and gastrointestinal bleeding.

Reference range
85–200 mg/dl

Alpha-1 antitrypsin deficiency
▶ In children
- Nonphysiologic neonatal jaundice
- Hepatitis of unclear origin in children
  ○ Hereditary, autosomal recessive alpha-1 antitrypsin deficiency

- In adults
  - Adult pulmonary emphysema
  - Adult hepatitis or cirrhosis of unclear origin
  - Cachexia
  - Malnutrition
  - Nephrotic syndrome
  - Pancreatitis

Increased
- Infection
- Neoplasm
  - Lymphoma
  - Cervical cancer
- Pregnancy
- Systemic lupus erythematosus
- Estrogen therapy

Alpha-Fetoprotein, See AFP → 16

ALT (Alanine aminotransferase)
See Aminotransferases → 23

AMA. See Antimitochondrial Antibodies (AMA) → 36

Amaurosis, See Vision Loss, Acute → 376

Amenorrhea
Absence of monthly menstruation, with primary and secondary forms.
See Gonadotropins → 158

Definitions
- Primary amenorrhea
  - No menstrual period by
    ○ Sixteen years old or
    ○ One year beyond family history
  - No secondary sexual characteristics by 14 years old
- Secondary amenorrhea
  - Previously regular cycles: 3 months of no menses
  - Previously irregular cycles: 6 months of no menses

See Dysmenorrhea → 109
See Polymenorrhea → 289
Physiologic amenorrhea
- Pre-menarche
- During pregnancy
- During lactation
- Postmenopausal
Primary amenorrhea
- Hypothalamus, central
  - Anovulation
  - Post-hormonal contraceptive Amenorrhea
  - Constitutional (family history)
  - Kallmann's syndrome
- Hypothalamico-hypophyseal
  - Hypothalamic and pituitary tumors
    ○ Craniopharyngioma
    ○ Dysgerminoma
    ○ Hyperprolactinemia/Prolactin-secreting tumors
  - Pituitary insufficiency
    ○ Empty sella syndrome
    ○ Pituitary tuberculosis
    ○ Pituitary schistosomiasis
  - Idiopathic gonadotropin deficiency
  - Early infantile brain damage
  - After trauma
  - Anorexia nervosa
  - Severe systemic diseases
  - Constitutional bradygenesis
- Dysgenesis of the genital organs
  - Mayer-Rokitansky-Küstner syndrome
  - Mullerian dysgenesis
  - Turner's syndrome
  - Swyer's synrome
  - Uterine hypoplasia
  - Uterine atresia
  - Hymenal atresia
  - Vaginal atresia/gynatresia
- Gonadal causes
  - Gonadal dysgenesis
  - Testicular feminization
- 17β-hydroxysteroid dehydrogenase deficiency

- Polycystic ovary syndrome
- Agonadism
- Hyperandrogenism
► Endocrine
- Hyper- and hypothyroidism
  ○ Diabetes mellitus
  ○ Homozygous adrenogenital syndrome

Secondary amenorrhea

Absence of menstruation (after previous normal cycles) for more than 3 months

► Hypothalamicohypophyseal causes
- Gonadotropin deficiency in tumors
- Postoperative gonadotropin deficiency (also after radiation treatment)
- Prolactinoma
- Functional gonadotropin deficiency
  ○ In stress situations
  ○ In anorexia nervosa
  ○ In athletes
  ○ Severe systemic diseases
- Anovulation
- Post-hormonal contraception (Post-Pill)

► Gonadal, ovarian causes
- Polycystic ovary syndrome (Stein-Leventhal syndrome)
- Turner's syndrome
- Hormone-active ovarian tumor
- Premature menopause
- Castration
  ○ Surgical
  ○ Radiation, irreversible
- After radiation, reversible
- During chemotherapy
- Autoimmune
- Myotonic dystrophy
- Postinfection
  ○ Mumps oophoritis
  ○ Severe pelvic inflammatory disease

► Adrenal causes
- Cushing's syndrome
- Androgengenital tumors
- Adrenocortical insufficiency

► Uterine and outflow tract abnormalties

- Female pseudohermaphroditism
  ○ Congenital adrenal hyperplasie
  ○ Exposure to maternal androgens in utero
- Hysterectomy
- Male pseudohermaphroditism
  ○ 5α-reductase deficiency
  ○ Complete and incomplete androgen insensitivity
  ○ Enzymatic defects in testosterone biosynthesis
- Asherman's syndrome
- Müllerian anomalies
  ○ Absence or anomalies of vagina, cervix. endometrium or endometrial cavity
  ○ Imperforate hymen
  ○ Labial agglutination or fusion
- Trauma
  ○ Cervical stenosis
  ○ Sclerosis of the uterine cavity
    - *Abortion*
    - *After uterine surgery (cesarian section, metroplasty, myomectomy)*
    - *Repeated or overzealous uterine curettage*
    - *Severe generalized pelvic infections*
    - *Tuberculous endometritis*
    - *Uterine shistosomiasis*
- Endometrial atrophy
- Vaginal stenosis

► Endocrine
- Prolactinoma
- Addison's disease
- Heterozygous adrenogenital syndrome
- Androgen-producing tumor
- Pituitary insufficiency
- Cushing's syndrome
- Sheehan's syndrome
- Hypothyroidism
- Hyperthyroidism
- Diabetes mellitus

► Intersexuality as a cause

- Transsexuality when taking androgens
- Hermaphroditism
- Testicular feminization
▶ Genital impairment as a cause
  - After hysterectomy
  - After curettage
  - Endometrial disorders
▶ Central impairment (with impairment of the hypothalamicohypophyseal tract)
  - Encephalitis
  - Meningitis
  - Craniocerebral trauma
  - CNS tumor
- Miscellaneous
  - Depression
  - Stress
  - Change of environment
  - Imprisonment
  - Addiction
  - Athletes; strenuous exercise
  - Body-building and use of androgens
  - Basic systemic disease
  - Post-hormonal contraception (Post-Pill)
  - Extreme obesity

Amentia, See Mental Retardation → 239, See Dementia → 96

Aminotransferases

Diagnostic, differentiation and progress assessment of: diseases of the liver, bile ducts, heart, skeleton and muscles. In clinical diagnosis of a fresh myocardial infarction the diagnostic sensitivity of **AST (GOT)** is 96 %, the specificity is 86 %. **ALT (GPT)** and AST are sensitive indicators of liver and bile duct diseases. The diagnostic sensitivity of the ALT is 83 %, the specificity opposite non-hepatopathies is 84 %. The diagnostic sensitivity of the AST in liver and bile duct diseases is 71 % and therefore not as good as the ALT. ALT is dissolved in the cytoplasm of the

hepatocytes. The extent of the increase correlates with the number of the affected cells. About 70 % of hepatocyte AST activity is localized in the mitochondria and about 30 % in the cytoplasm. AST activity levels and its relation to GPT is made in the form of the De-Ritis quotient: AST /ALT. Quotients < 1 indicate light liver damage, quotients > 2 more serious liver damage with necroses.

Reference range	
ALT (GPT)	0–23 U/l
AST (GOT)	0–19 U/l

Increased
▶ Liver and bile duct disorders
  - Acute hepatitis
  - Chronic active hepatitis
  - Alcoholic hepatopathy
  - Cirrhosis
  - Fatty liver
  - Cholangitis
  - Cholestasis
  - Primary biliary cirrhosis
  - Hepatic tumor (e.g. metastasis)
▶ Cardiac
  - Myocardial infarction
  - Pulmonary embolism
  - Perimyocarditis
  - Heart catheterization
  - Implantation of a cardiac pacemaker
  - Open heart surgery
  - Cardiac dysrhythmia
▶ Skeletal myopathies
  - Progressive myodystrophia
  - Myositis
  - Hypothyroid myopathy
  - Spasms, muscle injuries
  - Strong physical work
  - Malignant hyperthermia
  - Severe muscle trauma
  - Dermatomyositis
  - Polymyositis
▶ Miscellaneous
  - Epstein-Barr virus (EBV)

A
- Renal infarction
- Drugs
  - Amiodarone
  - Antibiotics
  - Antihypertensives
  - Heparin
  - Labetalol
  - Lovastatin
  - Narcotics
  - NSAIDs
  - Phenytoin
- Malignancy
- Seizure

Ammonia

Important indicator for early recognition, prevention and progress assessment of hepatic coma in patients with cirrhosis or acute decay of liver parenchyma. A relatively strong correspondence exists between the neurologic symptom complex and the ammonia level in the arterial plasma. In unconscious or disoriented patients a normal ammonia level rules out hepatic coma to a large extent. Patients with fatty liver, chronic active hepatitis or cor pulmonale can have elevated ammonia values with higher protein intake.

Reference range
19-82 µg/dl and/or 11-48 µmol/l (F)
25-94 µg/dl and/or 15-55 µmol/l (M)

Increased
▶ Hepatic failure
▶ Cirrhosis
▶ Hepatic encephalopathy
▶ Reye's syndrome
▶ Portacaval shunt
▶ Excessive protein intake
▶ (Chronic) infections
▶ Drugs
  - Diuretics
  - Methicillin
  - Polymixin B

Decreased
▶ Renal failure
▶ Drugs
  - Neomycin
  - Lactulose
  - Tetracycline

Amnesia

Impairment or lack of memory.

Causes
▶ Head trauma
  - Antegrade amnesia (after the event)
  - Retrograde amnesia (before the event)
  - Postconcussive syndrome
▶ Transient global amnesia (TGA)
  - Spontaneous
  - Minor trauma
  - Exertion
  - Emotional stress
▶ Korsakoff syndrome (thiamine deficiency in alcoholism)
▶ Degenerative diseases
  - Alzheimer's disease
  - Huntington's disease
▶ Cerebrovascular accident
  - Thalamus
  - Basal forebrain
  - Hippocampus
▶ Cerebral hypoxia
▶ Infections
  - Herpes simplex encephalitis
  - Meningitis
▶ Creutzfeldt-Jakob disease
▶ Hypoglycemia
▶ CNS neoplasm
▶ Postsurgical (e.g.lobectomy)
▶ Drugs
  - Alcohol
  - Midazolam
  - Benzodiazepines (Traveler amnesia)
▶ Psychosis

Amylase

Enzyme which splits polysaccharides.

In serum and urine of healthy persons. Pancreatic and salivary isoenzymes occur in almost the same activity ratio.

Serum reference range

60–180 U/l

Increased

▶ Pancreatic disorder
  • Acute pancreatitis
  • Pancreatic neoplasm
  • Pancreas abscess
  • Pancreas pseudocyst
▶ Other gastrointestinal/bowel disorder
  • Penetrating, perforated peptic ulcer
  • After ERCP
  • Acute cholecystitis
  • Intestinal obstruction
  • Intestinal infarction
  • Ascites
  • Appendicitis
  • Peritonitis
▶ Salivary gland inflammation
  • Parotitis (mumps)
▶ Drugs, toxins
  • Acute alcohol intoxication
  • Drug abuse
  • Morphine
▶ Macroamylasemia
▶ Malignancies (paraneoplastic hyperamylasemia)
  • Bronchial cancer
  • Esophageal cancer
  • Ovarian cancer
▶ Miscellaneous
  • Diabetic ketoacidosis
  • Ruptured ectopic pregnancy
  • Pulmonary infarction
  • Renal failure

Decreased

  • Advanced chronic pancreatitis
  • Hepatic necrosis

Amyloidosis

Characterized by increased deposition of amyloid fibers in the tissues. Amyloid fibers can consist of miscellaneous proteins that are either formed at an increased rate or broken down at a decreased rate. Amyloid deposits can lead to malfunctioning of the affected organs together with asthenia, weight loss and paresthesias.

Primary amyloidosis

Overproduction of immunoglobulin chains (AL: light chain–type amyloid)
▶ Multiple myeloma
▶ Monoclonal gammopathies

Secondary amyloidosis

AA: amyloid A, SAA: serum amyloid A
▶ Chronic infections
  • Osteomyelitis
  • Tuberculosis
  • Leprosy
  • Syphilis
  • Bronchiectases
▶ Chronic inflammations
  • Rheumatoid arthritis
  • Bechterew's disease
  • Collagen vascular disease
  • Ulcerative colitis

Hereditary amyloidosis

ATTR: Amyloid consisting of transthyretin

Amyloidosis in miscellaneous diseases

▶ Hemodialysis amyloidosis
▶ Familial Mediterranean fever
▶ Peripheral neuropathy
▶ Vitamin deficiencies
▶ Carpal tunnel syndrome
▶ Restrictive cardiomyopathy
▶ Acute myocarditis
▶ Myocardial fibrosis
▶ Nephrotic syndrome
▶ Renal failure
▶ Renal failure
  • Glomerulonephritis

- Drug/toxic nephropathy
- ▸ Rheumatoid polyarthritis
- ▸ Systemic lupus erythematosus
- ▸ Interstitial lung diseases

ANA

Antinuclear Antibody

Disease	ANA Frequency (%)
SLE	90-100
Disciform LE	21-50
Drug-induced lupus	95
Mixed connective tissue disease (MCTD)	100
Scleroderma	31-90
CREST syndrome	95
Rheumatoid arthritis	10-60
Felty's syndrome	60-110
Dermatomyositis	40
Autoimmune chronic hepatitis	45-100
Myasthenia gravis	35-50
Immune thrombocytopenia	50-70
Autoimmune thyroiditis	40-50
Leukemias	70
Infectious mononucleosis	30-70

Periarteritis nodosa, Raynaud's disease, Sjögren syndrome, cirrhosis
Normal titer less than 1:20 dilution

Mechanism
- ▸ IgG or IgM antinuclear antibody (ANA)
- ▸ Binds to nuclei or nuclear components
See Autoantibodies in Connective Tissue Diseases → 47

Positive in
- ▸ Rheumatologic
  - Systemic lupus erythematosus
  - Rheumatoid arthritis
  - Sjögren's syndrome
  - Mixed connective tissue disease
  - Necrotizing vasculitis
- ▸ Infections
  - Tuberculosis

- Chronic active hepatitis
- Subacute bacterial endocarditis
- HIV infection
- ▸ Miscellaneous
  - Type I diabetes mellitus
  - Multiple sclerosis
  - Pulmonary fibrosis
  - Silicone gel implants
  - Pregnant women
  - Advanced age
- ▸ Drugs (drug-induced SLE)
  - Carbamazepine
  - Chlorpromazine
  - Ethosuximide
  - Gold
  - Griseofulvin
  - Hydralazine
  - Isoniazid
  - Methyldopa
  - Minocycline
  - Penicillamine
  - Phenytoin
  - Primidone
  - Procainamide
  - Quinidine
  - Thiazides

Anacidity, Gastric

Absence of hydrochloric acid in the gastric juice.
- ▸ Advanced age
- ▸ Chronic gastritis
- ▸ Gastric carcinoma
- ▸ Polyposis ventriculi
- ▸ Pernicious anemia
- ▸ Hypochromic anemia
- ▸ Pellagra (niacin deficiency)
- ▸ Ulcerative colitis
- ▸ Addison's disease
- ▸ Gastric syphilis
- ▸ Gastric tuberculosis
- ▸ Intestinal parasites

Anal fistula
Rectal fistula, anorectal fistula
Tubelike tract at or near the anus; usually opening into the rectum above the internal sphincter with chronic seropurulent or mucus drainage from fistula.

Causes
▶ Perirectal abscess sequelae of rupture or surgery
▶ Anal fissure
▶ Crohn's disease
▶ Ulcerative colitis
▶ Anorectal carcinoma
▶ Local radiation therapy
▶ Infection
  • Tuberculosis (common)
  • Lymphogranuloma venereum
  • Syphilis
  • Gonorrhea
  • Actinomycosis
  • HIV
▶ Cryptitis
▶ Constipation
▶ Disease of the anal glands
▶ Thrombosed hemorrhoids

Anal pain, See Anorectal pain → 35

Anal tenesmus,
Painful spasm of the anal sphincter.
See Anorectal pain → 35

Anaphylaxis
Anaphylactic reaction
Severe allergic reaction with urticaria (hives), angioedema, hypotension and bronchospasm.

Common causes
▶ Drugs
  • Aspirin
  • Cephalosporin
  • Dextran
  • Glucocorticoids
  • Hymenoptera stings
  • Insulin
  • NSAIDs
  • Penicillins
  • Protamines
  • Radiocontrast media
  • Vaccines
▶ Food allergy
  • Eggs
  • Fish
  • Legumes
  • Milk
  • Nuts (especially peanuts)
  • Shellfish
  • Soybeans
▶ Latex allergy
▶ Medical products
  • Blood products
  • Sterilization agents
▶ Insect bites

DDx (pseudoanaphylactic reactions)
▶ Carcinoid syndrome
▶ After first contact with
  • Aspirin
  • Contrast media
  • Polymyxin
  • Pentamidine
▶ Globus hystericus
▶ Hereditary angioedema
▶ Pheochromocytoma
▶ Scombroid intoxication
▶ Systemic mastocytosis
▶ Vasovagal reactions
▶ Pulmonary embolism

ANCA, See Antineutrophil Cytoplasmic Antibodies (ANCA) → 37

Androgens, See Testosterone → 348

Anemia

Anemia is defined as an absolute reduction in the quantity of the oxygen-carrying pigment hemoglobin (Hgb) in the circulating blood. Anemia is further broadly subcategorized into acute and chronic.

Hemoglobin	
13–18 g/dl (m)	12–16 g/dl (f)
Hematocrit	
40–52% (m)	35–47 % (f)
Erythrocytes	
4.4–5.9 /pl (m)	3.8 –5.2/pl (f)

Acute anemia

The common pathway in life-threatening acute anemia is a sudden reduction in the oxygen-carrying capacity of the blood.

▶ Blood loss
- Traumatic injuries
- Massive upper or lower GI hemorrhage
- Ruptured ectopic pregnancy
- Ruptured aneurysms
- DIC

▶ Hemoglobinopathies
- Sickle cell anemia
- Thalassemias

▶ RBC enzyme abnormalities
- Glucose-6-phosphate dehydrogenase (G-6-PD) and pyruvate kinase (PK) deficiency

▶ Congenital coagulopathies
- Von Willebrand disease
- Hemophilia A (classic hemophilia)
- Hemophilia B (Christmas disease)

▶ Autoimmune hemolytic anemia
- Autoimmune diseases
  ○ Lupus
  ○ Lymphomas
  ○ Leukemias
  ○ Drug-induced

▶ Acquired platelet disorders
- Thrombotic thrombocytopenic purpura (TTP)
- Idiopathic thrombocytopenic purpura (ITP)

▶ Hemolytic-uremic syndrome (microangiopathic hemolytic anemia, thrombocytopenia, renal failure)

▶ Disseminated intravascular coagulation (DIC)

▶ Miscellaneous
- Abdominal trauma
  ○ Blunt
  ○ Penetrating
- Chronic anemia
- Sickle cell anemia
- Abdominal aneurysms
- Aortic dissection
- Diverticular disease
- Dysfunctional uterine bleeding
- Gastritis
- Peptic ulcer disease
- Hemolytic uremic syndrome
- Hemophilia, type A
- Hemophilia, type B
- Gastrointestinal bleeding (in kids)
- Ectopic pregnancy
- Hemorrhagic shock
- Thrombocytopenic purpura

Microcytic anemia (MCV ↓, MCH ↓)

▶ Iron deficiency
- Insufficient supply
- Insufficient resorption
  ○ Gastric/intestinal resection
  ○ Avitaminosis C
  ○ Gastric anacidity
  ○ Chronic diarrhea
  ○ Nontropical sprue
  ○ Inflammatory bowel disease
  ○ Enteritis
  ○ Intestinal tuberculosis
  ○ Excretory pancreatic insufficiency
  ○ Worm infestation
- Increased requirements
  ○ Growth
  ○ Pregnancy (400 mg/d)
  ○ Lactation period (720 mg/d)

- ○ Increased blood formation
- ○ Atransferrinemia
  - *Hereditary*
  - *Neoplastic*
- Iron loss
  - ○ Bleeding from the GI tract
    - *Hemorrhoids*
    - *Ulcer*
    - *Adenomas*
    - *Neoplastic*
    - *Angiodysplasias*
  - ○ Genital bleeding in women
  - ○ Urogenital tract
    - *Neoplasms*
    - *Hemosiderinemia: paroxysmal nocturnal hemoglobinuria*
    - *Artificial cardiac valves*
  - ○ Blood loss from other organs
    - *Oropharynx*
    - *Nose*
    - *Lung*
  - ○ Blood loss with Osler's disease
  - ○ Surgical, postoperative or traumatic blood loss
  - ○ Blood loss from hemodialysis
  - ○ Frequent blood samples
  - ○ Frequent blood donation
- Deferroxamin (over)treatment
▶ Anemia due to infection, inflammation, neoplastic
  - ○ Iron distribution disorder; ferritin usually increased
▶ Hemoglobinopathy
  - Thalassemia
  - Sideroachrestic anemia
▶ Myelopathies
  - Myeloproliferative syndrome
▶ Miscellaneous
  - Vitamin deficiency conditions
  - Protein deficiency
  - Hypothyroidism
  - Pituitary insufficiency
  - Lead intoxication
  - Atransferrinemia
▶ Iron utilization disorders (sideroachrestic

anemia)
- Hereditary
- Acquired
  - ○ Primary (idiopathic)
  - ○ Secondary
    - *Vitamin B_1 deficiency (beriberi)*
    - *Protein deficiency*
    - *Hypothyroidism*
    - *Neoplasms*
    - *Pituitary insufficiency*
  - ○ Acquired exogenously
    - *Alcohol*
    - *Lead*
    - *Tuberculostatics*
    - *Chloramphenicole*
    - *Chemotherapeutics*

Normochromic, normocytic anemia
▶ Acute hemorrhage
  - ○ Usually only hypovolemia at the outset; Hb drop only after several hours (note!)
▶ Hemolytic anemia
  - Corpuscular hemolytic anemia
    - ○ Congenital membrane defects
      - *Spherocytosis*
      - *Elliptocytosis*
      - *Acanthocytosis*
      - *Sickle cell anemia*
      - *Erythropoietic porphyrias*
      - *Congenital lipid disorders (e.g. α-, β-lipoproteinemia)*
    - ○ Enzyme defects
      - *Glucose-6-phosphate dehydrogenase deficiency*
      - *Pyruvate kinase deficiency*
      - *Defective glutathione metabolism (e.g. glutathione reductase)*
      - *Defective nucleotide metabolism (pyrimidine 5'-nucleotidase deficiency)*
    - ○ Impaired hemoglobin synthesis/ pathologic hemoglobins
      - *Hemoglobin S, C, D*
      - *Hemoglobinopathy from other unstable abnormal hemoglobins*

- *Thalassemia syndrome*
  ○ Acquired hemolytic anemia
    - *Paroxysmal nocturnal hemoglobinuria*
- Extracorpuscular hemolytic anemia
  ○ Immunohemolysis
    - *Isoimmunohemolytic anemia (e.g. Rh incompatibility; transfusion reactions)*
    - *Autoimmune hemolytic anemia (→ 47)*
    - *Drug-induced immunohemolysis*
  ○ Hemolysis in infectious diseases
    - *Malaria*
    - *Toxoplasmosis*
    - *Clostridia*
    - *Cholera*
    - *Sepsis*
    - *Babesiosis*
    - *Bartonellosis*
- Hemolytic anemia through physical, chemical-toxic noxa
  ○ Mechanical hemolysis
    - *Cardiac valve prosthesis*
    - *Microangiopathic hemolytic anemia (due to malignant tumors, hemolytic uremic syndrome, thrombotic thrombocytopenic purpura)*
  ○ Thermal erythrocyte damage
    - *Burns*
  ○ Uremia
  ○ Chemical substances
    - *Benzenes*
    - *Gasoline*
    - *Insect and snake venom*
    - *Bacterial toxins (Clostridium sepsis)*
  ○ Drugs
    - *Sulfonamides*
    - *Penicillin*
    - *Isoniazide*
    - *α-methyldopa*
    - *Chinidine*
    - *Phenacetin*
    - *Pyramidone*
    - *Chlorpromazine*
  ○ Hemolytic syndrome in metabolic disorders
    - *Zieve's syndrome (alcohol-toxic liver damage, hyperlipidemia, hemolytic anemia)*
    - *Hepatopathies (Wilson's disease and copper intoxication)*

▶ Renal anemia
  - Erythropoietin deficiency
  - Inhibition of erythropoiesis by inflammatory mediators
    ○ Uremic toxins
    ○ Cytokines from dialysis
  - Reduced erythrocyte survival time due to endogenous factors (uremic toxins)
  - Chronic occult blood loss
  - Osteomyelofibrosis
    ○ Hyperparathyroidism
  - Aluminum intoxication (in phosphate binders)
  - Iron deficiency
  - Vitamin B_{12} deficiency
  - Folic acid deficiency

▶ Bone marrow insufficiency
  - Aplastic anemia
    ○ Hypocellular bone marrow
    ○ Hypercellular bone marrow
  - Panmyelopathy
  - Suppression of blood-forming bone marrow
    ○ Malignant hematologic systemic disease
      - *Leukemias*
      - *Lymphomas*
      - *Myeloproliferative syndromes*
    ○ Lipid storage disorders
    ○ Bone marrow metastases of solid tumors
    ○ Infections and granulomas
      - *Tuberculosis*
      - *Sarcoidosis*

▶ Chronic systemic diseases
  - Uremia

- Chronic liver disease
► Chronic inflammation
  - Connective tissue disease
  - Chronic infection
► HIV infection
► Endocrine insufficiency
  - Hypothyroidism
  - Addison's disease
  - Hypogonadism
  - Panhypopituitarism
► Pure red cell aplasia
  - Acquired
    ○ Autoimmune diseases
  - Congenital
    ○ Blackfan-Diamond syndrome

Hyperchromic makrocytic anemia (MCV, MCH↑) due to lack of vitamin B_{12} and/or folic acid, pernicious anemia

► Increased demand
  - Pregnancy
  - Children
  - Increased hematopoiesis
    ○ Hemolytic anemia
  - Hemodialysis
  - Malignant tumors
  - Hyperthyroidism
► Insufficient supply
  - Malnutrition
    ○ Alcoholism
    ○ Vegetarianism
    ○ Malnutrition
► Malabsorption
  - Pernicious anemia
    ○ Absence of intrinsic factors
      - *Gastric resection*
      - *Hereditary atrophy of the gastric mucosa*
      - *Hypothyroidism polyendocrinopathy*
    ○ Intestinal diseases that affect the terminal ileum
      - *Receptor for vitamin B_{12} intrinsic factor complex missing from small intestine (nontropical sprue)*
      - *Sprue*
      - *Crohn's disease*
      - *Small intestine resection*
      - *Tumors of the small intestine*
      - *Drugs*
      - *Calcium chelating agent*
      - *Faulty pancreatic excretory function*
    ○ Increased consumption due to fish tapeworm
    ○ Bacterial overgrowth (e.g. in blind-loop syndrome)
► Increased excretion
  - Inadequate vitamin B_{12} binding in the serum
  - Liver disease
  - Kidney disease
► Enzyme defects
  - Methylmalonyl-CoA mutase
  - Vitamin-B_{12}-reductase
  - Other enzyme disorders
► Drugs
  - Folic acid antagonists
    ○ Methotrexate, trimethoprim, pyrimethamine
  - 5-FU
  - Triamterene
  - Trimethoprim
  - Aciclovir
  - Colchicine
  - Neomycin
  - Oral contraceptives

Macrocytic anemia without megaloblastic-type bone marrow changes

► Hematologic diseases
  - Acute leukemia
  - Myeloproliferative diseases
  - Malignant lymphomas
  - Multiple myeloma
  - Myelodysplasia
  - Aplastic anemia
► Miscellaneous
  - Chronic hepatopathy
  - Chronic nephropathy
  - Chronic inflammation /infection

A

- Ionizing radiation
- Intoxications

Aneurysm
Dilation of arteries.
Dilation of an artery due to an acquired or congenital weakness of the wall of the artery.

Causes
- Familial
  - Clustering of intracranial aneurysms
  - Polycystic kidney diseases
  - Osler-Weber-Rendu syndrome
  - Neurofibromatosis (Type I)
- Hypertension
- Lipid metabolism
- Trauma
- Infection, inflammation
  - Takayasu's arteritis
  - Giant-cell arteritis
  - Syphilis
  - Polychondritis
  - Reiter's syndrome
  - Behçet's syndrome
  - Rheumatoid arthritis
  - SLE
- Collagen disorder
  - Marfan's syndrome
  - Ehlers-Danlos syndrome

Risk Factors
- Cigarette smoking
- Arteriosclerosis
- Hypertension
- Lipid metabolism disorder
- Chronic obstructive pulmonary disease
- Increasing age
- Male sex

Thoracic aortic aneurysm
- Marfan's syndrome
- Ehlers-Danlos syndrome
- Trauma
- Infection
  - Syphilis
  - Other bacterial or mycotic infections
- Degenerative changes
  - Arteriosclerosis
  - Cystic medial necrosis
- Inflammation
  - Aortitis
  - Polychondritis
  - Behçet's syndrome
  - Kawasaki's syndrome
- Hypertension

Abdominal aortic aneurysm
- Atherosclerosis
- Lipid metabolism disorders
- Hypertension
- Aortic dissection
- Mycotic infection
- Cystic medial necrosis
- Ehlers-Danlos syndrome
- Marfan's syndrome
- Polycystic kidney diseases

Peripheral arteries
- Arteriosclerosis
- Takayasu's arteritis
- Trauma
- Syphilis
- Marfan's syndrome
- Kawasaki's syndrome

Coronary arteries
- Bacterial infection
- Atherosclerosis
- Ehlers-Danlos syndrome
- Congenital syphilis
- Scleroderma
- Polyarteritis nodosa
- Septic emboli
- Kawasaki's syndrome

Angina
Retrosternal pain, angina pectoris
See Chest Pain → 72
See Cardiac Risk Factor → 66
DDx onset
- Sudden onset
  - Angina
  - Myocardial infarction

- Aortic dissection
- Pulmonary embolus
- Esophageal rupture
- Spontaneous pneumomediastinum
- Spontaneous pneumothorax
▸ Gradual or variable onset
- Pericarditis
- Musculoskeletal chest pain
- Costochondritis
- Epidemic pleurodynia
- Mitral valve prolapse

Diagnostic hints
▸ Exertion or stress
- Angina
- Myocardial infarction
▸ Hypertension
- Aortic dissection
▸ Pleuritic (Deep breath or cough)
- Pulmonary embolus
- Pericarditis
- Spontaneous pneumomediastinum
- Musculoskeletal chest pain
- Cough fracture
▸ Swallowing or vomiting
- Esophageal rupture
- Spontaneous pneumomediastinum
▸ Supine position
- Pericarditis
- Spontaneous pneumomediastinum
▸ Movement
- Musculoskeletal chest pain
- Cough fracture

Evaluation
▸ High risk findings
- Chest pain
- History of known CAD
- Radiation of pain to left arm or neck
- Pain > 1 hr
- Diaphoresis
▸ Low risk findings
- Chest pain > 48 hr
- Chest pain fully reproduced with palpation
▸ Focus areas
- Identify non-cardiac cause

- Complications of MI

Indications for angiography in unstable angina
▸ Failure to stabilize with adequate therapy
▸ Recurrent pain
▸ Persistent pain
▸ Ischemia
▸ Previous revascularization
▸ Multiple admissions for undiagnosed chest pain
▸ High-risk findings
- Congestive heart failure
- Left ventricular dysfunction
- Mitral regurgitation
- Malignant ventricular arrhythmia
- Positive exercise stress test
- Positive stress imaging

Angiotensin-Converting Enzyme

Important enzyme in the renin-angiotensin-aldosterone system and the kallikrein-kinine system. ACE's effects are based on direct vasoconstrictive effect as well as increased catabolism of the vasodilatative bradykinines. ACE is found in the endothelial cells of the vascular system, particularly in the lungs and kidneys. Indicator in the diagnosis and progress of sarcoidosis.

Reference range
Adults: 8 to 52 U/L

Increased
▸ Sarcoidosis (Boeck's disease)
▸ Lung disease
- Smoker's bronchitis
- Allergic alveolitis
- Silicosis
- Asbestosis
- Tuberculosis
- Coccidioidomycosis
▸ Leprosy
▸ Berylliosis

A
▶ Virus hepatitis
▶ Biliary cirrhosis
▶ Alcoholic liver disease
▶ Gaucher's disease
▶ Kidney diseases
▶ Hyperparathyroidism
▶ Hyperthyroidism
▶ Diabetes mellitus
▶ Amyloidosis
▶ Multiple myeloma

Anion gap

Calculation of the anion gap is used for determination of the cause of metabolic acidosis. Chloride and bicarbonate usually constitute 85% of the anions in the serum; remaining anions (proteinate, sulfate, phosphate, organic anions) are called the anion gap. Important: If acidosis is caused by administration of chlorinated acids or loss of bicarbonate, the anion gap can be within the reference range.
Simplified calculation formula:
Na - (Cl + HCO3).

Reference range
8-16 mmol/l

Disorder	H^+	pH	HCO_3^-	pCO_2
Met. Ac.	↑	↓	↓↓*	(↓)
Met. Alk.	↓	↑	↑↑*	(↑)
Resp. Ac.	↑	↓	(↑)	↑↑*
Resp. Alk.	↓	↑	(↓)	↓↓*

* primary change
See Acidosis, Metabolic → 11
See Acidosis, Respiratory → 12
See Alkalosis, Metabolic → 18
See Alkalosis, Respiratory → 19

Decreased anion gap (< 6 mmol/l)
▶ Dilution
▶ Hypoalbuminemia
▶ Increased unmeasured cations

▶ Hypernatremia
▶ Hypermagnesemia
▶ Hypercalcemia
▶ Pheochromocytoma
▶ Pararoteinemia
▶ Muliple myeloma
▶ Hyperviscosity
▶ Lithium toxicity
▶ Laboratory error
  • Underestimation of serum sodium
  • Bromism

Increased anion gap
▶ Diabetic ketoacidosis
▶ Alcoholic ketoacidosis
▶ Starvation ketoacidosis
▶ Lactic acidosis
▶ Renal failure (acute/chronic)
▶ Drugs, toxins
  • Salicylate
  • Paraldehyde
  • Methanol
  • Ethylene glycol
▶ Hyperosmolar hyperglycemic nonketotic coma

Normal anion gap
▶ Bicarbonate loss
  • Enteral bicarbonate loss: diarrhea
  • Pancreatic fistula
▶ Fluid loss with pancreatitis
▶ Ureteroenterostomy
▶ Ileal stoma
▶ Drugs
  • Aldactone (in patients with cirrhosis)
  • Administration of HCL
  • Sulfamylon
  • Acetazolamide
  • Cholestyramine
▶ Recovery from diabetic ketoacidosis
▶ Carbonic anhydrase inhibitors
▶ Renal tubular acidosis
▶ Arginine and lysine during parenteral nutrition

Anisocoria

Pupils are not of equal size.
Note: "d" and "c" indicate whether the affected pupil is dilated (mydriasis) or contracted (miosis).

Local causes
▶ Drugs
  • Mydriatics (e.g. pilocarpine)
  • Miotics (e.g. atropine)
▶ Injury to the iris (d*)
▶ Inflammation
  • Keratitis (d)
  • Iridocyclitis (c*,d)
▶ Narrow angle glaucoma (d)
▶ Ischemia (with carotid artery insufficiency) (d)
▶ Diseases of the iris
  • Aniridia (d)
▶ Unilateral blindness due to:
  • Diseases of the optic apparatus (d)
  • Retinal causes (d)
▶ Ocular prosthesis

Paralysis of the pupillary sphincter (d)
▶ Infection
  • Syphilis
  • Herpes zoster
  • Tuberculosis
  • Meningitis
  • Encephalitis
  • Botulism
  • Diphtheria
▶ Intracranial neoplasms
▶ Cerebral aneurysm
▶ Cavernous sinus thrombosis
▶ Intracranial hematomas
▶ Degenerative neurologic disorders
  Toxic polyneuritis
  • Alcohol, lead, arsenic
  • Diabetes mellitus

Paralysis of the dilatator of the pupil (c)
  Horner's syndrome
  Neurofibromatosis
▶ Trauma

▶ Internal carotid artery aneurysm
▶ CNS causes
  • Multiple sclerosis
  • Syringomyelia
  • Neoplastic
▶ Congenital

Miscellaneous
▶ Tabes dorsalis
▶ Adie's syndrome (slow reaction to light, slow convergence response)
▶ Argyll-Robertson (reflex pupilloplegia, pupil unrounding)

Anisocytosis
See Erythrocyte, Morphology → 132

Anorectal pain

Anal pain, rectal pain
Local pain
▶ Anal fissure
▶ Vascular
  • Hemorrhoids
    ○ External hemorrhoid
    ○ Internal hemorrhoid
    ○ Thrombosed hemorrhoid
    ○ Infected hemorrhoid
  • Perianal thrombosis
▶ Abscess
  • Anorectal abscess
  • Perianal abscess
▶ Foreign body
▶ Fecal impaction
▶ Anal fistula (→ 27)
▶ Prolapse
  • Anal prolapse
  • Rectal prolapse
▶ Colonic endometriosis
▶ Dermatologic
  • Eczema
  • Psoriasis
▶ Inflammation
  • Pelvic inflammatory disease
  • Cryptitis
  • Papillitis

- Acute proctitis
- Prostatitis
▸ Neoplasm
  - Anal cancer
  - Rectal cancer
  - Metastases
▸ Neurologic
  - Compression of sacral nerves
  - Inflammation of sacral nerves
▸ Proctalgia fugax

Referred pain
▸ Coccygodynia
▸ Pelvic inflammatory disease
▸ Sacral nerve compression
▸ Tumor mass
▸ Infection, inflammation
  - Appendicitis
  - Diverticulitis
▸ Uterine myoma

Anorexia

Diminished appetite, aversion to food.
See Weight Loss → 382
See Malassimilation → 233
See Inappetence → 210

Risk factors
▸ Perfectionist
▸ Obsessive-compulsive personality
▸ Socially withdrawn
▸ High achiever

DDx
▸ Weigt loss (→ 382)
▸ Bulimia
▸ Affective disorder
  - Anxiety disorder
  - Major depression
▸ Schizophrenia

Antibody, antimitochondrial, See
Antimitochondrial Antibodies (AMA) → 36

Antibody, antineutrophil cytoplasmatic
See Antineutrophil Cytoplasmic
Antibodies (ANCA) → 37

Antibody, antinuclear, See ANA → 26

Antibody, antistreptococcal
See Antistreptococcal Antibodies → 37

Antibody, antithyroid microsomal. See
Antithyroid Microsomal Antibodies → 38

Antibody, antithyroglobulin
See TgAb → 349

Antibody, double stranded DNA
See Double Stranded DNA Antibody → 104

Antibody, single stranded DNA
See Single Stranded DNA Antibody → 333

Antibody, smooth muscle
See Smooth Muscle Antibody → 335

Antibody, TSH receptor
See TSH Receptor Antibody → 362

Antidiuretic hormone, See Diabetes
Insipidus → 99, See SIADH → 332

Antimitochondrial Antibodies (AMA)

Antibodies against mitochondrial
antigens, which can appear with or
without other autoantibodies and be
directed against a large number of
mitochondrial antigens, of which 6 are

more closely characterized (M1-M6). AMA are to a limited extent organ- and species-specific.

Increased:
- Hepatopathy (→ 226)
  - Primary biliary cirrhosis
  - Chronic active hepatitis
  - Cryptogenic cirrhosis
- Combined primary biliary cirrhosis and arthralgias in women
- Pseudo-lupus
  - Drug-induced lupus
- Rheumatoid arthritis
- Polymyalgia rheumatica

DDx of other collagen vascular disease

Type	Association
AMA-M1	Secondary syphilis
AMA-M2	Primary biliary cirrhosis
AMA-M3	Drug-induced lupus
AMA-M4	Hepatic disorders
AMA-M5	SLE
AMA-M6	Drug-induced hepatitis

Antineutrophil Cytoplasmic Antibodies (ANCA)

Antibodies bind to cytoplasmic region of neutrophils.

cANCA (cytoplasmatic)
- Wegener's granulomatosis (strongly associated)
- Crescentic glomerulonephritis (moderately associated)
- Polyarteritis nodosa (weakly associated)

pANCA (perinuclear)
- Crescentic glomerulonephritis (strongly associated)
- Microscopic polyangiitis
- Polyarteritis nodosa
- Systemic lupus erythematosus
- Inflammatory bowel disease
- Churg-Strauss vasculitis
- Wegener's granulomatosis

- Henoch-Schönlein purpura
- Temporal arteritis

ANCA (fluorescence pattern non–cANCA/–pANCA)
- Primary sclerosing cholangitis

Antistreptococcal Antibodies

Anti-streptolysin O titer, ASO/ASL

Antibodies against a whole series of streptococcal exoantigens can be found in the serum after or during an acute infection with β-hemolysing streptococci. Determination of such antibodies plays an essential role in acute infections of the body surfaces and certain organs, but the agents can also be identified bacteriologically (e.g. tonsil swab). In toxic and sensitizing secondary diseases, e.g. rheumatic fever, chorea minor, or acute glomerulonephritis, antistreptococcal antibodies are important progress parameters. A negative result does not rule out the presence of an existing or past streptococcal infection, particularly if antibody determination is the only test performed.

Reference range	
ASO/ASL	up to 200 IU (adults) up to 150 IU (children)
ADNase	up to 200 IU

Increased
- Streptococcal angina
- Rheumatic fever
- Acute glomerulonephritis
  - Membranoproliferative glomerulonephritis (20%)
  - Acute poststreptococcal glomerulonephritis (70%)
- Scarlet fever
- Erysipelas
- Rheumatic carditis
- Polyarteritis nodosa
- Streptococcal infection
- Tuberculosis

A

▶ Chronic hepatitis
▶ Hyperlipidemia with obesity
▶ Lipoid nephrosis

Decreased
▶ Newborns
▶ Antibody deficiency syndrome
▶ Nephrotic syndrome
▶ Exudative enteropathy

Antithrombin III

AT III is the physiologic inhibitor of the serum proteases of the coagulation system. Even subnormal concentrations indicate an imbalance, with hypercoagulability and thromboembolism risk.

Reference range

Level: 0.14–0.39 g/l

Activity: 70–120% of normal activity

See Disseminated Intravascular Coagulation → 104

Decreased
▶ Congenital heterozygous familial AT III deficiency
▶ Advanced hepatic failure
  • Cirrhosis
  • Toxic hepatic failure
▶ Sepsis
▶ Consumption coagulopathy
▶ Nephrotic syndrome
  • Protein loss (incl. AT III)
▶ Thrombolysis
▶ Exudative enteropathy (protein loss)
▶ Surgery involving large wound surfaces
▶ Post-traumatic
▶ Newborns
  • Physiologically reduced by approx. 30% in the first days of life
▶ Heparin therapy (initial phase)
▶ Oral contraceptives

Increased
▶ Warfarin therapy
▶ Cholestasis
▶ Post-myocardial infarction

Antithyroid Microsomal Antibodies

TMAb, thyroid antimicrosomal antibody, anti–microsomal antibody, microsomal antibody

Increased
▶ Thyroid disease
  • Hypothyroidism
    ○ Hashimoto's thyroiditis
    ○ Subclinical hypothyroidism
  • Granulomatous thyroiditis
  • Nontoxic nodular goiter
  • Thyroid carcinoma
▶ Autoimmune disorder
  • Autoimmune hemolytic anemia
  • Rheumatoid arthritis
  • Sjögren's syndrome
  • Systemic lupus erythematosus

Anuria, See Renal Failure, Acute → 315

Aortic Insufficiency

Aortic regurgitation

Acute
▶ Rheumatic fever
▶ Bacterial endocarditis
▶ Other valvular infection
▶ Aortic dissection
▶ Chest trauma
▶ Myxomatous aortic valve
▶ After prosthetic valve surgery

Chronic
▶ Rheumatic heart disease
  • Rheumatic fever
▶ Congenital heart disease
  • Bicuspid aortic valve
  • Septal defect
▶ Aneurysm
  • Aneurysm of valsalva's sinus
  • Dissecting aneurysm
▶ Aortitis
  • Bechterew's disease

- Syphilis
▶ Weight loss medications
▶ Rheumatolgic, collagen vascular disease
  • Systemic lupus erythematosus
  • Marfan's syndrome
  • Turner's syndrome
  • Pseudoxanthoma elasticum
  • Ankylosing spondylitis
  • Ehlers-Danlos syndrome
  • Polymyalgia rheumatica
  • Rheumatoid arthritis
  • Reiter's syndrome
▶ Miscellaneous
  • Bacterial endocarditis
  • Traumatic
  • Cystic medianecrosis of aorta
  • Hypertension
  • Arteriosclerosis
  • Myxomatous aortic valve
  • After prosthetic valve surgery

Aortic Stenosis
Valvular aortic stenosis
Narrowing of the aortic valve orifice.
Causes
▶ Congenital bicuspid valve
▶ Atherosclerosis
▶ Rheumatic fever
▶ Subacute bacterial endocarditis
DDx
▶ Supravalvular aortic stenosis
▶ Membranous supravalvular aortic stenosis
▶ Hypertrophic cardiomyopathy (IHSS)
▶ Mitral regurgitation

Aortic valve diseases
See Aortic Insufficiency → 38
See Aortic Stenosis → 39

AP, See Alkaline Phosphatase (AP) → 17

Aphasia
Impaired expression or comprehension of written or spoken language.
Aphasia is an acquired disorder of language due to brain damage and does not include developmental disorders of language or speech disorders that are limited to the motor apparatus of speech (dysarthria). Related disorders include alexia (disorder of reading), agraphia (disorder of writing), and apraxia (disorder of skilled movements).
Types
▶ Expressive aphasia (difficulty in expressing thoughts through speech or writing)
▶ Receptive aphasia (difficulty in understanding spoken or written language)
▶ Anomic or amnesia aphasia (difficulty in using correct names for particular things)
▶ Global aphasia (difficulty in almost all language functions due to severe damage to language areas of the brain)
Causes
▶ Cerebrovascular
  • Stroke (!)
  • Transient ischemic attacks (TIA)
  • Breaking aneurysm
  • Hemhorrage
  • Aortic arch syndrome (subclavian steal syndrome)
  • Thromboangitis obliterans
▶ Head trauma
  • Gunshot wound
  • Blows to the head
  • Other traumatic brain injury
▶ Miscellaneous
  • Encephalitis
  • Poliomyelitis
  • Temporal lobe abscess
  • Temporal lobe atrophy

- Brain tumors
- Senile dementia (Alzheimer's type)

Aplastic syndrome, See Anemia → 28

Appendicitis

Acute inflammation of the vermiform appendix often with anorexia, nausea or vomiting, abdominal pain (right lower quadrant: McBurney's point) and fever.

Frequent differential diagnoses
▶ Pelvic inflammatory disease (PID)
▶ Ovarian cyst
▶ Ruptured Graafian follicle
▶ Acute gastroenteritis
▶ No organic finding (!)

Luminal obstruction
▶ Fecaliths
▶ Hypertrophy of the lymphatic tissue
▶ Barium
▶ Vegetable
▶ Fruit seeds
▶ Foreign body
▶ Parasites (Ascariasis)
▶ Stricture

Arachnodactyly

Spider fingers
Abnormally long (spider-like) and slender hands and fingers. Feet and toes also often affected.

Causes
▶ Marfan's syndrome
▶ Achard syndrome (small receding mandible, broad skull, laxness of joints)
▶ Spondylocostal dysostosis
▶ Lutembacher's syndrome
▶ MASS syndrome
▶ Homocystinuria
▶ Van der Hoeve's syndrom(subtype of osteogenesis imperfecta)

Areflexia, See Renal Failure, Acute → 315

Arrhythmias
See Cardiac Dysrhythmias → 62

Arterial Bruit

Arterial murmur, bruit
▶ Arteriosclerosis
▶ Constricted arteries
  - Congenital
  - Intimal proliferation
  - Arteriosclerotic plaque
▶ Arterial aneurysm
▶ Thyroid artery dilation
▶ Arteriovenous fistula
▶ Aortic coarctation with large collaterals

Arterial Hypoxemia
See Blood Gas Analysis → 57

Pulmonary causes
▶ Restrictive lung disease (pCO_2 normal)
  - Pneumothorax
  - After pulmonary resection
  - Lung compression due to pleural effusion/tumor
▶ Diffusion impairment (pCO_2 normal or lowered)
  - Sarcoidosis
  - Lymphangitic metastases
  - ARDS
  - Hamman-Rich syndrome
▶ Distribution impairment (pCO_2 normal or lowered)
  - Pneumonia
  - Bronchial asthma
  - Emphysema
  - Atelectasis
  - Pulmonary infarction
  - Pneumoconiosis
  - Thoracic deformity
  - Neoplastic
  - Bronchial mucus obstruction

► Perfusion disorder (pCO_2 normal or decreased)
  ○ Pulmonary edema
  ○ Right-left shunt
► Miscellaneous
  • Mechanical ventilation
  • High altitude

Arthralgias, See Arthritis → 41

Arthritis

Articular rheumatism, arthralgia, joint disease, joint inflammation
Inflammation of a joint or a state characterized by inflammation of joints.

Monoarticular, oligoarticular
Monoarthritis, monoarticular joint pain
► Septic arthritis (see infection)
► Rheumatoid arthritis
► Juvenile rheumatoid arthritis
► Crystalline-induced arthritis
  • Gout
  • Pseudogout
  • Calcium oxalate
  • Hydroxyapatite
  • Calcium/phosphate crystals
► Trauma
► Hemarthrosis
► Degenerative joint disease
► Infection
  • Bacterial
    ○ Gonococcus
    ○ Staphylococcus
    ○ Pneumococcus
    ○ Tuberculosis
  • Viral
    ○ Hepatitis B
    ○ Rubella
    ○ Mumps
  • Fungal
  • Rickettsial
  • Parasitic
► Polyarticular rheumatic disease
  • Juvenile rheumatoid arthritis

  • Ankylosing spondylitis
  • Rheumatoid arthritis
  • Reiter's syndrome
  • Systemic lupus erythematosus
► Hematologic
  • Leukemia
  • Lymphoma
  • Bleeding disorders
    ○ Hemophilia
    ○ Von Willebrand's disease
    ○ Anticoagulant therapy
► Systemic
  • Psoriasis
  • Behçet's syndrome
  • Inflammatory bowel disease
    ○ Ulcerative colitis
    ○ Crohn's disesase
  • Pancreatitis
  • Pancreatic carcinoma
  • Whipple's disease
  • Familial Mediterranean fever
  • Storage disease
  • Acromegaly
  • Amyloidosis
► Neuropathic arthropathy
  • Tabes dorsalis
  • Diabetes mellitus
  • Syringomyelia
► Joint tumor
  • Hemangioma
  • Sarcoma
  • Pigmented villonodular synovitis
► Miscellaneous
  • Loose joint body
  • Foreign body
  • Palindromic rheumatism
  • Radiation
  • Relapsing polychondritis

Polyarticular
► Rheumatoid arthritis
► Juvenile rheumatoid arthritis
► Rheumatic fever
► Ankylosing spondylitis
► Collagen vascular disease
  • Systemic lupus erythematosus

A

- Polymyositis
- Dermatomyositis
- Scleroderma
- Mixed connective tissue disease
- Wegener's granulomatosis
- Polyarteritis nodosa
- Henoch-Schönlein purpura
- Polymyalgia rheumatica
▶ Systemic
- Psoriasis
- Sjögren's syndrome
- Reiter's syndrome
- Behçet's syndrome
- Inflammatory bowel disease
  ○ Ulcerative colitis
  ○ Crohn's disease
- Whipple's disease
- Pancreatitis
- Pancreatic carcinoma
- Familial Mediterranean fever
- Sarcoidosis
- Amyloidosis
- Acromegaly
- Hemochromatosis
- Wilson's disease
- Hypothyrroidism
- Hyperlipoproteinemia
▶ Hematologic
- Leukemia
- Lymphoma
- Multiple myeloma
- Hemophilia
- Hemoglobinopathies
▶ Hypersensitivity, autoimmune
- Serum sickness
- Hyperglobulinemic purpura
- Hypogammaglobulinemia
- Alpha-interferon induced
▶ Storage disease
- Gaucher's disease
- Fabry's disease
▶ Infection
- Bacterial
  ○ Neisseria gonorrhoeae
  ○ Streptococcus pneumoniae

○ Streptococcus pyogenes
○ Other streptococcus species
○ Staphylococcus aureus
○ Enterobacteriaceae
○ Haemophilus influenzae
○ Gram-negative bacilli
○ Lyme arthritis
○ Bacterial endocarditis
○ Tuberculosis
○ Reiter's syndrome
- Viral
  ○ Rubella
  ○ Parvovirus B19
  ○ Mumps
  ○ Varicella zoster virus
  ○ HIV
  ○ Hepatitis A virus
  ○ Hepatitis B virus
  ○ Hepatitis C virus
  ○ Arboviruses
  ○ Adenoviruses
  ○ Enteroviruses
  ○ EBV
  ○ Alphaviruses
- Fungal
- Rickettsial
- Parasitic
▶ Crystal deposition disease
- Gout
- Pseudogout
▶ Trauma
▶ Degenerative joint disease
▶ Joint tumor
- Hemangioma
- Sarcoma
- Pigmented villonodular synovitis
▶ Neuropathic arthropathy
- Tabes dorsalis
- Diabetes mellitus
- Syringomyelia
▶ Miscellaneous
- Relapsing polychondritis
- Palindromic rheumatism
- Erythema nodosum
- Renal transplant

- Tietze's syndrome
- Hypertrophic osteoarthropathy
- Intermittent hydrarthrosis
- Acute tropical polyarthritis
- Radiation

Arthropathy, See Arthritis → 41

Ascites

Accumulation of peritoneal fluid in the abdominal cavity.

Most common causes (90%)
▶ Cirrhosis (→ 78)
▶ Malignancy
▶ Congestive heart failure
▶ Tuberculosis

Causes by location
▶ Peritoneal source
- Tuberculosis
- Bacterial, fungal or parasitic disease
- Cancer (malignant ascites)
- Vasculitis
- Whipple's disease
- Familial mediterranean fever
- Endometriosis
- Starch peritonitis
▶ Extra-peritoneal source
- Cirrhosis (cirrhotic ascites)
- Congestive heart failure
- Budd-Chiari syndrome
- Hypoalbuminemia
  ○ Nephrotic syndrome
  ○ Protein-losing enteropathy
  ○ Malnutrition
- Hypothyroidism
- Ovarian disease (e.g. Meigs' syndrome)
- Pancreatic disease
- Chylous ascites

Classification I
▶ Mechanical ascites/portal hypertension
- Prehepatic block
  ○ Splenic vein thrombosis
  ○ Portal vein occlusion
    - *Thrombosis*

- *Tumor*
  ○ Arterioportal shunt
- Intrahepatic block (approx. 75 % of cases)
  ○ Pre-sinusoidal
    - *Myeloproliferative diseases*
    - *Wilson's disease*
    - *Liver metastases*
    - *Schistosomiasis*
  ○ Sinusoidal
    - *Cirrhosis*
    - *Chronic hepatitis*
    - *Fatty liver*
  ○ Post-sinusoidal
    - *Veno-occlusive diseases*
    - *cirrhosis*
    - *Drugs*
- Posthepatic blockage
  ○ Budd-Chiari syndrome (occlusion of the hepatic veins by thromboses or tumor compression)
  ○ Right ventricular failure
  ○ Constrictive pericarditis
▶ Malignant ascites
- Neoplastic
▶ Inflammatory ascites
- Bacterial peritonitis
▶ Pancreatogenic ascites
- Pancreatitis with irritation of the peritoneum
▶ Hypoalbuminemic ascites
- Nephrotic syndrome
- Exudative enteropathy

Classification II
▶ Without peritoneal irritation
- Portal ascites in:
  ○ Cirrhosis
  ○ Hepatic failure
  ○ Alcoholic hepatitis
  ○ Congested liver
    - *Heart failure*
    - *Right ventricular failure*
    - *Tricuspid insufficiency*
    - *Constrictive pericarditis*
    - *Obstruction of the inferior vena*

cava
- *Obstruction of the hepatic vein (Budd-Chiari syndrome)*
- *Cardiomyopathy*
  ○ Occlusion of the portal vein
- *Thrombosis*
- *Tumor*
  ○ Polycystic liver
  ○ Vitamin A overdose
  ○ Arteriovenous fistula
  ○ Idiopathic
- Hypoalbuminemia (→ 16)
  ○ Cirrhosis
  ○ Nephrotic syndrome
  ○ Severe hypoalbuminemia
  ○ Enteral protein loss syndrome
- *Mucosal diseases with increased protein exudation*
- *Intestinal lymphatic blockage*
- *Whipple's disease*
  ○ Malnutrition
- Chylous ascites
  ○ Rupture of abdominal lymph vessels
- *Trauma*
- *Surgery*
  ○ Obstruction of lymph vessels
- *Secondary in malignant diseases*
- *Tuberculosis*
- *Filariasis*
  ○ Hereditary lymphangiectasia
- Cardiac ascites
  ○ Right ventricular failure
  ○ Constrictive pericarditis
- Miscellaneous
  ○ Increased sodium reabsorption in cirrhosis through secondary hyperaldosteronism (increased synthesis of aldosterone and reduced hepatic catabolism of aldosterone)
  ○ Hypothyroidism
  ○ Amyloidosis
  ○ Mesenteric vein thrombosis
  ○ Hypothyroidism
  ○ Ovarian disorders
- *Meigs' syndrome*

- *Ovarian overstimulation*
▶ With peritoneal involvement
- Infections
  ○ Mycobacterial
  ○ Bacterial
- *Primary (spontaneous bacterial peritonitis [SBP] with cirrhosis)*
- *Secondary (rupture of visceral organs: intestines, gall bladder)*
  ○ Fungal
- *Oral candidiasis*
- *Histoplasmosis*
- *Cryptococcosis*
  ○ Parasites
- *Schistosomiasis*
- *Ascariasis*
- *Enterobiasis*
  ○ AIDS
- Neoplastic
  ○ Liver metastases/ intra-abdominal tumors/malignant ascites
- *Ovaries*
- *Pancreas*
- *Stomach*
- *Colon*
- *Lymphoma*
- *Peritoneal carcinomatosis*
- *Hepatocellular carcinoma*
- *Mesothelioma*
- *Lymphatic diseases*
- *Carcinoid*
- *Multiple myeloma*
- *Mastocytosis*
- Pancreatitis
- Miscellaneous
  ○ Peritoneal vasculitis
  ○ Systemic lupus erythematosus
  ○ Henoch-Schönlein purpura
  ○ Eosinophilic peritonitis
  ○ Familial Mediterranean fever
  ○ Whipple's disease
  ○ Uremia
  ○ Granulating peritonitis
- *Sarcoidosis*
  ○ Gynecologic

- *Endometriosis*
- *Ruptured dermoid cyst*
- *Peritoneal lymphangiectasis*

Classification III (Labs)
► Cell-rich ascites
- Granulocytes > 1000/ml
  ◦ Purulent peritonitis (evidence of bacteria)
- Lymphocyte > 70%
  ◦ Tuberculous peritonitis
- Malignant cells
  ◦ Peritoneal carcinomatosis
  ◦ Malignant tumors
► Chylous ascites
- Obstruction of the lymphatic drainage
  ◦ Tuberculosis
  ◦ Lymphomas
  ◦ Filariae
  ◦ Neoplastic
► Hemorrhagic ascites
- Erythrocytes > 10000/ml
  - *Neoplasm (malignant ascites)*
  - *Peritoneal carcinomatosis*
  - *Hepatocellular carcinoma*
  - *Ovarian cancer*
  ◦ Pancreatitis
  ◦ Tuberculous peritonitis
► High-protein ascites/Exudate
- Protein content > 2.5 g/l
  ◦ Peritonitis
  ◦ Collagen vascular disease
  ◦ Malignant tumors
  ◦ Peritoneal carcinomatosis
  ◦ Ileus (→ 206)
► Low-protein ascites/Transudate
- Protein content < 2.5 g/l
  ◦ Cirrhosis
  ◦ Hepatic failure
  ◦ Hypothyroidism
  ◦ Portal vein thrombosis
  ◦ Budd-Chiari syndrome (stenosis or occlusion of the hepatic vein)
  ◦ Malignant tumors
  ◦ Hepatic metastases
  ◦ Nephrotic syndrome

◦ Obstruction of the inferior vena cava
► Malignant ascites
- Cholesterol > 46 mg/dl
- Fibronectin > 50 µg/dl
- LDH > 300 U/l
- Cytology
► Pancreatogenic ascites
- Increased amylase
- Increased lipase
► Ascites fluid assorted labs
- Culture and cytology

Classification IV
► Exudate (Serum to ascites albumin gradient <1.1)
- Peritonitis
- Pancreatitis
- Vasculitis
- Neoplasm (malignant ascites)
- Abdominal trauma with ruptured lymphatics
- Amyloidosis
- Struma ovarii
- Intestinal lymphatic blockage
  ◦ Lymphangiectasis
  ◦ Malignant lymphoma
- Sarcoidosis
- Hypothyroidism
- Transected lymphatics after porta-cava shunt surgery
- Talc or starch powder peritonitis after surgery
- Tuberculous peritonitis
- Neoplastic diseases involving the peritoneum
► Transudate (Serum to ascites albumin gradient >1.1)
- Constrictive pericarditis
- Congestive heart failure
- Cirrhosis
- Primary (spontaneous bacterial peritonitis [SBP] with cirrhosis)
- Myelofibrosis
- Meig´s syndrome
- Viral hepatitis
- Nephrotic syndrome

- Budd-Chiari syndrome
- Disorders simulating ascites
- Pancreatic pseudocyst
- Hydronephrosis
- Ovarian cyst
- Mesenteric cyst
- Obesity

Aspartate-Aminotransferase
See Aminotransferases → 23

AST (Aspartate-Aminotransferase)
See Aminotransferases → 23

AT III, See Antithrombin III → 38

Ataxia

Lack of coordination, loss of coordination, incoordination, irregularity of voluntary movements, coordination impairment, clumsiness, wobbliness.

Inability to coordinate muscle activity during voluntary movement, so that smooth movements occur. Often due to disorders of the cerebellum or the posterior columns of the spinal cord.
See Gait Abnormalities → 149

Cerebellar, spinal and systemic
▶ Vitamin B_{12} deficiency!
▶ Malabsorption syndrome
▶ Drugs, toxins
  - Alcohol!
  - Benzodiazepines
  - Barbiturates
  - Morphine
  - Carbon monoxide
▶ Endocrine, metabolic
  - Paraneoplastic
  - Hypothyroidism
  - Diabetic neuropathy
  - α-β-lipoproteinaemia (clinical picture as in sprue, with retinitis pigmentosa and ataxia)
▶ Neoplasm
  - Fisher's syndrome
    ○ Cerebellar neoplasm
  - Acoustic neurinoma
  - Paraneoplastic
▶ Neurologic
  - Cerebellar cortex atrophy
  - Multiple sclerosis
  - Cerebellar abscess
  - Circulation disorders in the brain stem area
  - Diseases of the vestibular apparatus
  - Infectious causes
  - Hemorrhagic pseudoencephalitis
    ○ Cirrhosis
    ○ Alcoholism
    ○ Wernicke's encephalopathy
  - Cerebellar heredoataxia
  - Ataxia-teleangiectasia
  - GM2-gangliosidoses
  - Mitochondrial cytopathy
  - Spinocerebellar ataxia
  - Familial periodic ataxia
  - Arnold-Chiari syndrome
  - Graefe-Sjögren's syndrome
  - Hartnup syndrome
  - Wilson's disease
  - Westphal's disease (hepatolenticular degeneration occurring in puberty)
  - Mann syndrome
  - Myelin damage
    ○ Encephalitis
    ○ Measles
    ○ Chicken pox
    ○ Smallpox
  - Spinal cord compression and pressure on the dorsal nerve roots
  - HIV infection
  - Marinescu-Garland syndrome
  - Basilar impression/vertebral-basilar artery ischemia
  - Polyneuritis
  - Friedreich's ataxia
  - Tabes dorsalis

- Multiple sclerosis
► Miscellaneous
- Acanthocytosis

Cerebral ataxia (contralateral clinical picture)
► Thalamic syndrome
► Epiphyseal tumor
► Parietal lobe lesion
► Temporal lobe lesion
► Trauma
► Tumor
► Arteriosclerosis
► Infectious diseases
► Frontal lobe lesion
► Hemorrhage
► Ischemia
► Morgagni's syndrome

Atrial fibrillation
See Cardiac Dysrhythmias → 62

Autoantibodies in Connective Tissue Diseases

Disease	ANA Frequency (%)
SLE	90–100
Disciform LE	21–50
Drug-induced lupus	95
Mixed connective tissue disease (MCTD)	100
Scleroderma	31–90
CREST syndrome	95
Rheumatoid arthritis	10–60
Felty's syndrome	60–10
Dermatomyositis	40
Autoimmune chronic hepatitis	45–100
Myasthenia gravis	35–50
Immune thrombocytopenia	50–70
Autoimmune thyroiditis	40–50
Leukemias	70

Infectious mononucleosis	30–70
Periarteritis nodosa, Raynaud's disease, Sjögren syndrome, cirrhosis	

Disease:	Antibodies against
SLE	anti-double-stranded DNA
	anti-single-stranded DNA
	anti-ribonucleoprotein (RNP)
	anti-NA
	anti-Sm
	anti-Ro/SSA
	anti-La/SSB
	anti-histone (medicamentous LE)
Scleroderma	anti-NA
	anticentromere
	anti-Scl-70
	anti-ribonucleoprotein (RNP)
Polymyositis/ dermato-myositis	anti-Jo-1
	anti-Ku-1
	anti-Pm-1
MCTD	anti-ribonucleoprotein (RNP)
Sjögren's syndrome	anti-Ro/SSA
	anti-La/SSB
Wegener's granuloma-tosis	ANCA
CREST syndrome	anticentromere

Autoimmune Hemolytic Anemia
AIHA

Anemias resulting from an increased rate of erythrocyte destruction due to immune attacks against own erythrocyte membrane antigens.
► Warm autoimmune hemolytic anemia (→ 381)
► Cold agglutinin disease (cold reactive IgM autoantibodies) (→ 79)
► Paroxysmal cold hemoglobinuria (complement activating IgG) (→ 278)
► Drug-induced hemolytic anemia
See Anemia → 28

Azoospermia, Oligospermia

Azoospermia, aspermia: absence of living spermatozoa in the semen, failure of spermatogenesis.

Oligospermia: subnormal concentration of sperms in the ejaculate (< 20 million/ml). See Impotence → 208

Pretesticular azoospermia
► Ejaculatory dysfunctions
  • Psychosexual dysfunction
  • Prior urologic surgery
  • Drugs
  • Neurologic disease
► Hypogonadotropic hypogonadism (pituitary FSH and LH deficiency)
► Anabolic steroid hormone abuse (body building)
► Hypothyroidism
► Hemochromatosis

Testicular azoospermia
► Cryptorchidism (undescended testes)
► Androgen resistance syndromes
► 5-alpha reductase deficiency
► Congenital anorchism
► Infection of testes (orchitis)
  • Mumps
  • Testicular tuberculosis
  • Syphilis
  • Other bacterial infections
► Sertoli only syndrome
► Vascular disorder
  • Trauma
  • Torsion (twisting)
  • Varicocele
► Traumatic damage
► Testicular tumor
► Gonadotoxins
  • Alcohol
  • Radiation
  • Heat
  • Chemotherapeutics
  • Excessive heat
  • Drugs

Posttesticular azoospermia
► Obstructive lesions of the
  • Epididymis
  • Vas deferens
  • Ejaculatory ducts
► Vasectomy
► Retrograde ejaculation
  • Postoperative conditions
  • Impaired nerve function

Babinski Reflex
Babinski's sign, Babinski's phenomenom
Extension of the great toe and abduction of the other toes when stimulating the external portion (the outside) of the sole. Normal in younger children. After about 2 years old indicative of pyramidal tract involvement.

Positive in:
► Stroke
► Subarachnoid hemorrhage
► Head injury
► Spinal cord injury
► Spinal cord tumor
► Multiple sclerosis
► Funicular myelosis
► During generalized tonic-clonic seizure
► Brown–Sequard syndrome
► Friedreich's ataxia
► Brain tumor
  • brain stem
  • cerebellum
  • corticospinal tract
► Amyotrophic lateral sclerosis
► Syringomyelia
► Wallenberg's syndrome
► Familial periodic paralysis
► Infectious diseases
  • Meningitis
  • Poliomyelitis (some forms)
  • Rabies
  • Tabes dorsalis
  • Tetanus
  • Tuberculosis (spine TB)

▶ Hypoglycemia
▶ Hepatic encephalopathy
▶ Pernicious anemia

Back Pain
Backache, cervical/lumbar pain
Pain in the spine or muscles of the back.
Common causes
▶ Idiopathic lumbago
▶ Discopathy
▶ Trauma due to lifting
Vertebral causes
▶ Postural imbalance
  • Anteroposterior
    ○ Pregnancy
  • Lateral
    ○ Scoliosis
    ○ Leg length discrepancy
▶ Trauma
  • Lumbar sprain
  • Lumbar strain
  • Vertebral fracture
  • Subluxation of joints
▶ Disc herniation
▶ Spondylitis, Sacroiliitis
  • Ankylosing spondylitis
  • Spondylitis in colitis
  • Psoriatic arthritis
  • Reiter's syndrome
  • Behçet's syndrome
▶ Spondylosis
▶ Rheumatoid arthritis
▶ Polymyalgia rheumatica
▶ Fibromyalgia
▶ Spinal stenosis
  • Congenital
  • Degenerative
  • Posttraumatic
  • Paget's disease
  • Renal osteodystrophy
  • Iatrogenic
    ○ Postlaminectomy
    ○ Postchemonucleolysis
▶ Infection, inflammation

• Disc space infection
• Reiter's disease
• Borreliosis
• Herpes zoster
• Osteomyelitis
• Spondylodiscitis
• Epidural abscess
• Arachnoiditis (!)
▶ Congenital
  • Spina bifida
  • Spondylolysis
  • Spondylolisthesis
▶ Spinal or vertebral tumor
  • Benign
    ○ Meningioma
    ○ Hemangioma
  • Malignant
    ○ Osteogenic Sarcoma
    ○ Multiple myeloma
  • Metastasis
▶ Hyperparathyroidism
▶ Osteochondrosis
▶ Osteoporosis
▶ Osteomalacia
▶ Scheuermann's disease
▶ Hypomobility
▶ Hypermobility
▶ Facet syndrome
Extravertebral causes
▶ Idiopathic (very frequent)
  • Musculoligamentary
  • Psychosomatic
▶ Referred pain
  • Cardiac, pulmonary
    ○ Coronary ischemia
    ○ Pleuritis
    ○ Pleurodynia
    ○ Pneumonia
    ○ Pulmonary embolia
  • Abdominal
    ○ Pancreatitis
    ○ Pancreas carcinoma
    ○ Cholelithiasis
    ○ Ulcer disease
  • Renal

B

- ◦ Nephrolithiasis
- ◦ Pyelonephritis
- ◦ Polycystic kidney disease
- Vascular
  - ◦ Aortic aneurysm
  - ◦ Leriche's syndrome
- Neurogenic
  - ◦ Intraspinal processes
  - ◦ Herpes zoster
- Myogenic
  - ◦ Myopathies
  - ◦ Myositis
  - ◦ Myotendinosis
- Gynecologic
  - ◦ Tumor
  - ◦ Endometriosis
- Hematologic
  - ◦ Sickle cell disease
  - ◦ Myelofibrosis
- Retroperitoneal
  - ◦ Abscess
  - ◦ Hematoma
  - ◦ Fibrosis
  - ◦ Tumor
- Coxarthrosis
- Gonarthrosis
- Foot deformity
- Abnormally flexible ribs

Pain along the entire vertebral column
▶ Skeletal system
- Without neurologic failures
  - ◦ Osteoporosis
  - ◦ Cushing's disease
  - ◦ Osteomalacia
  - ◦ Spondylarthritis
  - ◦ Paget's disease
  - ◦ Primary/secondary hyperparathyroidism
  - ◦ Scoliosis
  - ◦ Abnormalities
  - ◦ Idiopathic
- Neurologic failure possible
  - ◦ Malignant processes of vertebral body

Neck pain (cervical spine)
▶ Skeletal system
- Without neurologic failures
  - ◦ Degenerative skeletal changes
  - ◦ Distortions
- Neurologic failures possible
  - ◦ Osteolytic processes
    - – *Malignancy*
    - – *Bacterial inflammations*
  - ◦ Fractures
  - ◦ Injury of disci and ligaments
▶ Other cause
- Without neurologic failures
  - ◦ Polymyalgia rheumatica
- Neurologic failures possible
  - ◦ Meningitis
  - ◦ Subarachnoid hemorrhage

Upper back pain (thoracic spine)
▶ Skeletal system
- Without neurologic failures
  - ◦ Degenerative skeletal changes
  - ◦ Scoliosis
  - ◦ Incorrect posture
  - ◦ Scheuermann's disease
- Neurologic failures possible
  - ◦ Osteolytic processes
    - – *Malignancy*
    - – *Bacterial inflammations*
  - ◦ Fractures
- With neurologic failures
  - ◦ Spinal tumor
  - ◦ Epidural abscess
▶ Other cause
- Without neurologic failure
  - ◦ Coronary heart disease
  - ◦ Myocardial infarction
  - ◦ Aortic aneurysm
  - ◦ Pleuritis
  - ◦ Mediastinitis
  - ◦ Ulcer disease
- With neurologic failures
  - ◦ Herpes zoster

Low back pain, lumbar pain (lumbar spine/ os sacrum)
▶ Skeletal system

- Without neurologic failures
  - Degenerative skeletal changes
  - Lumbago syndrome
  - Bechterew's disease
  - Sacroileiitis
- Neurologic failures possible
  - Osteolytic processes
    - *Malignancy*
    - *Bacterial inflammations*
  - Fractures
  - Spondylolisthesis
- With neurologic failure
  - Lumbal discopathy
  - Syndrome of the tight spinal canal
  - Dysraphia
► Other cause
- Without neurologic failures
  - Pancreas affections
  - Aortic aneurysm
  - Gynecologic diseases
  - Chronic ureteral obstruction
  - States of functional pain
- Neurologic failure possible
  - Retroperitoneal tumors

Barrel Chest

A thorax permanently resembling the shape of a barrel, typical for emphysema.

Causes
► Emphysema
► Chronic bronchitis (with emphysema)
► Osteomalacia
► Congested lung
► Asthma
► Lung cyst

Basophilic Leukocytes

Reference range

0.5% (least common leukocyte)

Increased (Basophilia)
► Hypothyroidism
► Allergic diathesis
► Chronic inflammatory processes

- Ulcerative colitis
- Chronic sinusitis
- Asthma
- Chronic sinusitis
► Infections
- Viral infections
  - Chicken pox
  - Influenza
- Tuberculosis
► Hodgkin's lymphoma
► Myeloproliferative syndromes, hematologic
- Polycythemia vera
- Chronic myelogenous leukemia
- Idiopathic thrombocythemia
- Osteomyelosclerosis
► Endocrine
- Hypothyroidism
- Increased estrogen
  - Estrogen therapy
- Diabetes mellitus
► Miscellaneous
- Following splenectomy
- Mastocytosis
- Radiation exposure

Decreased
► Stress
► Hypersensitivity reaction
► Corticosteroids
► Pregnancy
► Hyperthyroidism

Bilirubin

During physiologic catabolism of hemoglobin in the reticuloendothelial system, water-insoluble indirect (unconjugated) bilirubin is formed, which then binds to albumin in the blood. In the liver, water-soluble direct bilirubin is then formed through conjugation, which reaches the intestine via the gall bladder, where it is transformed by bacteria into urobilinogens. 80% of urobilinogen is excreted in the feces and 20% goes into enterohepatic circulation. Only approx. 1% is discharged through the kidneys. An increase in urobilinogens results in increased excretion of urobilinogens in the urine. If total bilirubin is > 2 mg/dl, **jaundice** of the conjunctiva, skin and mucosa results.

Reference range
Total bilirubin 0.3–1.0 mg/dl (5.1–17 µmol/l)

Classification I
▶ Primarily direct bilirubin (conjugated bilirubin, obstructive jaundice)
- Hepatic disorders
  - Viral hepatitis A, B, C, D, E
  - Epstein-Barr virus (EBV)
  - Cytomegalovirus (CMV)
  - Hepatitis due primarily to hepatotropic viruses
  - Autoimmune hepatitis
  - Acute alcoholic hepatitis
  - Hepatotoxic liver damage
  - Liver cell carcinoma
  - Cholangitis
  - (Decompensated) cirrhosis of miscellaneous genesis
  - Biliary tract obstruction
  - Storage diseases
  - Liver abscess
- Congested liver
  - Congestive heart failure
- Shock
- Sepsis
- Hepatic trauma
- Sarcoidosis
- Amyloidosis
- Postoperative jaundice
- Total parenteral nutrition
- Extrahepatic cholestasis (→ 75)
  - Biliary atresia
  - Cystic fibrosis
  - Cholecystitis
  - Choledocholithiasis
  - Neoplasm
    - *Gallbladder tumors*
    - *Bile duct tumors*
    - *Pancreas tumors*
    - *Lymphoma*
    - *Metastases*
  - External compression
  - Strictures (common bile duct, primary sclerosing cholangitis, AIDS with cryptosporidium infection)
  - Pancreatitis
  - Parasites (Ascariasis)
- Intrahepatic biliary obstruction
  - Primary biliary cirrhosis
  - Primary sclerosing cholangitis
  - Liver allograft rejection
- Graft-versus-host disease
- Hereditary
  - Dubin-Johnson syndrome
  - Rotor's syndrome
  - Gilberts disease
- Drugs, toxins
  - Corticosteroids
  - Chemotherapeutics
  - Halothane
  - Indomethacin
  - Methyldopa
  - Phenothiazines
  - Tetracyclines
- During pregnancy
  - Benign recurring cholestasis
  - HELLP syndrome
  - Eclampsia
  - Hyperemesis gravidarum
- Neonatal patients
  - Sepsis
  - Intrauterine viral infections
  - Neonatal hepatitis
  - Intrahepatic and extrahepatic biliary atresia
  - Biliary tract obstruction
    - *Choledochal cyst*
    - *Abdominal mass*
    - *Annular pancreas*
  - Trisomy 18
  - Galactosemia
  - Tyrosinemia
  - Hereditary (Dubin-Johnson, Rotor's

syndrome)
- Hypermethioninemia
- Alpha-1 antitrypsin deficiency
- Cystic fibrosis
- Following hemolytic disease of the newborn syndrome
- Hypopituitarism
- Hypothyroidism

▶ Primarily indirect (unconjugated bilirubin/hemolytic jaundice)
- Hemolytic anemia
  - Sickle cell anemia
  - Spherocytosis
  - Thalassemia
  - Glucose-6-phosphate dehydrogenase deficiency
  - Transfusion reaction
  - Drug-induced
  - Autoimmunohemolysis
- Pernicious anemia
- Conditions following hemorrhage
- Polycythemia vera
- Sepsis
- Hyperbilirubinemia after portocaval shunt insertion
- Gilbert's syndrome
- Jaundice of newborn
- Fetal erythroblastosis
- Kernicterus
- Blood transfusion in premature infants
- Hyperthyroidism
- Gilbert's syndrome
- Crigler–Najjar syndrome
- Lucey-Discroll syndrome
- Hyperbilirubinemia after heart surgery
- Primary hyperbilirubinemia

Classification II
▶ Prehepatic
- Congenital hemolytic anemia
  - Hemoglobinopathy
  - Wilson's disease
  - Spherocytosis
- Acquired hemolytic anemia
  - Drugs

- Zieve's syndrome
- HELLP syndrome
- Malaria
- Autoantibodies
- Congenital anemia
  - Glucose-6-phosphate dehydrogenase deficiency
  - Primaquine
  - Fava beans
  - Hemolysis after quinine

▶ Intrahepatic
- Liver parenchyma disorders
  - Wilson's disease
  - Porphyrias
  - Alcoholic liver damage
  - Hemochromatosis
- Hepatitis
  - Concomitant hepatitis with bacterial, viral, parasitic infections
  - Viral hepatitis
  - Inflammatory bowel disease
  - Alcohol
  - Drugs
- Sepsis
- Shock
- Congested liver
  - Right ventricular failure
  - Budd-Chiari syndrome (stenosis or occlusion of the hepatic vein)
  - Constrictive pericarditis
- Functional hyperbilirubinemia
  - Gilbert's disease
  - Crigler–Najjar syndrome
  - Dubin-Johnson syndrome
  - Rotor's syndrome

▶ Intrahepatic cholestasis (impaired bile secretion in the liver)
- Cholestatic course of viral hepatitis
- Drug-induced cholestatic jaundice
  - Phenothiazines
  - Sex hormones
  - Thyroid depressants
- Fatty liver
- Pregnancy cholestasis
- Idiopathic postoperative jaundice

B

- Mechanical drainage impairment
  - Liver cancer.
  - Cholangiocellular carcinoma
  - Liver metastases
  - Liver cysts
  - Echinococcosis
  - Amebiasis
  - Liver abscess
  - Primary biliary cirrhosis
  - Primary sclerosing cholangitis
- Zieve's syndrome
- Reye's syndrome
- Drugs
► Extrahepatic
- Stenosing diseases of the extrahepatic bile ducts
  - Choledocholiths
  - Papillary stenosis
  - Carbonic anhydrase inhibitors
  - Tumors
  - Stricture
  - Parasites
- External compression of the cystic duct
  - Pancreatitis
  - Pancreatic cyst
  - Pancreatic cancer
  - Echinococcosis of the liver
  - Liver abscess
  - Duodenal abscess
  - Metastases
  - Lymphomas
  - Mirizzi's syndrome
- Miscellaneous
  - Parasitosis
  - Caroli's syndrome

Bilirubinuria

Presence of bilirubin in the urine. Normally bilirubin does not occur in the urine. If serum bilirubin is over threshold value (> 2 mg/100 ml), urine contains bilirubin and becomes dark. Bilirubinuria does not occur in pure hemolytic types of jaundice. Its presence, readily detected at the bedside with a commercial urine test strip, indicates hepatobiliary disease. Unconjugated hyperbilirubin is tightly bound to albumin, not filtered by the glomerulus, and absent from urine even with raised serum levels of unconjugated bilirubin. A positive test for urine bilirubin confirms that any raised plasma levels are from conjugated hyperbilirubinemia.

See Bilirubin → 51
See Cholestasis → 75

Causes

► Fetal erythroblastosis
► Biliary atresia
► Obstructive jaundice
► Cirrhosis
► Hepatitis
► Cholangitis
► Dubin-Johnson syndrome
► Rotor's syndrome
► Polycythemia vera

Bladder Discomfort

Causes

► Cystitis
► Stones
► Vesical diverticulum
► Infection
- Trichomonas
- Gonorrhea
- Tuberculosis
- Bilharziosis
► Foreign body
► Tumor
► Tumor infiltration
- Cervica carcinomal
- Rectal carcinoma
► Diabetes mellitus
► Myelitis
► Descensus uteri
► Drugs
- Isoniazid
- Phenothiazine

Bleeding, anovulatory

Metrorrhagia

Causes

▶ Immature hypothalamic-pituitary-ovarian axis
▶ Polycystic ovary syndrome (Stein Leventhal syndrome)
▶ Peri-menopause
▶ Nutrition
  • Obesity
  • Very low calorie diets
  • Nutritional status
  • Anorexia nervosa
▶ Intense exercise
▶ Norepinephrine (affects LH)
▶ Psychologic stress

Bleeding, cerebral

See Bleeding, Intracranial → 56

Bleeding, Genital

Vaginal bleeding

See Bleeding, anovulatory → 55

Causes

▶ Midcycle ovulatory bleeding
▶ Inadequate corpus luteum
▶ Vaginal or cervical disease
  • Cervical cancer
  • Vulvar cancer
  • Vaginal cancer
  • Vaginal varices
  • Cervical erosion
  • Trauma in the vaginal area
  • Prolapsed uterus
  • Colpitis senilis
  • Vaginal infections
▶ Uterine or endometrial disease
  • Endometriosis
  • Endometritis
  • Uterine adenomytosis
  • Endometrial polyps
  • Uterine leiomyomas

  • Neoplastic
  • Intrauterine device (IUD)
▶ Endocrine disorders
  • Hypothalamic or pituitary lesion
  • Adrenal disease
  • Thyroid disease
▶ Hemorrhaging during pregnancy (in the first three months of pregnancy, causes remain unknown in > 50%)
  • Abortion
  • Ectopic pregnancy
  • Hydatidiform mole
  • chorionepithelioma
  • Premature placental abruption
  • Placenta previa
  • Lacerated placenta
  • Ruptured uterus
  • Vaginal infections or trauma
  • Cervicitis
  • Cervical polyp
  • Cervical neoplasms
  • Postcoital hemorrhage
  • Velamentous insertion
  • Rupture hemorrhage
    ○ Labia
    ○ Vaginoperineum
▶ Hemorrhage after childbirth
  • Rupture hemorrhage
    ○ Labia
    ○ Vaginoperineum
  • Endometriosis
  • Follicle persistence
  • Adherent placental residue
  • Fibrinogen deficiency
  • Atonic secondary bleeding
▶ Spotting (genital organ bleeding that is not bound to the normal cycle as well as postmenopausal hemorrhages)
  • Organic bleeding disorders
    ○ Carcinoma (vaginal, cervical, endometrial)
    ○ Myoma
    ○ Cervical polyp
    ○ Varicosis of the vagina
    ○ Injuries

○ IUD
○ Cervical ectopia
○ Infections
  - *Colpitis*
  - *Adnexitis*
  - *Endometritis)*
○ Stress/psychogenic factors
- Endocrine impairment
  ○ Corpus luteum deficiency syndrome
  ○ Follicle persistence
  ○ Estrogen-progestogen therapy
  ○ Estrogen breaktrough bleeding
  ○ Granulosa cell tumor
  ○ Chorionepithelioma

Bleeding, Intracranial

Subarachnoid hemorrhage, SAH
Bleeding within the subarachnoid space
(CSF filled space between the middle
membrane and the brain itself). Approx.
10% of intracranial bleedings.
▶ Causes
  • Trauma
  • Nontraumatic
    ○ Ruptured intracerebral aneurysm
    ○ Arteriovenous malformation
    ○ Mycotic aneurysm
    ○ Bacterial endocarditis
    ○ Hemorrhagic diathesis
    ○ Leukemia
    ○ Brain tumor
    ○ Infections
▶ Disorders associated with aneurysm
  • Polycystic kidney disease
  • Fibromuscular dysplasia (FMD)
  • Other connective tissue disorders
  • Other aneurysms
  • Hypertension
  • Smoking
  • Alcoholism

Extradural hemorrhage
Bleeding between the skull and the dura
mater. Approx. 30% of intracranial
bleedings.

▶ Skull fracture (Rupture of the middle
  meningeal artery)
▶ Rarely hemorrhage from a fracture gap,
  injured venous sinus or arachnoid villi

Subdural hemorrhage
Bleeding from leaking blood veins that are
located between the dural and
arachnoidal membranes (the meninges).
Approx. 50% of intracranial bleedings.
▶ Usually due to head injury
▶ Types
  • Acute subdural hematoma (symptoms
    within 24 hours)
  • Subacute subdural hematoma
    (symptoms within two to 10 days)
▶ Risks
  • Head injury
  • Very young or advanced age
  • Chronic use of aspirin
  • Anticoagulant medication
  • Alcoholism
  • Any disorder that results in falling

**Intracerebral hemorrhage (cerebral
bleeding, hematencephalon)**
Bleeding within the brain due to rupturing
of an intracranial vessel, e.g. in the region
of the internal capsule. Approx. 10% of
intracranial bleedings.
▶ Causes
  • Trauma (brain injury in connection
    with epidural/subdural hematomas)
  • Abnormalities of blood vessels
    ○ Aneurysm
    ○ Angioma
  • Hypertension (hypertensive
    intracerebral hemorrhage)
  • Anticoagulant medication
  • Secondary bleeding
    ○ After cerebral infarction
    ○ Tumor
    ○ Angioma
    ○ Perinatal hemorrhage
▶ Risks
  • Hemophilia
  • Decreased platelet count

- Sickle cell anemia
- DIC
- Anticoagulant medication
- Hypertension
- Embolic strokes

Bleeding, puerperal
See Bleeding, Genital → 55

Bleeding tendency
See Hemorrhagic Diathesis → 176

Bleeding Time

Reference ranges
Range: 2 to 9.5 minutes

Increased
▶ Thrombocytopenia
▶ Disseminated intravascular coagulation
See Disseminated Intravascular
Coagulation → 104
▶ Platelet disorders
  • Bernard-Soulier
  • Glanzmann's
▶ Capillary wall abnormalities
▶ Von Willebrand's disease
▶ Drugs
  • Aspirin
  • Beta-lactamase antibiotics
  • Dextran
  • Moxalactam
  • NSAIDs
  • Streptokinase
  • Urokinase
  • Warfarin

Blindness, See Vision Loss, Acute → 376

Blood Gas Analysis
Determination of oxygen partial pressure
(pO_2), carbon dioxide partial pressure
(pCO_2), oxygen saturation and buffer
capacity in arterial blood. Partial

respiratory failure occurs when respiratory
exchange is disturbed such that an arterial
hypoxemia without hypercapnia takes
place. Global respiratory failure occurs
when hypercapnia also takes place due to
alveolar insufficiency.

Reference range

Oxygen partial pressure (pO_2)

arterial pO_2	70-10 mmHg
venous pO_2	35-40 mmHg

Oxygen saturation (SO_2)

arterial SO_2	< 95%
venous SO_2	70-75%

Carbon dioxide partial pressure (pCO_2)

arterial pCO_2	35-45 mmHg
venous pCO_2	40-50 mmHg

Serum bicarbonate (HCO_3)

arterial HCO_3	20-27 mmol/l
venous HCO_3	19-28 mmol/l

pH

arterial pH	7.35-7.45
venous pH	7.26-7.46

Base excess (BE)

arterial BE	-3.4 - +2.3 mmol/l
venous BE	-2 - -5 mmol/l

Disorder	H^+	pH	HCO_3^-	pCO_2
Met. Ac.	↑	↓	↓↓*	(↓)
Met. Alk.	↓	↑	↑↑*	(↑)
Resp. Ac.	↑	↓	(↑)	↑↑*
Resp. Alk.	↓	↑	(↓)	↓↓*

* primary change
See Alkalosis, Metabolic → 18
See Acidosis, Respiratory → 12
See Alkalosis, Metabolic → 18
See Alkalosis, Respiratory → 19

Blood glucose
See Hyperglycemia → 189

See Hypoglycemia → 199,
See Glucosuria → 155
See HbA1, HbA1c → 162

Blood, occult, in the feces
See Occult Blood → 262

Blood pressure
See Hypertension → 194
See Hypotension → 204

Blurred vision, See Vision, Blurred → 376

Bone Pain

Causes
▸ Injury
  • Fractures
  • Fractures without appropriate trauma
  • Other injuries
▸ Osteoporosis
▸ Osteomalacia
▸ Osteomyelitis
  • Tuberculosis
  • Syphilis
  • Brodie's abscess
▸ Aseptic bone necrosis
▸ Primary/secondary hyperparathyroidism
▸ Renal osteopathy
▸ Paget's disease
▸ Tumor
  • Multiple myeloma
  • Acute leukemia
  • Benign bone tumor
  • Malignant bone tumor
  • Metastases
    ∘ Bronchial carcinoma
    ∘ Breast cancer
    ∘ Prostate cancer
    ∘ Hypernephroma
    ∘ Thyroid cancer
▸ Cystic subcartilaginous osteolyses
▸ Fibrous dysplasia (Jaffé-Lichtenstein)
▸ Gaucher's disease

▸ Vitamin C deficiency (avitaminosis)
▸ Polio
▸ Drugs
  • Erythropoietin
  • GCSF
  • Warfarin
▸ Sickle cell anemia

Bradycardia
See Cardiac Dysrhythmias → 62

Brain Tumors

Primary brain tumors
▸ Infiltrative astrocytoma
▸ Pilocytic astrocytoma
▸ Oligodendroglioma
▸ Mixed oligoastrocytoma
▸ Glioblastoma multiforme (GBM)
▸ Ependymoma
▸ Medulloblastoma
▸ Meningioma
Secondary brain tumors (brain metastases)
▸ Lung cancer
▸ Breast cancer
▸ Melanoma
▸ Renal cancer
▸ Colon cancer
▸ Genital cancer

Breast Swelling

Breast mass, breast tumor
Breast swelling in women
▸ Pregnancy
▸ Premenstrual syndrome (PMS)
▸ Mastitis
  • Acute bacterial mastitis
  • Chronic mastitis
▸ Benign tumor
  • Fibroadenoma
  • Papilloma
▸ Breast cancer
▸ Hematoma

▶ Fat necrosis
▶ Duct ectasia
▶ Mammary adenosis
▶ Prolactinoma
▶ Contraceptive use

Breast swelling in men
See Gynecomastia → 160

Breath Odor

Bad breath, fetor oris, halitosis, ozostomia, stomatodysodia.
Foul odor from the mouth.

With coma
▶ Hepatic coma
▶ Uremic coma
▶ Diabetic coma
▶ Ketoacidotic coma

Without coma
▶ Teeth, mouth
  • Dental caries
  • Parodontosis
  • Poor dental hygiene
  • Stomatitis
  • Thrush
  • Tumor exulceration in the mouth
  • Dry mouth [xerostomia, (→ 384)]
    ○ Salivary gland disorder
    ○ Drugs
    ○ "Mouth breathing"
▶ Respiratory tract
  • Pharyngitis (See Sore Throat → 336)
  • Sinus infections
  • Atrophic rhinitis
  • Chronic bronchitis
  • Bronchiectasis
  • Lung abscess
  • Pneumonia
▶ Gastrointestinal tract
  • Esophagitis
  • Reflux esophagitis
  • Hiatus hernia
  • Esophageal diverticulum
  • Ulcer disease
  • Gastric carcinoma
  • Gastritis
  • Ileus (→ 206)
  • Gastrocolic fistula
  • Constipation
▶ External agents
  • Garlic
  • Onions
  • Strong spices
  • Coffee
  • Alcohol
  • Cigarette smoking
  • Chewing tobacco
▶ Other systemic disorder
  • Diabetes mellitus
  • Liver disease
  • Kidney disease
▶ Miscellaneous
  • Hyperemesis gravidarum
  • Fasting (ketone odor)
  • Cyanide
  • Botulism
  • Benzol
  • "Pseudohalitosis" (psychiatric)

Breathing, Vesicular

Decreased
▶ Lobar pneumonia
▶ Emphysema
▶ Pneumothorax
▶ Pleuritis
▶ Pleural effusion
▶ Pleural callosity

Increased
▶ Hyperventilation
▶ Bronchitis
▶ Bronchial asthma
▶ Around infiltration or atelectasis
  • Pneumonia
  • Tumor

Bronchial secretion, See Sputum → 339

Brudzinski's Sign

Physically demonstrable sign of meningitis. Severe neck stiffness causes involuntary hip flexion upon passive flexion of the head.

Causes
▶ Meningitis
▶ Encephalitis
▶ Subarachnoid hemorrhage

Bruits, See Carotid Bruit → 69, See Arterial Bruit → 40

Buffer capacity
See Blood Gas Analysis → 57

C-Peptide

Amino-acid chain connecting A and B chains of insulin in proinsulin. Removed in the conversion of proinsulin to insulin. The level of C-peptide is a gauge of how much insulin is being produced in the body.

Reference range
0.33–1.20 nmol/l

Decreased
▶ Low insulin production
▶ With elevated serum insulin: drug-induced hypoglycemia

Increased
▶ Insulinoma

Normal values in patients with insulin injections
▶ Patient still producing insulin

C-reactive protein, See CRP → 90

CA-125

Cancer (cell-surface) antigen found on derivatives of coelomic epithelium. Elevated levels are associated with ovarian malignancy (tumor marker) and benign pelvic disease such as endometriosis.

Reference range
< 35 U/ml

CA-125 elevation in malignant diseases
▶ Ovarian cancer (!)
▶ Pancreatic cancer
▶ Breast cancer
▶ Endometrial cancer
▶ Cervical cancer
▶ Hepatic tumor
  • Liver cancer
  • Metastases
▶ Colorectal cancer
▶ Gastric carcinoma
▶ Bronchial carcinoma

CA-125 elevation in non-malignant disorders
▶ Pelvic inflammatory disease
▶ Endometriosis
▶ (Tuberculous) peritonitis
▶ Pelvic irradiation
▶ Pancreatitis
▶ Cholecystitis
▶ Acute hepatitis
▶ Cirrhosis
▶ Renal failure
▶ Uterine fibroids
▶ Pregnancy
▶ Post-Menopause

CA-19-9

Tumor marker.

Reference range
< 37 U/ml

Malignant disease
▶ Increased in
  • Colorectal cancer

- Pancreatic cancer
- Gastric carcinoma
- Biliary tract carcinoma
▸ Mildly elevated in
  - Liver carcinoma
  - Bronchial carcinoma
  - Breast cancer
  - Ovarian cancer
  - Uterine cancer

Non-malignant diseases
▸ Cirrhosis
▸ Pancreatis
▸ See Pleural Effusion → 286
▸ Diseases of the biliary tract
  - Choledocholithiasis
  - Cholecystitis

Cabot's ring bodies
See Erythrocyte, Morphology → 132

Cachexia, See Weight Loss → 382

Calcification, Intracranial (x-ray)

Infection
▸ Congenital tuberculosis
▸ Tuberculoma

Vascular
▸ Aneurysm of the internal carotid artery
▸ Sturge-Weber syndrome

Neoplasm
▸ Endothelioma of the dura
▸ Plexus papilloma

Miscellaneous
▸ Organic cerebral psychosyndrome
▸ Pseudohypoparathyroidism
▸ Calcified pituitary (usually without significance)

Calcitonin

Hormone produced in the C cells of the thyroid gland, regulating blood calcium together with parathyroid hormone (PTH) and vitamin D.

Reference range

< 50 pg/ml

Increased
▸ Malignant diseases
  - Medullary thyroid cancer (!!)
  - Lung cancer
  - Insulinomas
  - VIPomas
▸ Non-malignant diseases
  - Newborns
  - Pregnancy
  - Renal failure
  - Zollinger-Ellison syndrome (associated with MEN)
  - Pernicious anemia

Calcium

Calcium (Ca) is required for the proper functioning of numerous intracellular and extracellular processes, including muscle contraction, nerve conduction, hormone release, and blood coagulation. In addition Calcium plays a unique role in intracellular signaling and is involved in the regulation of many enzymes.

Reference range

| Total calcium: | 1.25-2.75 mmol/l |
| Ionized calcium | 1.1-1.4 mmol/l |

The maintenance of Ca homeostasis, therefore, is critical. 55% of calcium is ionized in the plasma, 40% bound to protein, and 5% bound to organic acids. The concentration of ionized calcium, which represents the biologically active form depends on the pH value and albumin concentration. Equation for estimation of ionized calcium:

- Ionized calcium = measured calcium (mmol/l) 0.025 x albumin (g/l) + 1.0
- Calcium + ((Normal Albumin - Serum Albumin) x 0.8))
- Calcium / (0.6 + (Total Protein/8.5))

See Hypercalcemia → 187
See Hypocalcemia → 198

Carbon dioxide partial pressure
See Blood Gas Analysis → 57

Carcinoembryonic antigen
See CEA → 70

Cardiac Dysrhythmias
Cardiac arrhythmias
Any abnormality in rate, regularity, or sequence of cardiac activation. Patients frequently complain of palpitations.
Common causes
- Myocardial infarction
- Drugs
- Myocarditis
- Thyroid disease
- Electrolyte imbalance
- Cardiomyopathy
- Cardiac dilatation

Types
- Sinus bradycardia, bradyarrhythmia
- Atrioventricular block (AV block)
- Bundle-branch block, right
- Sinoatrial block (SA block)
- Supraventricular tachycardias
- Sinus tachycardia
- Atrial fibrillation, flutter
- Reentry supraventricular tachycardias
- Premature ventricular contractions (PVCs)
- Ventricular tachycardia

Sinus bradycardia, bradyarrhythmia
- Physiologic
  - Physical training (athletes with high cardiac ejection fraction)
  - Physiologic at night (35-40/min possible)
  - Vagotonia
  - Carotid sinus syndrome
    - Hypersensitive carotid sinus
    - Vagal nerve stimulation (carotid sinus pressure through torsional head movement, vomiting, abdominal pain etc. leads to bradycardia or asystolia)
  - Vasovagal syncope
- Cardiac
  - CHD
  - Myocardial infarction
  - Perimyocarditis
  - Sick sinus syndrome (SSS)
    - Hypothyroidism
    - Chronic hepatopathy
    - Amyloidosis
    - Typhoid fever
    - Brucellosis
    - Hypercapnia
    - Hypoxia
  - Catheterization of the heart
- Drugs
  - Antiarrhythmics
  - Betablockers
  - Calcium antagonists
  - Cimetidine
  - Digitalis
- Miscellaneous
  - Wandering atrial pacemaker
  - Ventricular rhythm
  - Impairment of cardiovascular center
    - Increased intracranial pressure
    - Tumors
    - Meningitis
    - Sepsis
  - Hyperkalemia
  - Hypocalcemia
  - Hypothyroidism

- Hypothermia
- Hypoxia

Atrioventricular block (AV block)
▶ Cardiac
- CHD
- Myocardial infarction
- Perimyocarditis
- Rheumatic fever
- Infectious mononucleosis
- Sarcoidosis
- Amyloidosis
- Cardiac inflammation
  ○ Diphtheria
  ○ Sarcoidosis
  ○ Lyme disease
▶ Drugs
- Anti-arrhythmics
- Betablockers
- Calcium antagonists
- Cimetidine
- Digitalis
▶ Cardiac valve disease
- Aortic stenosis
- Congenital heart disease
▶ Increased vagal tonus

Bundle-branch block, right
Intraventricular block due to interruption of conduction in the right bundle branch manifested in the ECG by prolongation of the QRS complex (> 0.12 s)
▶ Right ventricular strain
- Vitium
  ○ Atrio-septal defect
  ○ Tetralogy of Fallot
- Acute pulmonary embolism
- Cor pulmonale
▶ Coronary heart disease
▶ Myocardial infarction
▶ Myocarditis
▶ Cardiomyopathy
▶ Idiopathic
- Lenègre's disease
- Lev's disease

Sinoatrial block (SA block)
▶ Cardial

○ Sick sinus syndrome
  - *Idiopathic*
  - *Cardiomyopathy*
○ CHD
○ Myocardial infarction
○ Perimyocarditis
- Drugs
  ○ Antiarrhythmics
  ○ Betablockers
  ○ Calcium antagonists
  ○ Cimetidine
  ○ Digitalis
▶ Bradyarrhythmia absoluta
- Chronic atrial fibrillation with bradycardic frequency of the ventricle in faulty atrioventricular conduction

Tachycardic cardiac dysrhythmias
Heart rate > 90/min.
▶ Main tachyarrhythmias
- Sinus tachycardia
- Atrial extraysystoles
- Atrial flutter
- Atrial fibrillation
- Atrial tachycardia
- Reentry tachycardias
- Preexcitation syndromes
- Ventricular extraysystoles
- Ventricular tachycardia
- Torsade de pointes.

Supraventricular tachycardias
Supraventricular tachyarrhythmias may be regular or irregular. Atrial fibrillation is the most frequently seen. The majority of sustained regular tachyarrhythmias are probably due to re-entry mechanisms.
▶ Sinus tachycardia
▶ Atrial fibrillation, flutter
▶ Reentry supraventricular tachycardias

Sinus tachycardia
Tachycardia originating from the sinus node. Heart rate 100-160/min, mostly regular. A normal QRS complex follows every P wave.
▶ Physiologic
- Infants, small children

- Physical or emotional stress
- Increased sympathicotonia
▶ Drug, stimulants
  - Adrenaline
  - Alcohol
  - Atropine
  - Beta$_2$-sympathomimetics
  - Caffeine
  - Cocaine
  - Nicotine
  - Theophylline
▶ Miscellaneous
  - Perimyocarditis
  - Heart failure
  - Cor pulmonale
  - Hypovolemia
  - Anemia
  - Shock
  - Acidosis
  - Fever
  - Hyperthyroidism
  - Pheochromocytoma
  - Orthostasis

Atrial fibrillation, flutter

Atrial fibrillation is an atrial rhythm that is ineffective, chaotic, irregular and rapid, with a frequency of > 350/min (350-600/min). Most frequent form of supraventricular tachyarrhythmia, often seen in the elderly and generally asymptomatic. Atrial flutter is a supraventricular arrhythmia in which the atria contract at a rate of 250-350/min. In atrial fibrillation/flutter the atrium loses the ability to pump, which can lead to a hemodynamically effective reduction of the cardiac output up to 20%. Due to the filter function of the AV-node only a part of the atrial excitation is conducted onto the ventricle. This can result in very different stroke volumes with pulse deficit. With increasing tachyarrhythmia, the cardiac output drops

▶ Cardiac valve disease
  - Rheumatic heart disease
  - Mitral stenosis
  - Mitral regurgitation
  - Mitral valve prolapse
  - Tricuspid stenosis
  - Tricuspid insufficiency
▶ Non-valvular cardiac disease
  - Coronary heart disease
  - Myocardial infarction
  - Cardiomyopathy
  - Left-ventricular failure
  - Hypertension
  - Myocardial infarction
  - Myocarditis
  - Pericarditis
  - Sick sinus syndrome
  - Preexcitation syndromes (Wolff-Parkinson-White syndrome)
  - Tachycardia-bradycardia syndrome
  - After aortocoronary bypass
  - Blunt heart injury
  - Atrio-septal defect
  - Atrial tumors (myxoma)
  - Storage diseases
    - Amyloidosis
▶ Systemic
  - Hypoxemia
  - Hyperthyroidism
  - Hypothyroidism
  - Arterial hypertension
  - Pulmonary embolism
  - Obstructive lung disease
  - Restrictive lung disease
  - Pneumonia
  - Pheochromocytoma
  - Cerebrovascular accident
  - Multiple sclerosis
  - Electrolyte imbalance (decompensated)
  - Fever
  - Hypovolemia
  - Hypothermia
  - Vomiting
▶ Drugs, toxins
  - Alcoholism ("holiday heart syndrome")
  - Amphetamine

- Betasympathomimetics
- Caffeine
- Cocaine
- Digitalis intoxication in hypokalemia
- Nicotine
▶ Idiopathic

Reentry supraventricular tachycardias
▶ AV node reentry tachycardia without preexcitation
- Congenital
- Mitral valve prolapse
- Cardiomyopathy
- Hyperthyroidism
▶ AV reentry tachycardia with preexcitation complex (Wolff-Parkinson-White syndrome):
- Congenital
- Emotional excitation
- Heavy exercise
- Drugs
  ◦ Nicotine
  ◦ Tea
  ◦ Coffee
  ◦ Cocaine

Premature ventricular contractions (PVCs, Extrasystoles)
Premature ventricular depolarization arising from an ectopic focus in the ventricles. Extra beats with a broad (> 0.12s) and bizarre QRS complex.
▶ Physiologic
- In healthy persons
- Emotional stress
- Strain induced
▶ Cardiovascular
- CHD
- Myocardial infarction
- Cardiac valve disease
- Perimyocarditis
- Hypertension
- Heart failure
- After heart catheterization
- After heart surgery, trauma
- Pulmonary embolism
- Cor pulmonale

- Electro-accident
- Long QT syndromes
- Cardiomyopathies
  ◦ Diabetes mellitus
  ◦ Glycogen storage diseases
  ◦ Amyloidosis
  ◦ Hemochromatosis
  ◦ Addison's disease
  ◦ Cirrhosis
  ◦ Intoxication
  ◦ Protein deficiency
▶ Extracardial
- Hyperthyroidism
- Infections and fevers
  ◦ Diphtheria
  ◦ Perimyocarditis
  ◦ Brucellosis
  ◦ Scarlet fever
- Hypercalcemia
- Hypokalemia
- Acidosis
- Meteorism
▶ Electrolyte imbalance
- Potassium
- Calcium
▶ Drugs, toxins
- Alcohol
- Antiarrhythmics
- Caffeine
- Catecholamines
- Chloroform
- Digitalis
- Ether
- Halothan
- Nicotine
- Theophylline
- Tricyclic antidepressants
▶ Miscellaneous
- Rheumatic fever
- Diaphragmatic eventration
- Scleroderma
- Pheochromocytoma
- Vitamin B_{12} deficiency

Ventricular tachycardia
Tachycardia originating from a ventricular

focus and lasting > 30 s with broad QRS complexes at a rate of > 90 beats/min. The ventricular ectopic beats can be of a single morphology (uniform ventricular tachycardia), of different morphologies.

Caution: ventricular tachycardias are life threatening.

► Myocardial infarction
► CHD
► Cardiomyopathy
► Ventricular aneurysm
► Electrolyte deficiencies
  • Hypokalemia
  • Hypocalcemia
  • Hypomagnesia
► Sympathomimetics
  • Caffeine
  • Methamphetamine
  • Cocaine

Torsades des pointes
"Twisting of the points. A ventricular tachycardia with a long QT interval and a short-long-short sequence in the beat preceding its onset. Risk factor for sudden death.

► Myocardial infarction
► Congenital
  • Romano-Ward symdrome (autosomal dominant)
  • Lange-Nielsen syndrome (autosomal recessive)
► Drugs
  • Amiodarone
  • Disopyramide
  • Ketanserin
  • Non-sedative antihistamines
  • Phenothiazine
  • Procainamide
  • Sotalol
  • Terfenadine
► Electolyte imbalance
  • Hypokalemia

Ventricular fibrillation
Fine, rapid, fibrillary movements of the ventricular muscle replacing the normal

contraction.
► Increased catecholamine levels
► Improper sympathetic stimulation
► Electrolyte imbalances
► Hypoxia
► Acid-base disturbances
► Proarrhythmic drugs
► Hyperthermia
► Hypothermia
► Prolonged QT syndromes

Cardiac murmurs
See Heart Murmur, Continuous → 169
See Heart Murmur, Diastolic → 169
See Heart Murmur, Systolic → 170

Cardiac Risk Factor
Coronary Risk Factor
► Hypercholesterolemia
  • LDL cholesterol > 130 mg/dl
  • HDL cholesterol < 40 mg/dl
► Hypertension (> 140/90 mmHg)
► Cigarette smoking
► Diabetes mellitus
► Age
  • Men > 45
  • Women > 45 (early menopause)
  • Women > 55 (normal onset menopause)
► Family history of premature coronary artery disease (myocardial infarction, stroke, sudden death)
► Obesity
► Sedentary living
► Type A personality
► Lack of supportive primary relationship
► Other cardiac risk factors
  • Increased apolipoprotein B (LDL core)
  • Decreased apolipoprotein A-1 (HDL core)
  • Hypertriglyceridemia
  • Hyperhomocysteinemia
  • Decreased serum folate
  • Increased c-reactive protein

- Increased fibrinogen
- Chronic obstructive lung disease
- Chronic renal failure
- Infections
- Low birth weight
- ACE DD genotype
- Insulin resistance syndrome
- Oral contraceptive use
- Immunosuppressive posttransplant
- Alcohol (> 3oz/day)
- Syndrome X (hypertriglyceridemia, hypertension, insulin resistance, centripetal obesity)

Cardiac Valve Disease, Acquired

Frequency of acquired cardiac valve disease in descending order
▶ Mitral regurgitation (→ 241)
▶ Aortic stenosis (→ 39)
▶ Combined mitral vitium
▶ Combined aortic vitium
▶ Aortic regurgitation (→ 38)
▶ Mitral stenosis (→ 242)
▶ Tricuspid regurgitation (→ 359)
▶ Tricuspid stenosis
▶ Pulmonary valve vitium
▶ Aortic regurgitation, associated with aortic stenosis

Cardiogenic shock, See Shock → 329

Cardiomyopathy

Diseases of the myocardium that are not the result of CHD, valve disease, pericardial disease or pulmonary/systemic hypertension.
Primary cardiomyopathies
▶ Idiopathic
▶ Familial
▶ Endomyocardial fibrosis
▶ Eosinophilic endomyocardial disease
Secondary Cardiomyopathies
▶ Infection

- Viral
  ○ Adenoviruses
  ○ Arboviruses
  ○ CMV
  ○ Coxsackie virus B1–B5
  ○ Coxsackie virus A
  ○ ECHO viruses
  ○ Epstein-Barr virus
  ○ Flavivirus
  ○ Hepatitis viruses
  ○ HIV viruses
  ○ Influenza virus
  ○ Measles virus
  ○ Mumps virus
  ○ Poliovirus
  ○ Psittacosis
  ○ Rabies virus
  ○ Varicella-zoster virus
- Bacterial
  ○ Beta-hemolyzing streptococci
  ○ Borrelia burgdorferi
  ○ Brucella
  ○ Diphtheria
  ○ Enterococci
  ○ Pertussis
  ○ Rheumatic fever
  ○ Rickettsia
    - *Rocky Mountain spotted fever*
    - *Q fever*
    - *Typhoid fever*
  ○ Spirochetes
    - *Syphilis*
    - *Leptospirosis*
    - *Lyme disease*
  ○ Staphylococcus
  ○ Syphilis
  ○ Tetanus
  ○ Tuberculosis
  ○ Tularemia
  ○ Typhoid fever
- Fungal
  ○ Aspergillosis
  ○ Actinomycosis
  ○ Blastomycosis
  ○ Coccidioidomycosis

- ◦ Cryptococcosis
- ◦ Histoplasmosis
- ◦ Oral candidiasis
- Protozoal
  - ◦ Amebiasis
  - ◦ Echinococcosis
  - ◦ Leishmaniasis
  - ◦ Malaria
  - ◦ Sacrosporidiosis
  - ◦ Toxoplasmosis
  - ◦ Trypanosomiasis (Chagas' disease)
- Helminths
  - ◦ Ascariasis
  - ◦ Cysticercosis
  - ◦ Echinococcosis
  - ◦ Filariasis
  - ◦ Schistosomiasis
  - ◦ Trichinosis

▶ Collagen vascular disease
- Rheumatoid arthritis
- Systemic lupus erythematosus
- Polyarthritis nodosa
- Scleroderm
- Dermatomyositis
- Giant cell myocarditis
- Kawasaki's disease

▶ Drugs, toxins
- Acetazolamide
- Adriamycin
- Alcohol
- Bleomycin
- Catecholamines
- Chemotherapeutics
- Chloroquin
- Chlorthalidone
- Cobalt
- Cocaine
- Cyclophosphamide
- Daunorubicin
- Doxorubicin
- Drugs
- Emetin
- Hydrochlorothiazide
- Indomethacin
- Lead

- Lithium
- Methyldopa
- Penicillin
- Phenothiazine
- Phenylbutazone
- Phenytoin
- Reserpine
- Spironolactone
- Sulfonamides
- Sulfonyl ureas
- Tetracycline
- Tricyclic antidepressants

▶ Endocrine, metabolic
- Hyperthyroidism
- Hypothyroidism
- Pheochromocytoma
- Hyperparathyroidism
- Acromegaly
- Cushing's disease
- Diabetes mellitus
- Vitamin deficiency
  - ◦ Vitamin B
  - ◦ Vitamin C
  - ◦ Niacin
  - ◦ Selen
- Vitamin D overdose
- Obesity
- Uremia
- Gout
- Oxalosis
- Porphyria
- Electrolyte imbalances

▶ Allergic
- Cardiac transplant rejection
- Drug-induced

▶ Infiltrative, granulomatous
- Tumor
  - ◦ Sarcomas
  - ◦ Rhabdomyomas
  - ◦ Myxomas
  - ◦ Angiomas
- Metastasis
  - ◦ Leukemia infiltration
- Sarcoidosis
- Amyloidosis

- Hemochromatosis
▶ Neuromuscular
  - Muscular dystrophy
  - Myotonic dystrophy
  - Friedreich's ataxia
  - Refsum´s disease
▶ Hematologic
  - Leukemia
  - Sickle cell anemia
  - Polycythemia vera
  - Thrombotic thrombocytopenic purpura
▶ Physical
  - Hypothermia
  - Heatstroke
  - Trauma
  - Electrical shock
  - Lightning strike
  - Irradiation
  - Chronic tachycardia
▶ Hereditary disorders
  - Glycogen storage disorders
  - Niemann-Pick disease
  - Hand-Schüller-Christian-syndrome
  - Fabry's disease
  - Gaucher's disease
  - Whipple's disease
  - Mucopolysaccharidosis
  - Gangliosidosis
  - Hunter's syndrome
  - Hurler's syndrome
  - Carnitine deficiency
▶ Miscellaneous
  - Postpartal cardiomyopathy
  - Idiopathic

Carotid Bruit

Carotid murmur
▶ Aortic stenosis
▶ Arteriosclerosis
▶ Arterial aneurysm
▶ Thyroid artery dilation
▶ Arteriovenous fistula
▶ Aortic coarctation

▶ After trauma to the carotid artery
▶ Vascular angioma in the skull
▶ Fever
▶ Hyperthyroidism

Carpal tunnel syndrome

Most common nerve entrapment syndrome, characterized by nocturnal hand paresthesia and pain, sometimes sensory loss and wasting in the median hand distribution. Women more affected than men, often bilateral. Caused by entrapment of the median nerve within the carpal tunnel.

Causes
▶ Idiopathic
▶ Tenosynovitis of flexor tendons
▶ Fibrosis of flexor tendons
▶ Trauma
  - Cut on flexor side of the wrist
  - Crushing injury to flexor side of the wrist
  - Fracture
    ◦ Colles'
    ◦ Scaphoid bone
  - Luxation
  - Occupational trauma
▶ Tumor
  - Hematoma
  - Benign tumor
  - Wrist ganglion
▶ Endocrine, metabolic
  - Acromegaly
  - Amyloidosis
  - Diabetes mellitus
  - Estrogens
  - Gout
  - Hypothyroidism
  - Mucopolysaccharidoses
  - Paget's disease
  - Paraproteinemia
  - Uremia
▶ Rheumatologic
  - Degenerative arthritis

- Dermatomyositis
- Rheumatoid arthritis
- Scleroderma
- Systemic lupus erythematosus
▶ Granulomatous
- Tuberculosis
- Sarcoidosis
- Leprosy
▶ Pregnancy
▶ Congestive heart failure

Cavitary Lesion on Chest X-Ray

Causes
▶ Necrotizing infection
- Bacteria
  - Staphylococcus aureus
  - Streptococcus pyogenes
  - Streptococcus pneumoniae
  - Pseudomonas aeruginosa
  - Haemophilus influenzae
  - Legionella
  - Actinomyces
- Mycobacteria
  - Mycobacterium tuberculosis
  - Mycobacterium kansasii
- Fungi
  - Coccidioides immitis
  - Blastomyces hominis
  - Histoplasma capsulatum
  - Aspergillus
  - Mucor
- Parasitic
  - Echinococcus
  - Entamoeba histolytica
  - Paragonimus westermanni
▶ Cavitary infarction
▶ Septic embolism
- Staphylococcus aureus
- Anaerobes
▶ Vasculitis
- Wegener's granulomatosis
- Periarteritis
▶ Neoplasm
- Bronchial carcinoma

- Metastases
- Lymphoma
▶ Miscellaneous
- Cysts
- Bullae
- Pneumatocele
- Lung abscess
- Sequestration
- Empyema
- Bronchiectasis
- Emphysema bubble
- Foreign body
- Diaphragmatic hernia
- Mediastinal hernia
- Esophageal diverticulum
- Calcified heart wall/aortic aneurysm
- Rib abnormality

CEA

Carcinoembryonic antigen, cancer antigen.

Carcinoembryonic antigen (CEA) is a protein-polysaccharide complex found in colon carcinomas (tumor marker) and in normal fetal intestine, pancreas, and liver.

Reference range
< 3 µg/l

Increased
▶ Malignant diseases
- Colorectal tumors
- Medullar thyroid carcinoma
- Breast cancer
- Gastric carcinoma
- Pancreatic cancer
- Bronchial carcinoma
- Ovarian cancer
- Cervical cancer
▶ Non-malignant diseases (concentration usually below 4x the upper limit)
- Inflammatory liver diseases
- Alcoholic cirrhosis
- Pancreatitis
- Inflammatory bowel disease
- Smoking

• Pulmonary emphysema

Cerebrovascular Accident
CVA., cerebral infarction, stroke

Sudden development of focal neurologic deficits related to impaired cerebral blood supply. In more than 80% of cases, a cerebral infarction (primary ischemic insult) is the cause, in approx. 20% an intracerebral hemorrhage (primary hemorrhagic insult). Mortality is approx. 50% after 6 months, and about 30% of the survivors need daily care.

Cerebral ischemia
▶ Thrombosis
• Atherosclerosis
• Dissection
  ◦ Carotid
  ◦ Vertebral
  ◦ Intracranial arteries (traumatic/spontaneous)
• Arteritis
  ◦ Temporal arteritis
  ◦ Polyarteritis nodosa
  ◦ Takayatsu´s arteritis
  ◦ Wegner´s granulomatosis
  ◦ Behçet's syndrome
  ◦ Systemic lupus erythematosus
  ◦ Meningitis (bacterial, fungal, protozoan, parasitic)
• Venous sinus thrombosis
  ◦ Infections of face, ear, sinus
• Hematologic disorders
  ◦ Thrombotic thrombocytopenic purpura
  ◦ Polycythemia vera
  ◦ Sickle cell disease
  ◦ Factor C deficiency
  ◦ Factor S deficiency
  ◦ Antiphospholipid antibodies
  ◦ Diffus intravascular coagulation
▶ Embolism
• Artery-to-artery
  ◦ Carotid bifurcation
  ◦ Aortic arch
  ◦ Distal vertebral artery
  ◦ Arterial dissection
• Cardioembolic
  ◦ Dysrhythmia
    - Atrial fibrillation
    - Sick sinus syndrome
  ◦ Structural heart disease
    - Valvular lesions (mitral stenosis, mitral valve prolapse)
    - Mechanical valve
    - Bacterial endocarditis
    - After myocardial infarction (mural thombus)
    - Dilated cardiomyopathy
  ◦ Complication of cardiac surgery
  ◦ Paradoxic embolism
    - Atrial septal defect
    - Patent foramen ovale
    - Spontaneous echo contrast
▶ Associated to
  ◦ Carcinomas
  ◦ Oral contraceptives
▶ Vasoconstriction
• Reversible cerebral vasoconstriction after
  ◦ Trauma
  ◦ Migraine
  ◦ Eclampsia
  ◦ Radiation
• Cerebral vasospasm after subarachnoid hemorrhage
▶ Hypotension in presence of atherosclerotic carotid disease
• Hypovolemia
• Stokes-Adams attack

Intracerebral bleeding
▶ Hypertension
▶ Non-hypertensive causes
• Aneurysm
• Arteriovenous malformation
• Hemorrhagic disorders
  ◦ Coagulopathy
  ◦ Thrombocytopenia
  ◦ Disseminated intravascular

coagulation
  ○ Anticoagulant therapy
- Tumor hemorrhage
- Intracranial trauma
- Connective-tissue disease
  ○ Lupus erythematosus
  ○ Polyarteritis nodosa
- Leukemia
- Pertussis

Risk factors
▸ Hypertension
▸ Hypothyroidism
▸ Obesity
▸ Diabetes mellitus
▸ Coronary artery disease
▸ Aortic arch plaque
▸ Family history of ischemic stroke
▸ Age > 65
▸ Women affected > men
▸ Race: Afro-American, hispanic
▸ Hypercholesterolemia
▸ Hypertriglyceridemia
▸ Increased apolipoprotein-a
▸ Oral contraceptive use
▸ Cigarette smoking
▸ Sedentary living
▸ See Cardiac Risk Factor → 66

DDx
▸ Head trauma
▸ Encephalitis
▸ Meningitis
▸ Hypertensive encephalopathy
▸ Postcardiac arrest ischemia
▸ Intracranial mass
  • Epidural hematoma
  • Subdural hematoma
  • Intracranial tumor
▸ Migraine (with neurologic deficits)
▸ Seizure (with neurologic deficits)
▸ Metabolic disorder
  • Hyperglycemia (nonketotic hyperosmolar coma)
  • Hypoglycemia
  • Uremia
  • Myxedema

• Toxins
▸ Psychiatric disorder
▸ Shock

Ceruloplasmin

Acute-phase and transport protein. Ceruloplasmin varies with the α_2-globulin fraction in electrophoresis. It transports copper from the liver to copper-utilizing tissues. About 90% of serum copper binds to ceruloplasmin. Faulty transport of copper through ceruloplasmin can result in toxic liver damage with release of copper into the serum. The results are: liver damage, damage to other organs from copper deposition: renal tubules, CNS (neurologic and psychiatric symptoms), Kayser-Fleischer ring and others. See Copper → 85.

Reference range
20–60 mg/dl

Increased ceruloplasmin
▸ Wilson's disease
▸ Acute inflammation
▸ Obstructive jaundice
▸ Cholestasis
▸ Pregnancy
▸ Contraceptives
▸ Hodgkin's lymphoma
▸ Tumor

Decreased ceruloplasmin
▸ Wilson's disease
▸ Menkes' syndrome (inherited copper deficiency)
▸ Nephrotic syndrome
▸ Exudative enteropathy
▸ Malnutrition
▸ Malabsorption

Chest Pain

See Angina → 32

Nonpleuritic chest pain
▸ Cardiac

- Coronary heart disease
- Myocardial infarction
- Stable and unstable angina pectoris
- Aortic aneurysm
- Mitral valve prolapse
- Hypertrophic cardiomyopathy
- Pericarditis
- Myocarditis
- Pericardial tamponade
- Functional cardiac problems
- Cor pulmonale
- Bland–White–Garland syndrome
▶ Vascular
- Aortic aneurysm/dissection
- Pulmonary embolism
▶ Pulmonary
- Pulmonary embolism, infarction
- Pleuritis
- Pleurodynia
- Pneumonia
- Bronchitis
- Pneumothorax
- Neoplasm
  - Bronchogenic carcinoma
  - Mesothelioma
  - Metastatic tumor
▶ Mediastinal
- Mediastinal tumors
  - Lymphoma
  - Thymoma
- Mediastinitis
- Mediastinal emphysema
▶ Esophageal disease
- Esophageal spasm
- Esophagitis
- Achalasia
- Mallory-Weiss syndrome
- Esophageal rupture
- Foreign body
- Carcinoma
- Diverticula
▶ Abdominal diseases with pain radiating into the thorax, GI causes
- Abdominal distension
  See Ileus → 206

- Biliary
  - Cholecystitis
  - Cholelithiasis
  - Impacted stone
  - Neoplasm
- Gastrointestinal
  - Plummer-Vinson syndrome
  - Hiatal hernia
  - Gastritis
  - Peptic ulcer disease
  - Pancreatitis
- Subphrenic abscess
- Splenic infarction
▶ Musculoskeletal
- Vertebrogenic thoracic pain
- CS/TS osteochondrosis
- Bechterew's disease
- Tietze's syndrome
- Periostitis
- Intercostal myositis
- Thoracic outlet syndrome
▶ Neurologic
- Herpes zoster
- Tabes dorsalis
- Neurofibroma
- Degenerative changes of the cervical spine
- Intercostal neuralgia
▶ Functional, psychiatric
- Hyperkinetic heart syndrome
- Extrasystoles
- Endocrinologic
  - Hyperthyroidism
  - Hypothyroidism
  - Pheochromocytoma attack
  - Conn's syndrome
  - Acromegaly
  - Diabetes mellitus
  - Hypoglycemia
- Anxiety disorders
- Depression

Pleuritic chest pains
▶ Cardiac
- Pericarditis
- Postpericardiotomy (Dressler's

syndrome)
- ▶ Pulmonary
  - Pulmonary embolism
  - Pulmonary infarction
  - Pleuritis
  - Pneumothorax
  - Hemothorax
  - Pneumonia
  - Empyema
  - Lung abscess
  - Bronchiectasis
  - Tuberculosis
  - Bronchial carcinoma
  - Pleural mesothelioma
  - Carcinomatous effusion
- ▶ Gastrointestinal
  - Liver abscess
  - Pancreatitis
  - Whipple's disease
    - ○ Associated pericarditis
    - ○ Associated pleuritis
- ▶ Abdomnal
  - Subdiaphragmatic abscess
  - Splenic infarction
  - Splenic enlargement
- ▶ Mediastinal
  - Mediastinitis
  - Trauma
  - Retropharyngeal abscess
  - Tracheoesophageal fistula
- ▶ Musculosceletal
  - Costochondritis
  - Chest wall trauma
  - fractured rib
  - Interstitial fibrosis
  - Myositis
  - Strain of pectoralis muscle
  - Herpes zoster
  - Soft tissue tumor
  - Bone tumor
- ▶ Miscellaneous
  - HIV infection
  - Collagen vascular disease with pleuritis
  - Familial Mediterranean fever

- Neurotic

Cheyne-Stokes Respiration
Periodic respiration
Regularly alternating periods of apnea and hyperpnea due to impairment of the medullary respiratory center.
Causes
- ▶ Heart failure
- ▶ Cerebrovascular disorder
  - Cerebral stroke
- ▶ Subdural hematoma
- ▶ Uremic coma
- ▶ Hypoxia
- ▶ Drugs, toxins
  - Benzodiazepines
  - Opiates

Chloride
The major anion found in the fluid outside of cells and in blood. It usually follows sodium passively if its concentration changes. Thus it is also regulated by aldosterone.

Reference range
98–106 mmol/l

Hypochloremia
- ▶ Water losses
  - Intestinal loss
    - ○ Gastric suction (NG suction)
    - ○ Vomiting (bulimia nervosa)
    - ○ Diarrhea
  - Renal losses
    - ○ Salt-losing nephritis
    - ○ Renal failure
  - Excessive sweating
  - Respiratory losses
  - Burns
- ▶ Drugs
  - Bicarbonate
  - D5W (excessive IV)
  - Diuretics
    - ○ Ethacrynic acid

- Furosemide
- Thiazide diuretics
• Glucocorticoids
► Mineralocorticoid elevation
  • Hyperaldosteronism
  • Cushing's syndrome
  • ACTH-secreting tumors
  • Overconsumption of licorice (mineralocorticoid effect)
► Metabolic, endocrins
  • Hyponatremia (→ 336)
  • Pseudohyponatremia
  • Adrenal insufficiency (Addison)
  • Diabetic coma
  • SIADH
• Congestive heart failure (edema)

Hyperchloremia
► Artifact (low anion gap)
► Respiratory alkalosis
► Metabolic, endocrine
  • Hypernatremia (→ 336)
  • Metabolic acidosis (→ 11)
  • Hyperparathyroidism (→ 275)
► Renal
  • Renal tubular acidosis
  • Nephrotic syndrome
  • Renal failure
► Drugs
  • Acetazolamide
  • ACTH
  • Ammonium chloride
  • Arginine chloride
  • Boric acid
  • Bromide intoxication (Pseudohyperchloremia)
  • Estrogens
  • Lysine chloride
  • Na^+Cl^- (excess IV)
  • Triamterene
► Gastrointestinal
  • Prolonged diarrhea
  • Dehydration
  • Loss of pancreatic secretion
  • Ileal loops
  • Ureteral colonic anastamosis

Cholecystitis
Inflammation of the gallbladder
Calculous cholecystitis (cholelithiasis)
► Female gender
► Race: Scandinavians > Afro-Americans
► Obesity
► Rapid weight loss
► Hormonal therapy in women
► Pregnancy
► Increasing age
Acalculous cholecystitis
► Biliary stasis (→ 75)
  • Seriously ill patients
  • Major surgery
  • Severe trauma
  • Burns
  • Sepsis
  • Long-term TPN
  • Prolonged fasting
► Miscellaneous
  • Myocardial infarction
  • Other cardiac disease
  • Sickle cell disease
  • Diabetes mellitus
  • Salmonella infection
  • AIDS with
    ○ Cytomegalovirus
    ○ Cryptosporidiosis
    ○ Microsporidiosis
Idiopathic

Cholestasis
Retention of substances normally excreted into bile due to reduced bile formation or flow. Leading to **jaundice** (icterus), pruritus and increase of cholestatic enzymes. See Bilirubin → 51
Intrahepatic cholestasis (impaired bile flow in the liver)
► Hepatocellular
  • Viral hepatitis
  • Alocoholic hepatitis

- Chronic active hepatitis
- Alpha-1 antitrypsin deficiency
- Leptospirosis
- Toxic, allergic
- Drugs
  - Anabolic steroids
  - Chemotherapeutics
  - Methamizol
  - Oral antihypoglycemics
  - Oral contraceptives
  - Phenothiazines
  - Tranquilizers
- Metabolic
  - Hemochromatosis
  - Wilson's disease
▶ Hepatocanalicular
- Drugs
- Sepsis
- Toxic shock syndrome
- Postoperative
- Total parenteral nutrition
- Neoplasm
- Sickle cell anemia
- Amyloidosis
- Primary sclerosing cholangitis
- Biliary atresia
- Familiar progressive cholestasis
- Alagille syndrome
▶ Ductular
- Primary biliary cirrhosis
- Sarcoidosis
▶ Functional cholestasis
- Pregnancy cholestasis
- Intermittent cholestasis
▶ Vascular
- Budd–Chiari syndrome (stenosis or occlusion of the hepatic vein)
- Ischemia of other origin
▶ Impaired secretion due to lack of transport pumps
- Cystic fibrosis
- Bylers syndrome
- Dubin-Johnson syndrome
▶ Impaired bile acid synthesis
▶ Idiopathic postoperative jaundice

▶ Mechanical drainage disorder
- Liver cancer
- Cholangiocellular carcinoma
- Liver metastases
- Liver cysts
- Echinococcosis
- Amebiasis
- Liver abscess
- Primary biliary cirrhosis
- Primary sclerosing cholangitis
▶ Zieve's syndrome
▶ Reye's syndrome

Extrahepatic cholestasis
▶ Stenosis of the extrahepatic bile ducts
- Bile duct calculi
- Stenosis of the bile papilla
- Carbonic anhydrase inhibitors
- Neoplastic
  - Bile duct carcinoma
  - Papillary carcinoma
- Stricture
- Parasites
- Biliary atresia
- Bile duct cysts
▶ External compression of the bile duct from outside
- Mirizzi's syndrome (benign obstruction of the hepatic ducts due to spasm and/or fibrous scarring of surrounding connective tissue; often associated with a stone in the cystic duct and chronic cholecystitis)
- Pancreatitis
- Pancreatic cyst
- Pancreatic cancer
- Echinococcosis of the liver
- Liver abscess
- Duodenal abscess
- Metastases
- Lymphomas
▶ Miscellaneous
- Cholecystectomy
- Choledochotomy with T-tube drainage
- Pancreatoduodenectomy
- After ulcer surgery

- Primary and secondary sclerosing cholangitis
- Infectious causes
  ○ Relapsing cholangitis
  ○ Pericholedochal infection (e.g. liver abscess)
  ○ Hydatid cyst
  ○ Cryptosporidiosis
  ○ Parasitosis
- Caroli's syndrome (congenital cystic dilation of the intrahepatic bile ducts, sometimes associated with intrahepatic stones and biliary obstruction)
- Idiopathic relapsing cholestasis
- After liver transplantation
- Rare congenital causes

Cholesterol
See Coronary Risk Factor → 66
See Hypercholesterolemia → 188
See HDL Cholesterol → 162
See LDL Cholesterol → 218

Cholinesterase
Catalyzing the hydrolysis of acylcholines.

Reference range
3000-8000U/l

Decreased serum cholinesterase
▶ Liver damage
  • Hepatitis
  • Cirrhosis
  • Drug-toxicity
  • Tumors, metastases
▶ Nephrotic syndrome
▶ Acute infection
▶ Chronic malnutrition
▶ Myocardial infarction
▶ Obstructive jaundice
▶ Congenital deficiency
▶ Ulcerative colitis
▶ Drugs, intoxication
  • E-605
  • Endoxan

- Oral contraceptives
- Organophosphates
- Prostigmin
- Streptokinase
▶ Pregnancy

Increased serum cholinesterase
▶ Coronary heart disease
▶ Fatty liver
▶ Hyperthyroidism
▶ Exudative enteropathy with albumin loss
▶ Beginning stage of alcohol-toxic cirrhosis
▶ Obesity
▶ Diabetes mellitus

Chvostek's Sign
Spasm of the orbicularis oculi or oris muscle by a slight tap over the facial nerve.

In tetany (→ 348)
▶ Hypoparathyroidism
▶ Hyperventilation
▶ Hypocalcemia
▶ Hypomagnesemia

Chylothorax
Chylopleura, chylous hydrothorax.
Presence of lymphatic fluid in the pleural space due to leakage from the thoracic duct or other vessel.

Nontraumatic
▶ Malignancies
  • Lymphomas
  • Nonlymphomatous malignancies
▶ Miscellaneous
  • Cirrhosis
  • Tuberculosis
  • Filariasis
▶ Congenital chylothorax (in neonates)
▶ Idiopathic
Traumatic
▶ Iatrogenic

▶ Nonsurgical penetrating trauma

Cirrhosis
Progressive disease of the liver with diffuse damage to hepatic parenchymal cells.
See Liver diseases → 226
See Fatty Liver → 142
See Cholestasis → 75
See Hepatomegaly → 179
Alcohol abuse
Infection
▶ Viral hepatitis (A, B, B/D, C, E, F)
▶ Schistosomiasis
Biliary
▶ Primary biliary cirrhosis
▶ Primary sclerosing cholangitis
▶ Secondary biliary cirrhosis (Obstruction of extrahepatic bile ducts)
Cryptogenic
▶ Posthepatitic cirrhosis
▶ Postnecrotic cirrhosis
Autoimmune disease
▶ Autoimmune cholangiopathy
▶ Autoimmune hepatitis
Drugs, toxins
▶ Alcohol
▶ Amiodarone
▶ Arsenic
▶ Beryllium
▶ Halothane
▶ Isoniazid
▶ MAO inhibitors
▶ Methotrexate
▶ Methyldopa
▶ Nitrofurantoin
▶ Pesticides
▶ Phosphorus
▶ Vinyl chloride
Congestive
▶ Right ventricular failure
• Constrictive pericarditis
• Cor pulmonale

• Mitral stenosis
• Tricuspid insufficiency
▶ Obstruction of the hepatic vein (Budd-Chiari syndrome)
Metabolic
▶ Hemochromatosis
▶ Wilson's disease
▶ Alpha-1 antitrypsin deficiency
▶ Glycogen storage diseases
▶ Galactosemia
▶ Hereditary fructose intolerance
▶ Hereditary tyrosinosis
▶ Hypervitaminosis A
▶ Thalassemia
▶ Sickle cell disease
▶ Porphyria cutanea tarda
▶ Abetalipoproteinemia
▶ Cystic fibrosis
Miscellaneous
▶ Sarcoidosis
▶ Granulomatous cirrhosis
▶ Congenital hepatic fibrosis
▶ Indian childhood cirrhosis
▶ Nutritional (intestinal bypass)
▶ Steatohepatitis (nonalcoholic)

CK, CK-MB, See Creatine Kinase (CK) → 88

Claudicatio; See Peripheral Arterial Occlusive Disease → 282

Clubbing
Thickening and widening of the extremities of the digits due to proliferation of distal tissues, especially the nail-beds with abnormally curved and shiny nails (→ 250).
Pulmonary disease
▶ Infection
• Bronchiectasis
• Lung abscess
• Tuberculosis
• Empyema

- Neoplasm
  - Bronchial carcinomas
  - Pulmonary metastases
  - Mesothelioma
  - Hepatoma
- Emphysema
- Cystic fibrosis
- Pulmonary fibrosis, silicosis
- Arteriovenous malformations
- Pulmonary artery sclerosis

Cardiovascular disease
- Cyanotic congenital heart disease
- Endocarditis (subacute bacterial)
- Heart failure

Gastrointestinal diseases
- Ulcerative colitis
- Crohn's disease
- Celiac sprue

Liver diseases
- Cirrhosis
- Chronic obstructive jaundice
- Liver tumors

Miscellaneous disorders
- Cerebrovascular insult
- Thyrotoxicosis
- Pachydermoperiostosis

Idiopathic

Coagulation
See Bleeding Time → 57
See Thromboplastin time → 352
See Partial Thromboplastin Time → 278

Coagulation disorder
See Hemorrhagic Diathesis → 176

Cobalamin, See Vitamin B12 → 378

Cold Agglutinin Disease
Cold reactive autoimmune hemolytic anemia
Cold hemagglutin disease is a reactive autoimmune hemolytic anemia associated with IgM antibodies to red blood cells. These antibodies react best at low temperature. The red cells become coated with IgM antibodies in the cooler peripheral circulation. Complement is activated when the blood warms up resulting in intravascular hemolysis. See Anemia → 28
Causes
- Idiopathic
- Secondary
  - Non-Hodgkin's lymphoma
  - Mycoplasma pneumoniae infection
  - Infectious mononucleosis

Collapsing Pulse
Bounding pulse
Pulse with fast upstroke and fast downstroke.
- Aortic regurgitation
- Hyperkinetic circulation
- Hyperthyroidism
- Anemia
- Essential hypertension
- See Pulse pressure → 308

Color sensation impairment
See Dysopias → 109

Coma
Reduced consciousness
Impairment of perception and behavior that can occur in very different degrees. Clinically, three degrees of severity of quantitative disturbances of consciousness (impaired vigilance) are distinguished: somnolence, stupor and coma.

Coma is denoted by absolute unconsciousness of extended duration. Classification is made by means of the Glasgow coma scale, for example (→ 154)

See Confusion → 81
See Mental Retardation → 239
See Dementia → 96
See Delirium → 95

Common causes
► Psychoses
► Encephalitis
► Cerebral masses
► Endocrine encephalopathies
► Subarachnoid hemorrhage
► Syncopes
► Intoxication
► Heatstroke

Important DDx
► Brain stem syndromes without genuine loss of vigilance
  • Apallic syndrome
  • Locked-in syndrome
► Qualitative disturbances of consciousness
  • Consciousness shift
  • Narrowed consciousness

Mnemonic "AEIOU–TIPS"
► Alcohol
► Encephalitis (other CNS causes: epilepsy, tumor)
► Insulin
► Opiates (drugs)
► Uremia (other metabolic causes: hypernatremia, hepatic failure, thiamine deficiency)
► Trauma
► Infection
► Psychiatric
► Syncope

Without focal or lateralizing neurologic signs, normal brainstem functions
► Drugs, toxins
  • Alcohol
  • Amphetamines
  • Analgesics
  • Antiepileptics
  • Caffein
  • Carbon monoxide
  • Corticosteroids
  • Digitalis
  • Hypnotics
  • Lead
  • Lithium
  • Methyl alcohol
  • Metoclopramide
  • Narcotics
  • Organophosphates
  • Salicylates
  • Sedatives
  • Tricyclic antideprssants
► Drug withdrawal
  • Alcohol
  • Sedatives
► Endocrine, metabolic
  • Diabetic acidosis
  • Hypoglycemia
  • Addisonian crisis
  • Pheochromocytoma crisis
  • Pituitary insufficiency
  • Diabetes insipidus
  • Thyrotoxic crisis
  • Hypothyroid coma
  • Hepatic coma
  • Uremia
  • Porphyria
  • Profound nutritional deficiency
  • Thiamindeficiency!
  • Hypo-/Hypernatremia
  • Hypo-/Hyperkaliemia
  • Hypo-/Hypercalcemia
  • Hypo-/Hypermagnesemia
  • Hypo-/Hyperphosphatemia
  • Hypoxia
  • Hypercarbie
  • Severe metabolic acidosis/alkalosis
  • Lactic acidosis
    ∘ Biguanides
  • Hypo-/Hyperosmolality
  • Hypo-/Hyperthermia

▶ Severe infections
- Meningitis
- Endocarditis
- Septicemia
- Pneumonia
- Malaria
- Typhoid fever
- Rheumatic fever
- Creutzfeldt-Jakob disease
- Progressive multifocal leukoencephalopathy

▶ Central nervous system disorders
- Head trauma
  ○ Concussion
- Bilateral subdural hematoma
- Hydrocephalus
- Eclampsia
- Postictal state
- Migraine
- Carcinomatosis meningitis
- Hypertensive encephalopathy
- Wernicke's encephalopathy
- Reye's syndrome

▶ Diffuse cerebral hypoxia
- Pulmonary causes
- Blood pressure disorders
- Hypertensive encephalopathy
- Cerebrovascular disease
- Shock
- Cardiac causes
  ○ Congestive heart failure
  ○ Cardiac dysrhythmias

▶ Psychiatric diseases
- Acute psychosis
  ○ Catatonia
  ○ Postoperative
  ○ Postpartum
- Hysterical coma

With focal or lateralizing neurologic signs, normal brainstem functions
▶ Subdural hematoma
▶ Epidural hematoma
▶ Intracerebral hemorrhage
▶ Tumor with edema
▶ Brain abscess with edema

▶ Cerebral infarction with edema
▶ Herpesvirus encephalitis
▶ Focal seizure
▶ Thrombocytopenic purpura

Brainstem lesion with multiple abnormal reflexes
▶ Brain hemorrhage
▶ Brain tumor
▶ Cerebral infarction
▶ Brain abscess
▶ Acute hemorrhagic leukoencephalitis
▶ Disseminated encephalomyelitis
▶ Migraine of basilar artery
▶ Severe drug overdose

Coma scale
See Glasgow Coma Scale → 154

Conduction deafness. See Hearing Loss, Hearing Impairment → 165

Confusion

Mental dysfunction, disorientation, delirium.

Inability to think with normal speed or clarity with lack of attention and disorientation. See Dementia → 96,
See Coma → 79,
See Mental Retardation → 239

Causes
▶ Alcohol intoxication
▶ Low blood sugar
▶ Head trauma, concussion
▶ Delirium tremens (alcoholic withdrawal after sustained intoxication)
▶ Hypoxemia
- Chronic pulmonary disorders
▶ Hypercapnia
▶ Fluid and electrolyte imbalance
- Dehydration
- Hyponatremia
- Hypomagnesemia
- Hyperkalemia

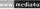

- Hypercalcemia
► Nutrition
  - Niacin deficiency (pellagra)
  - Thiamine deficiency
  - Vitamin C deficiency
  - Vitamin B$_{12}$ deficiency
► Environmental
  - Hyperthermia (fever)
  - Heat stroke
  - Hypothermia
► Drugs, toxins
  - Alcohol
  - Atropine
  - Barbiturates (withdrawal)
  - Chloroquine
  - Cimetidine
  - CNS depressants
  - Cardiac glycosides
  - Heavy metal poisoning
  - Imipramine
  - Indomethacin
  - Lidocaine
  - Narcotics (withdrawal)
  - Scopolamine
► Infections
  - Encephalitis
  - HIV infection
  - Severe infectious diseases
► Cerebrovascular
  - Arteriosclerosis
  - Basilar artery thrombosis
► Brain tumor
► Seizures
► Metabolic disorders
  - Hepatic encephalopathy
  - Uremia
  - Acute hepatic porphyria
► Illnesses in advanced age
► Sleep deprivation

Congenital Abnormalities

Preventable causes
► Diet, vitamin deficiencies
  - Folic acid deficiency

- Vitamin A deficiency
- Low calcium
- Herbals
  - Butterbur
  - Coltsfoot
  - Golden seal
  - Groundsel
  - Ragwort
► Drugs
  - Alcohol
  - Anticonvulsants
  - Caffeine
  - Cocaine
  - Diazepam
  - Heroin
  - Marijuana
  - Petrol sniffing
  - Cigarette smoking
  - Tetracyclines
  - Warfarin
► Infections
  - Chickenpox
  - Cytomegalovirus
  - HIV
  - Listeria
  - Rubella
  - Syphilis
  - Toxoplasmosis
► Radiation
► Maternal diabetes mellitus

Congenital Heart Disease

Causes
► Genetic syndromes
  - Down's syndrome
  - Trisomy 13
  - Turner's syndrome (XO)
  - Marfan syndrome
  - Noonan syndrome
  - Ellis-van Creveld syndrome
► Viral infection
  - Rubella
► Drugs, toxins
  - Alcohol use (of the mother)

- Chemotherapeutics
- Immunosuppressives
- Retinoic acid (acne)
- Thalidomide
▶ Miscellaneous
- Radiation
- Lack of oxygen

Types
▶ Defects without shunt
- Aortic stenosis (AS)
- Coarctation of the aorta (CoA)
- Pulmonic stenosis (PS)
▶ Acyanotic defects with L to R shunt
- Atrial septal defect (ASD)
- Ventricular septal defect (VSD)
- Patent ductus arteriosus (PDA)
- Endocardial cushion defect (ECD)/ Atrioventricular canal (AV canal)
- Aorticopulmonary window (APW)
- Ruptured sinus of Valsalva aneurysm
▶ Cyanotic defects with R to L shunt
- Tetralogy of Fallot
- Tricuspid atresia
- Truncus arteriosus
- Transposition of great arteries (TGA)
- Hypoplastic left heart syndrome (HLHS)
- Total anomalous pumonary venous return
- Pulmonary atresia
- Double outlet right ventricle (DORV)
- Single ventricle
- Common atrium

Conjunctivitis, See Red Eye → 311

Constipation
Difficult stool passage with decreased stool frequency (< 3 stools per week).
Gastrointestinal disorders
▶ Colonic extraluminal obstruction
- Intraabdominal/pelvic tumors
  ○ Peritoneal carcinomatosis
  ○ Urogenital tumor (uterus, ovaries)

- Volvulus
- Hernia
- Rectocele, enterocele
- Ascites
- Adhesions
- Pregnancy
▶ Colonic intraluminal obstruction
- Colorectal carcinoma
- Benign colonic tumors
- Endometriosis
- Diverticulitis
- Diverticular stricture
- Colonic stricture
- Chronic ulcerative colitis
- Eosinophilic colitis
- Infections
  ○ Chronic amebiasis
  ○ Lymphogranuloma venereum
  ○ Syphilis
  ○ Tuberculosis
- Ischemic colitis
- Postoperative disorder
- Intussusception
- Corrosive enemas
▶ Anorectal disorders
- (Ulcerative) proctitis
- Perianal abscess
- Fissures
- Fistulas
- Rectal ulcer
- Lymphogranuloma venereum
- Postoperative disorder
- Rectal, anal carcinoma
- Rectal prolapse
- Anal atresia, malformation, stenosis
- Hereditary internal anal sphincter myopathy
- Hemorrhoids
- Descending perineum syndrome

Neuromuscular
▶ Aganglionic megacolon (Hirschsprung's disease)
▶ Amyloidosis
▶ Brain tumor
▶ Cerebrovascular accident

- Chagas disease
- Dermatomyositis
- Diabetic autonomic neuropathy (diabetes)
- Intestinal pseudoobstruction
- MEN 2b
- Meningocele
- Multiple sclerosis
- Muscular dystrophies
- Neurofibromatosis
- Paraplegia
- Parkinson's disease
- Scleroderma
- Senile dementia
- Spinal lesions
- Tabes dorsalis

Metabolic, endocrine
- Diabetes mellitus
- Glucagonoma
- Hypokalemia (laxative abuse)
- Hypercalcemia
- Hypothyroidism
- Panhypopituitarism
- Pheochromocytoma
- Porphyria
- Primary aldosteronism (Conn's syndrome)
- Pseudohypoparathyroidism
- Uremia

Drugs
- Analgesics
- Antacids
  - Aluminum hydroxide
  - Calcium carbonate
- Anticholinergics
- Anticonvulsants
- Antidepressants
- Antihypertensives
- Antiparkinsonian
- Antipsychotics
- Antispasmodics
- Barium sulfate
- Benzodiazepines
- Bismuth
- Calcium channel blockers

- Cation-containing agents
- Calcium supplements
- Cholestyramine
- Diuretics
- Ferrous sulfate
- Ganglionic blockers
- Heavy metal poisoning
- Ion-exchange resins
- Laxative abuse
- MAO inhibitors
- Opiates
- Phenothiazines
- Sucralfate
- Vinca alkaloids

Functional
- Diet
  - Fasting, reduced food intake
  - Low-residue diet
  - Low fluid intake
  - Lack of fiber
  - Chronic laxative/enema abuse
- Fecal impaction
- Repressed urge to defecate
- Travel constipation
- Change of environment
- Extended bed rest
- Emotional stress
- Idiopathic obstipation
- Irritable bowel syndrome

Behavioral, psychiatric disorder
- Depression
- Eating disorder
- Obsessive/compulsive disorder
- Psychosis

Constipation and Diarrhea, Alternating

Causes
- Colon cancer
- Intestinal polyposis
- Diverticulosis
- Intestinal tuberculosis
- Megacolon

Convulsions, See Epilepsy → 128

Coombs' test

Evidence of incomplete antibodies that stick to erythrocytes (direct Coombs') or circulate freely in the serum (indirect Coombs'). Coombs reagent is anti-human globulin antibody. It binds to human IgG antibody and C3 complement. Produced in rabbits by immunization

Direct Coombs: Is IgG or complement bound to red blood cell?

Indirect Coombs: Is antibody against red blood cell present in serum?

Direct Coombs test positive
▶ Autoimmune hemolytic anemia
▶ Gilbert's syndrome
▶ Transfusion reaction
▶ Infectious diseases
  • Infectious mononucleosis
  • Cytomegalic disease
  • Viral pneumonia
▶ Collagenosis
▶ Systemic lupus erythematosus
  • Chronic polyarthritis
▶ Neoplasm
  • Hodgkin's lymphoma
  • Lymphadenosis
  • Lymphosarcoma
▶ Therapy with α-methyldopa

Indirect Coombs test positive
▶ Rh incompatibility due to incomplete antibodies in the mother's serum
▶ DDx otherwise same as direct Coombs test

Copper

Reference range
80–140 µg/dl

See Ceruloplasmin → 72

Increased copper
▶ Tumor
  • Bronchial carcinoma
  • Breast cancer
  • Prostate cancer
▶ Acute and chronic infections
▶ Liver disease with cholestasis
▶ Intrauterine device

Decreased copper
▶ Malabsorption
▶ Nephrotic syndrome
  • Loss of ceruloplasmin
▶ Wilson's disease
▶ Menkes' syndrome (Inherited copper deficiency)

Cor Pulmonale

Hypertrophy or dilation of the right ventricle resulting from a disorder of the respiratory system.

Causes
▶ Lung disease
  • Chronic obstructive pulmonar disease (COPD)
  • Chronic bronchitis
  • Interstitial lung diseases
  • Pulmonary emphysema
  • Pulmonary fibrosis
  • Bronchiectases
  • Cystic fibrosis
  • Bronchopulmonary dysplasia following neonatal RDS
  • Scleroderma
  • After pulmonary resection
▶ Hypoxic
  • Chronic bronchitis
  • Emphysema
  • Chest wall dysfunction
  • Obesity
  • Sleep apnoe
  • Neuromuscular disease
  • Alveolar hypoxia in chronic high altitude exposure
▶ Pulmonary vascular disorder
  • Pulmonary embolism (relapsing)
  • Primary pulmonary hypertension

- Vasculitis from systemic disease
  - Necrotizing and granulomatous arteritis
  - Drug-induced lung disease (e.g. amiodarone)
  - Collagen vascular disease
- Tumor embolism
- Sickle cell anemia
- Schistosomiasis
- Sarcoidosis
- Pulmonary capillary hemangiomatosis
- Veno-occlusive lung disease
▶ Parenchymal disease with loss of vascular surface area
  - Emphysema
  - alpha1-antitrypsine deficiency
  - Bronchiectasis
  - Diffuse intestinal disease
    - ARDS
    - Collagen vasscular disease
    - Pneumoconiose
    - Sarcoid
    - Idioathic pulmonary fibrosis
    - Histiocytosis X
    - Tuberculosis
    - Chronic fungal infection
    - Hypersenitivity pneumonitis
▶ Vascular
  - Arterial hypertension causes
    - Collagen vascular disease
    - Portal hypertension
    - Human immunodeficiency virus (HIV) infection
    - Drugs (appetite suppressants)
    - Persistent pulmonary hypertension of the newborn
  - Venous hypertension causes
    - Disease of the left atrium
    - Disease of the left ventricle
    - Central pulmonary vein compression
      - *Fibrosing mediastinitis*
      - *Adenopathy*
      - *Tumor masses*
▶ Ventilation disorder
  - Impairment of the respiratory center

- Neuromuscular disease of the lung
  - ALS
  - Myasthenia gravis
  - Poliomyelitis
  - Guillain-Barré syndrome/ Polyradiculitis
  - Bilateral diaphragmatic paralysis
- Severe kyphoscoliosis
▶ Drugs
  - Appetite suppressants
▶ Cardiac disease
  - Left ventricular failure
  - Mitral valve disease
  - Left atrial myxoma
  - Congenital heart disease

Coronary Artery Disease

Acute coronary syndrome, myocardial infarction.

Atherosclerotic causes

See Coronary Risk Factor → 66

Nonatherosclerotic causes

▶ Emboli
  - Thrombi from
    - Left atrium
    - Left ventricle
    - Prosthetic valves
    - Catheter (angiography)
  - Endocarditis
  - Atrial myxoma
  - Air emboli
▶ Mechanical obstruction
  - Chest trauma
  - Dissection
    - Aorta
    - Coronary arteries
▶ Increased vasomotor tone
  - Variant angina
  - Raynaud's disease
  - Nitrate withdrawall
▶ Vasculitis
  - Collagen vascular disease
  - Takayasu's disease
  - Luetic aortitis

- Miscellaneous
  - Anomalous origin of coronary artery
  - Aortic stenosis
  - Hypertrophic cardiomyopathy
  - Hypotension
  - Hematologic disorder
  - Cocaine

Cortisol

Pay attention to the circadian rhythm of secretion (Cortisol 8 am: 4-19. Cortisol 4 pm: 2-15). Great variation due to pulsatile secretion.

Reference range

5-25 µg/dl morning
3-12 µg/dl evening

See Cushing's Syndrome → 91
See Addison's Disease → 14

Increased (hypercortisolism)

- Cushing's disease
- Adrenal cortex adenoma
- Adrenal cortex carcinoma
- Ectopic ACTH production
  - Small-cell lung cancer
  - Chronic renal failure
  - Pregnancy
- Drugs
  - Alcohol
  - Corticosteroids
  - Oral contraceptives
- Depression
- Familial cortisol resistance
- Pregnancy

Decreased (hypocortisolism)

- Adrenal cortical insufficiency (Addison's disease)
- Anterior pituitary dysfunction
- Congenital adrenal hyperplasia
- Waterhouse-Friderichsen syndrome
- Cancer metastasis
- Tuberculosis
- Amyloidosis
- Hemochromatosis

Cough, Chronic

Most common causes

- Sinusitis
- Allergic rhinitis
- Asthma
- Gastroesphogeal reflux
- Chronic bronchitis (smoking)
- Bronchiectasis
- Post-viral (hyperresponsiveness)
- Post-bronchitic (hyperresponsiveness)

Causes

- Asthma, allergic
  - Cough variant asthma (CVA)
  - Allergic rhinitis
  - Atopic rhinitis
  - Post-viral (hyperresponsiveness)
  - Post-bronchitic (hyperresponsiveness)
- Pulmonary
  - Bronchiectasis
  - Cystic fibrosis
  - Foreign body
  - Fungal lung infection
  - Ciliary dyskinesia
  - Interstitial lung disease
  - Emphysema
  - Sarcoidosis
  - Tuberculosis
  - Other chronic lung disease
- Infection
  - Pertussis
  - Tuberculosis
  - Parasitic infection
  - Bordetella pertussis
  - Chlamydia trachomatis
  - Fungal lung infection
  - Sinusitis
  - Chronic bronchitis
  - Adenoiditis
  - Croup
  - Opportunistic infections
- Aspiration
  - Gastroesophageal reflux disease (GERD)

- Tracheoesophageal fistula
- Laryngotracheal cleft
- Esophageal immotility
- Vocal cord paralysis
- Achalasia
- Pharyngeal discoordination
- Neurologic disorders
▶ Foreign body in
- Bronchus
- Nose
- Larynx
- Trachea
- Ear
▶ Neoplasm, intrathoracic mass
- Subglottic hemangioma
- Papillomatosis
- Bronchogenic carcinoma
- Pulmonary neoplasm
- Esophageal cancer
- Lymphangitis carcinomatosis
- Thoracic aneurysm
- Goiter
- Mediastinal lymphadenadenopathy
- Cervical mass
▶ Otologic
- Cerumen
- Ear foreign body
- Infection
- Neoplasm
- Hair in the ear canal
▶ Drugs, toxins, environment
- ACE inhibitors
- Alcoholism
- Betablockers
- Low humidity
- Occupational inhalation of bronchial irritants
- Overheating
- Smoking
▶ Cardiovascular
- Congestive heart failure
- Left ventricular failure
- Rheumatic heart disease
- Mitral valve stenosis
▶ Congenital

- Aortic arch anomalies
- Subglottic stenosis
- Tracheomalacia
- Bronchogenic cyst
- Foregut cyst
- Esophageal duplication
- Tracheal stenosis
- Bronchial stenosis
- Bronchial web
▶ Psychogenic
- Psychogenic cough
▶ Miscellaneous
- Frequent vomiting
- Post-cerebrovascular accident

Creatine Kinase (CK)

Enzyme catalyzing the reversible transfer of phosphate from phosphocreatine to ADP, forming creatine and ATP. Certain isozymes are elevated in plasma following myocardial infarctions. See Troponin I and Cardiac Troponin T → 361

Isoenzymes
▶ MB: heart
▶ MM: skeletal muscle
▶ BB: brain, bowel infarction, neoplasm (prostate, GI, breast, ovary, lung, brain)

Increased total CK and CK–MB ratio
▶ Myocardial infarction
▶ Cardiogenic shock
▶ Perimyocarditis
▶ Right ventricular failure
▶ Valvular defects
▶ Heart surgery
▶ Cardiac contusion

Increased total CK
▶ Vigorous exercise
▶ Intramuscular injections
▶ Malignant hyperthermia
▶ Rhabdomyolysis
▶ Myositis
▶ Crush injury or trauma
▶ Surgery
▶ Muscular spasm

- Epileptic attack
► Arterial embolism
► Hyperthermia
► Muscular dystrophy
  - Duchenne's
  - Becker's
  - Leyden-Moebius
  - Ocular
► Pulmonary infarction
► Acute aortic dissection
► Myotonic dystrophy
► Myasthenia gravis
► Neurogenic muscular atrophy
► Intoxication
► Alcoholism
► Inflammatory myopathies
  - Polymyositis
  - Dermatomyositis
  - Viral myositis
  - Bacterial and viral myositis
► Endocrine myopathies
  - Hypothyroidism
► Increased total CK in damage to other tissues
  - Liver, pancreas and GI diseases
  - Pregnancy and labor
  - Malignant tumors
  - Hyperthyroidism
  - Thyrotoxic crisis

Creatinine

Creatinine is formed in the muscles and released into the blood. Creatinine synthesis thus depends on the individual muscular mass. With normal kidney function it is almost completely excreted through glomerular filtration. Only a limitation of the glomerular filtration rate (GFR) < 50% leads to an increase in serum creatinine. With acute kidney function impairment, an increase in creatinine occurs only after a delay.

Indication: acute or chronic kidney diseases, pathologic urine findings, monitoring of kidney diseases, intensive care, postoperative, patients, followup of therapy with potentially nephrotoxic substances, muscle traumas, burns, degenerative muscle processes, hypertension, extrarenal diseases (diarrhea, vomiting, Excessive sweating), hemodialysis, metabolic disorders (diabetes, hyperuricacidemia), diseases with elevated protein metabolism (multiple myeloma, acromegaly).

Reference range

M: 0.84-1.36 mg/dl	
F: 0.66-1.17 mg/dl	

Increased creatinine
See Renal Failure, Acute → 315

Influencing factors
► Sex (women < men)
► Age (decreasing after age 20)
► Muscle mass (decreased muscular mass can cause (falsely!) low serum creatinine levels)
► Pregnancy (reduced creatinine)
► Hyperglycemia (osmotic diuresis with reduced creatinine levels)
► Obesity, ascites
► Proteinuria
► Time of day (highest in the afternoon)

Creatinine Clearance

Measurement of the clearance of endogenous creatinine, used for evaluating the glomerular filtration rate (GFR).

Estimating Creatinine Clearance

Creatinine clearance for **males** (ml/min) = $\{[(140 - (\text{age in years})] * (\text{body weight in kg}) / (72 * (\text{serum creatinine in mg/dL})\}$ mL/min
Creatinine clearance for **females** (ml/min) = $\{[(0.85) * (140 - (\text{age in years})] * (\text{body weight in kg}) / (72 * (\text{serum creatinine in mg/dL})]\}$ mL/min
(Method of Cockcroft and Gault, 1976)

Reference range

50-140 ml/min

Increased

▶ Pregnancy
▶ Exercise

Decreased

▶ Renal insufficiency
▶ Acute or chronic kidney disease
▶ Nephrotic syndrome
▶ Drugs
  • Antibiotics
  • Cimetidine
  • Procainamide
  • Quininidine
▶ Diabetes mellitus
▶ Heart failure

Influencing factors

▶ Sex (women < men)
▶ Age (decreasing after age 20)
▶ Muscle mass
▶ Pregnancy
▶ Hyperglycemia (osmotic diuresis)
▶ Obesity, ascites (less CC)
▶ Proteinuria (increased CC)
▶ Time of day (highest in the afternoon)

CRP

C-reactive protein

Acute-phase protein. Formed in the liver. Rises more than 6 hours after triggering stimulus. Peaks within 50 hours. Short half life of 5-7 hours. CRP rapidly declines after condition resolves. CRP is supposed to recognize endogenous toxic materials released in the event of tissue damage, bind these and initiate their removal. When bound to microbes it acts as an opsonin and activates macrophages and complement. CRP is a better indicator for an inflammatory response than other acute-phase proteins due to its rapid increase and shorter half-life.

Reference range

Adults: < 5 mg/l

Increased

▶ Infections
  • Bacteria
  • Viruses
  • Parasites
  • Fungi
▶ Myocardial infarction
  • Increased C-reactive protein predictive of CAD
▶ Rheumatic, collagen vascular disease
  • Rheumatoid arthritis
  • Juvenile arthritis
  • Bechterew's disease
  • Degenerative joint diseases
  • Psoriasis arthropathy
  • Reiter's syndrome
  • Pseudogout
  • Systemic lupus erythematosus
  • Sjögren's syndrome
  • Dermatomyositis
  • Polymyositis
  • Polymyalgia rheumatica
  • Wegener's granulomatosis
  • Vasculitis
▶ Miscellaneous
  • Inflammatory bowel disease
  • Malignant tumors
  • Leukemia
  • Acute pancreatitis
  • Postoperatively

Crystalluria

Excretion of crystalline material in the urine.

Uric acid crystals and urates

▶ Gout
▶ Purine-rich food
▶ Fever
▶ Malignant diseases
▶ Drugs
  • Chemotherapeutics
  • Pyrazinamide

Calcium oxalate
▶ Food containing oxalate
▶ Oxalosis

Cholesterol crystals
▶ Chylous urine

Cystine crystals
▶ Cystinuria

Leucine and tyrosine crystals
▶ Severe liver disease

Struvite crystals
▶ Urinary tract infection

Cushing's Syndrome

Constellation of symptoms and signs caused by an excess of cortisol hormone. There are ACTH-dependent (80%) and ACTH-independent (20%) forms.

ACTH–independent Cushing
▶ Iatrogenic hypercortisolism
  • Long-term glucocorticoid therapy (most common cause)
▶ Adrenal Cushing
  • Adrenal adenoma
  • Adrenal hyperplasia
  • Adrenal carcinoma
▶ Miscellaneous
  • Alcoholism
  • Depression
  • Severe acute or chronic illness

ACTH–dependent Cushing
▶ Central Cushing
  • Pituitary ACTH secreting adenoma (usually microadenomas)
  • Hypothalamic hyperfunction (increased corticotropin-releasing hormone)
▶ Ectopic ACTH production
  • Small cell carcinoma of the lung
  • Pancreatic islet cell carcinoma
  • Carcinoids of the
    ○ Lungs
    ○ Gut
    ○ Thymus
    ○ Pancreas
    ○ Ovary
  • Medullary thyroid carcinoma
  • Pheochromocytoma
  • Other tumors
▶ Ectopic corticotropin-releasing hormone-screting tumor
  • Bronchial carcinoid
  • Gangliocytoma
  • Medullary thyroid carcinoma
  • Oat cell carcinoma of the lung
  • Prostatic carcinoma
  • Pheochromocytoma

Cyanosis

Methemoglobinemia
Bluish or purplish tinge to the skin and mucous membranes due to an increase of the reduced hemoglobin of about 5 g/dl. Distiguish between pulmonary and cardiac cyanosis as well as central and peripheral cyanosis. Central cyanosis is due to a respiratory failure, a right-left shunt or a reduced oxygen partial pressure in the breath (high altitude). In peripheral cyanosis there is an increased oxygen consumption in the peripheral tissue due to a reduced or decelerated blood flow.

Central cyanosis
▶ Pulmonary disease (respiratory failure)
  • Chronic bronchitis
  • Pneumonia
  • Asthma
  • Emphysema
  • Bronchiectasis
  • Atelectasis
  • Tuberculosis
  • Pulmonary fibrosis
  • Pulmonary embolism
  • Pulmonary edema
  • Lung tumor
  • Pulmonary hypertension
  • Sclerosis of the pulmonary artery
  • Pleural effusion

- Valvular pneumothorax
- Foreign-body aspiration
- Shock lung
- Cystic disease of the lung
- Fibrosing alveolitis
- Pneumoconiosis
- Mediastinitis
- Pickwickian syndrome
- Central or peripheral respiratory paralysis
  - Intoxication
  - Poliomyelitis
  - Polyneuropathy
- Intrapulmonary arteriovenous aneurysms
▶ Cardiac (mixed blood cyanosis)
  - Cardiac defect with right-left shunt
    - Fallot's tetralogy
    - Patent ductus arteriosus
    - Double-outlet ventricle
    - Single ventricle
    - Transposition of the great vessels
    - Complex vitium with shunt reversal to right-left
      - *Ventricular septal defect*
      - *Atrio-septal defect*
▶ Primary alveolar hypoventilation
▶ Central or peripheral respiratory paralysis

Hemoglobin cyanosis (cyanosis in abnormal hemoglobin without O_2 transport ability. Rare cause)
▶ Methemoglobinemia (danger of death only over 70 %, Heinz' bodies)
  - Congenital
    - Diaphorase deficiency
    - Congenital methemoglobinemia
  - Acquired
    - Nitrites
    - Sodium nitroprusside
    - Sodium thiocyanite
    - Nitrates
    - Sulfonamides
    - Azulfidine
    - Phenacetin

  - Nitrobenzene
  - Nitrogases
  - Toxic-hemolytic anemia through hydrogen peroxide
  - Phenylhydrazine
▶ Sulfhemoglobinemia
  - Sulfonamide
  - Phenacetin

Peripheral cyanosis (usually cardiac exhaustion and usually a late symptom)
▶ Reduced cardiac output
  - CHD
  - Hypertensive cardiac disease
  - Valvular defect
  - Shunt vitium
  - Cardiomyopathy
  - Inflammatory cardiac diseases
  - Cardiac dysrhythmia
  - Pericardial effusion
  - Pericardium callosity
  - Heart tumors
  - Endomyocardial fibrosis
▶ Venous stasis
▶ Cold exposure
▶ Raynaud´s phenomenon

Cylindruria

Presence of renal cylinders or casts in the urine.

Hyaline casts
▶ Spntaneous
  - After physical exercise
  - After kidney palpation
▶ Heart failure
▶ Congested kidney
  - Right ventricular failure
  - Venous stasis
▶ Infection with fever
▶ Kidney diseases

Granular casts
▶ Kidney diseases
  - Acute glomerulonephritis
  - Chronic glomerulonephritis
  - Nephrotic syndrome

- Toxic nephropathy
  - Cadmium
  - Carbon tetrachloride
  - Contrast media
  - Bismuth
  - Mercury
  - Methyl alcohol
  - Uranium
▶ Pneumonia
▶ Sepsis

Leukocyte casts
▶ Pyelonephritis
  • Purulent
  • Chronic pyelonephritis
▶ Interstitial nephritis
▶ Glomerulonephritis

Red cell cast
▶ Renal tumor
▶ Renal infarct
▶ Necrotizing papillitis
▶ Renal tuberculosis
▶ Trauma
▶ Glomerulonephritis
▶ Collagen vascular disease
▶ Acute interstitial nephritis
▶ Cystic kidneys
▶ Amyloidosis

Epithelial cell casts
▶ Interstitial nephritis
▶ Chronic glomerulonephritis
▶ Chronic pyelonephritis
▶ Acute tubular insufficiency

Waxy casts
▶ Severe pyelonephritis
▶ Severe glomerulonephritis
▶ Acute renal failure
▶ Chronic renal failure
▶ Amyloidosis

Fatty casts
▶ Nephrotic syndrome
▶ Glomerular sclerosis

Cystic kidney diseases
See Renal Cysts → 314

Cystitis, See Dysuria → 114

δ-Aminolevulinic Acid

Proof of δ-aminolevulinic acid in the urine is used for immediate guideline with clinical suspicion of porphyria (in addition to porphobilinogens, porphyrins → 290). Important in the DDx of acute abdomen of unclear origin.

Normal values

20ml collected urine (for immediate diagnostic in the laboratory)
<7.5 mg/24h urine

Indication
▶ Acute hepatic porphyria
  • Acute intermittent porphyria
  • Porphyria variegata
  • Hereditary coproporphyria
▶ Chronic hepatic porphyria
▶ Drug damage to the liver
  • Barbiturates
▶ Lead poisoning

D-dimer
See Fibrin Degradation Products → 145

Deafness. See Hearing Loss, Hearing Impairment → 165

Death, See Sudden Death → 343,
See Karnofsky Performance Scale → 216

Deep vein thrombosis
See Thrombophilia → 351

Dehydration
Exsiccation

Decrease in body water. Water content of the adult is approx. 60% of the body weight, of which 2/3 is intracellular and 1/3 extracellular (interstitial and intravascular fluid). Clinical symptoms of dehydration include thirst, dry mucosa, tachycardia, hypotension, empty cervical veins, oliguria and tendency to collapse. In the laboratory it can result in a relative increase in hematocrit, serum proteins, hemoglobin and urea. Deviations from isotonia are usually linked to serum sodium levels because **serum osmolality** is mostly dependent on serum sodium. Serum osmolality (SO) = 2* [serum sodium + potassium] + glucose [mg/dl/18] + urea [mg/dl/6]

Isotonic dehydration
SO: normal; SS: normal; ECS: normal
▶ Chronic vomiting
▶ Chronic diarrhea
▶ Hemorrhage, blood loss
▶ Ascites and pleural puncture
▶ Fistula drains
▶ Displacement of fluid into transcellular (third) space
  • Ileus (→ 206)
  • Peritonitis
  • Ascites
  • Pancreatitis
▶ Loss through the skin
  • Burns
  • Large wounds
  • Exudative dermatosis
▶ Loss through the kidneys
  • Polyuric phase of renal failure
  • Salt-loss nephritis
  • Diuretic therapy
  • Addison's disease
  • Adrenal failure
  • Renal tubular acidosis
  • Saluretics
▶ Decreased intake of water and electrolytes
  • Ileus (→ 206)
  • Peritonitis

Hypotonic dehydration
SO: reduced; SS: reduced; ECS: reduced; increased intracellular volume

▶ Miscellaneous
  • See also isotonic dehydration
  • Massive vomiting
  • Massive or chronic diarrhea
  • Excessive sweating with substitution of water poor in sodium chloride
  • Diuretic therapy
  • Duodenal secretion
  • Pancreatic or gall bladder fistula
  • Inhibited sodium resorption in the intestine in chronic inflammatory intestinal diseases
  • After ascites puncture
  • Steatorrhea with binding of sodium to fatty acids
▶ Decreased reabsorption of sodium in the kidney
  • Chronic renal failure with GFR < 20 ml/min with excessive strain on the remaining glomerula
  • Polyuric phase of renal failure
  • Salt-loss nephritis
  • Tubular kidney impairment
  • Renal tubular acidosis
  • Adrenal failure
  • Addison's disease
  • Hypoaldosteronism
  • Extreme hypertension with secondary pressure natriuresis
  • Bartter's syndrome
▶ Cerebrally regulated salt loss
  • Brain tumors
  • Polio
  • Encephalitis
▶ Intoxication
  • Vitamin D
  • Sublimate

Hypertonic dehydration
SO: increased; SS: increased; ECS: extreme decrease; intracellular volume decrease
▶ Insufficient water supply
  • Hydropenia
  • Desert
  • Athletes
  • Inability to hydrate in:

- ○ Coma
- ○ Esophageal stenoses
- ○ Dysphagia
▶ Water loss via:
  • Skin
    ○ Burns
    ○ Excessive sweating
    ○ Fever
  • Lungs
    ○ Fever
    ○ Extreme hyperventilation
  • Kidneys
    ○ Chronic renal failure
  • Gastrointestinal tract
    ○ Vomiting
    ○ Diarrhea
    ○ Fistulas in inflammatory bowel disease
▶ Impaired concentration capacity of the kidneys
  • Renal/central diabetes insipidus
  • Osmotic diuresis
    ○ Diabetes mellitus
  • Nephrotoxic drugs
  • Polycystic kidneys
  • Pyelonephritis
  • Interstitial nephritis
  • Sickle cell disease
  • Electrolyte imbalance
    ○ Hypercalcemia
    ○ Hypokalemia
  • High urea content in the blood from protein catabolism
▶ Excessive supply of osmotically effective fluids
  • I.v. hypertonic solutions
  • Per tube (highly concentrated protein and glucose solutions)
▶ Lack of thirst
  • Advanced age
  • Psychoses
  • Unconsciousness
▶ ADH deficiency
▶ Secondary hyperaldosteronism
  • Heart failure

- • Cirrhosis
▶ Cholera
▶ Vomiting

Dehydro-3-Epiandrosterone
DHEA
Main secretory product of the suprarenal cortex with unclear physiologic significance.
Increased
▶ Anovulation
▶ Polycystic ovaries
▶ Hirsutism
▶ Hyperprolactinemia
▶ Adrenogenital syndrome
▶ Androgen-producing tumor
▶ Ovarian tumors
▶ Adrenal cortex tumors
Decreased
▶ Menopause

Delirium
In delirium, hallucinatory episodes, agitation and disorientation occur in addition to impaired consciousness
Exogenous causes
▶ Withdrawal of alcohol, barbiturates or other sedatives after chronic intoxication
▶ Drug intoxication
  • Atropine
  • Benzodiazepines
  • Camphor
  • Ergotamine
  • Scopolamine
▶ Toxins
  • Methyl alcohol
  • Organophosphates
  • Heavy metals
▶ Thiamine deficiency
Neurologic causes
▶ Bacterial meningitis (tuberculosis)
▶ Viral encephalitis (HIV)

- Subarachnoid hemorrhage
- Cerebral contusion
- Cerebral masses

Miscellaneous causes
- Pneumonia
- Typhoid fever
- Rheumatic fever
- Septicemia
- After hypoxia
- Postoperative and postconcussive states
- Thyrotoxicosis
- Hypoglycemia
- Acidosis
- Hepatic encephalopathy

Delta wave
See ECG, U-, Delta Wave → 122

Dementia
Mental deficiency, oligophrenia
The usually progressive loss of cognitive and intellectual functions, without impairment of perception or consciousness; caused by a variety of disorders, most commonly structural brain disease. Dementia is characterized by disorientation, impaired memory, judgment and intellect, and a shallow labile affect. Prevalence in the USA is about 8-10% of persons in the age group > 65 years and about 25% of persons in the age group > 85 years.
See Mental Retardation → 239, coma (→ 79), confusion (→ 81).

Diagnostic criteria
- Amnesia
  - Short-term memory impairment (e.g. three objects after 5 minutes)
  - Long-term memory impairment (e.g. events of the day before)
- Impairment of abstract thinking
- Limited judgment ability
- Orientation disturbances
- Impairment of other higher cognitive

functions
  - Aphasia (speech disturbance)
  - Apraxia (impaired motions)
  - Agnosia (loss of comprehension)
  - Acalculia (inability to perform calculations)
  - Personality changes

Frequently associated problems
- Delirium
- Depression
- Psychotic symptoms
  - Delusion
  - Hallucinations
- Behavioral disorders

Criteria for the severity of dementia
- Mild: reduced performance in the household or in social activities, but independent personal hygiene and judgment are retained.
- Medium: independent life is dangerous and intermittent monitoring necessary.
- Severe: serious loss of independence, with permanent care and monitoring necessary.

Most common causes
- Alzheimer's disease
- Alcoholism
- Vascular dementia
  - Multi-infarct
  - Diffuse white matter disease (Binswanger's)
- Parkinson's disease
- Drug intoxication

Less common causes
- Vitamin deficiencies
  - Thiamine (B1, Wernicke's encephalopathy)
  - B_{12} (pernicious anemia)
  - Nicotinic acid (pellagra)
  - Folic acid
- Endocrine and other organ disorders
  - Hypothyroidism
  - Hyperthyroidism
  - Hyperparathyroidism

- Hypoparathyroidism
- Adrenal insufficiency
- Cushing´s syndrome
- Hepatic failure, encephalopathy
- Renal failure
- Pulmonary failure
- Phenylketonuria
- Hepatolenticular degeneration (Wilson's disease)
- Hemochromatosis

▶ Chronic infections, inflammations
- Chronic meningitis
  ○ Tuberculosis
  ○ Borreliosis
- Syphilis, neurosyphilis
- HIV encephalopathy
- Postinfectious encephalitis (Postencephalitis)
- Papovavirus (progressive multifocal leukoencephalopathy)
- Prion (Creutzfeldt-Jakob disease)
- Sarcoidosis
- Whipple's disease

▶ Toxic disorders
- Drugs, intoxication
  ○ Anticonvulsants
  ○ Antihypertensives
  ○ Antihistamines
  ○ Betablockers
  ○ Digoxin
  ○ Psychopharmaceutics
- Heavy metals
  ○ Mercury
  ○ Lead
- Dialysis dementia (aluminum)

▶ Psychiatric disorders
- Depression
- Schizophrenia
- Conversion reaction

▶ Degenerative disorders
- Huntington's disease
- Pick's disease (frontal temporal dementia)
- Diffuse Lewy body disease
- Diffuse supranuclear palsy (Steel-Richardson syndrome)
- Multisystem degeneration (Shy-Drager syndrome)
- Hereditary ataxias
- Amyotrophic lateral sclerosis
- Frontal lobe dementia
- Cortical basal degeneration
- Multiple sclerosis

▶ Vascular disorders
- Multi-infarct dementia
- Lacunar state
- Diffuse white matter disease (Binswanger's)
- Inadequate circulation and oxygen supply in:
  ○ Chronic obstructive lung disease
  ○ Chronic heart failure
  ○ Cardiac dysrhythmias

▶ Head trauma, CNS damage
- Dementia pugilistica
- Chronic subdural hematoma
- Postanoxia
- Normal-pressure hydrocephalus
- Generalized paralysis
- Dementia with epilepsy

▶ Neoplasms
- CNS tumor
- Metastases

▶ Miscellaneous
- Vasculitis, systemic lupus erythematosus
- Acute intermittent porphyria
- Recurrent nonconvulsive siezures

▶ Pediatric disorders
- Hallervorden-Spatz disease
- Subacute sclerosing panencephalitis
- Metabolic disorders
  ○ Wilson's disease
  ○ Leukodystropies
  ○ Lipid storage diasease

DDx of dementia

▶ Pseudodementias
- Hypomania
- Depression
- Schizophrenia

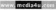

- Hysteria
► Korsakoff's syndrome
► Aphasia
► Lack of motivation, particularly in advanced age

Depigmentation, See Depigmentation, hypopigmentation, leukoderma → 203
See Hypomelanosis → 203

Depression

Diagnostically unspecific description for affective impairment, exhibited in a depressive syndrome with sadness, lack of motivation, lack of interest, guilt, feeling of worthlessness, loss of libido, eating and sleep disturbances.

Classification I

► Major depression
Severe, episodic impairment with accompanying neurovegetative symptomatic complex
► Bipolar impairment
Intermittent manic phases during the depressive phase, not necessarily distinguishable from major depression.
► Dysthymic disease
Chronic and not as severe as major depression. Frequently associated with a personality disorder.
► Cyclothymic disease
Less severe, frequently with melancholia
► Organic depression
Organic encephalopathy
► Adjustment disorder
► Seasonal affective disorder
Autumn depression

Classification II

► Endogenous depression
► Neurotic depression
► Reactive depression
► Age-related depression
► Menopause
► Premenstrual syndrome

Organic causes of depression
► Drugs, toxins
  • Alcohol abuse
  • Analgetics
  • Antibiotics
  • Antihypertensives
  • Clonidin
  • Cocaine
  • Corticosteroids
  • Digitalis
  • Ethionamid
  • Griseofulvin
  • H_2 blockers
  • Indomethacin
  • Isoniacid
  • L-Dopa
  • Methyldopa
  • Oral contraceptives
  • Phenylbutazon
  • Procainamid
  • Propanolol
  • Reserpin
  • Sulfonamides
  • Tranquillizer (withdrawal)
► Endocrine, metabolic
  • Hypothyroidism
  • Thyrotoxicosis
  • Cushing's syndrome
  • Hyperparathyroidism
  • Addisson's disease
  • Hypercalcemia
  • Hyponatremia
  • Hypokalemia
  • Diabetes mellitus
  • Pernicious anemia
  • Chronic renal failure/Dialysis
► Neurologic
  • Stroke
  • Subdural hematoma
  • Multiple sclerosis
  • Brain tumor
  • Parkinson's disease
  • Alzheimer's disease
  • Huntington's chorea
  • Epilepsy

- Dementia
- Frontal brain lesion
► Infections
  - Viral infection
    ◦ Mononucleosis
    ◦ Influenza
    ◦ Viral hepatitis
    ◦ HIV infection
  - Syphilis
► Malnutrition
  - Vitamin B_{12} deficiency
  - Pellagra
► Miscellaneous
  - Neoplasm (pancreatic cancer)
  - Myocardial infarction
  - Postoperative (heart surgery)
  - Steroid withdrawal therapy
  - Parturition
  - Altitude sickness

DHEA
See Dehydro-3-Epiandrosterone → 95

Diabetes Insipidus

Chronic excretion of very large amounts of pale urine of low specific gravity, resulting from inadequate output of pituitary antidiuretic hormone (ADH, arginine vasopressin, AVP), causing dehydration and excessive thirst.

Central (pituitary) diabetes insipidus
Release of insufficient AVP. Thirst experiment: no increase of urine osmolality; after stimulation with DDAVP increase to > 750 mosmol/kg H_2O
► Head trauma
► Postoperative
  - Posthypophysectomy
► CNS tumor
  - Craniopharyngeoma
  - Adenomas
  - Metastases
  - Lymphoma, leukemia
  - Granulomas

► Infections
  - (Basilar) meningitis
  - Encephalitis
  - Toxoplasmosis
► Inflammation
  - Sarcoidosis
  - Tuberculosis
  - Lymphocytic neurohypophysitis
  - Wegener's granulomatosis
  - LE
  - Scleroderma
► Chemical toxins
► Vascular disorders
  - Sheehan's syndrome
  - Stroke
  - Aneurysm
  - Aortocoronary bypass
  - Hypoxic encephalopathy
► Congenital pituitary malformations
► Genetic

Nephrogenic diabetes insipidus
Renal resistance to antidiuretic action of AVP. No increase of the urine osmolality after thirst experiment and DDAVP
► Drugs
  - Alcohol
  - Aminoglycosides
  - Amphotericin B
  - Barbiturates
  - Cisplatin
  - Diuretics
  - Foscarnet
  - Lithium
  - Rifampicin
► Metabolic
  - Hypercalcemia
  - Hypokalemia
► Urinary tract obstruction
  - Ureter
  - Urethra
► Hematologic/vascular disorder
  - Sickle cell diseasae
  - Acute tubular necrosis
► Tumor
  - Granuloma

- Sarcoma
- ► Infiltration
  - Amyloidosis
- ► Polycystic kidneys
- ► Pregnancy
- ► Genetic

Primary polydipsia
Inhibition of AVP secretion due to excessive fluid intake. Thirst experiment: normal increase of the urine osmolality
- ► Psychogenic
  - Schizophrenia
  - Obsessive-compulsive disorder
- ► Dipsogenic (abnormal thirst)
  - Granulomas
  - Tuberculous meningitis
  - Headtrauma
  - Multiple sclerosis
  - Drugs
    ○ Carbamazepine
    ○ Lithium
- ► Iatrogenic

Diabets insipidus during pregnancy
Probably splitting of AVP through hydrolysis

Diabetes mellitus
See Hyperglycemia → 189

Diaphragmatic Dysfunction

Anatomic defects
- ► Congenital
  - Bochdalek hernia
  - Morgagni hernia
  - Eventration of the diaphragm
  - Diaphragmatic agenesis
- ► Acquired
  - Traumatic rupture
  - Penetrating injuries
  - Idiopathic
  - Iatrogenic
    ○ Surgery
    ○ Other invasive procedures

Innervation defects
- ► Cerebrovascular accident
- ► Spinal cord disorders
  - Trauma (cervical spinal cord)
  - Syringomyelia
  - Poliomyelitis
  - Motor neuron disease
- ► Phrenic nerve neuropathy
  - Trauma to the phrenic nerve
    ○ Surgery
    ○ Radiation
    ○ Tumor
  - Guillain-Barré syndrome
  - Brachial plexus neuritis
  - Diabetes mellitus
  - Nutritional neuropathy
  - Alcohol abuse
  - Vasculitic neuropathy
  - Lead and poison neuropathy
  - Infection-related nerve injury
    ○ Diphtheria
    ○ Tetanus
    ○ Typhoid
    ○ Measles
    ○ Botulism
- ► Myasthenia gravis
- ► Muscular disorders
  - Myotonic dystrophies
  - Duchenne muscular dystrophy
  - Metabolic myopathies
  - Polymyositis
- ► Idiopathic

Diaphragmatic Elevation

Abdominal causes
- ► Obesity
- ► Pregnancy
- ► Hepatomegaly
- ► Splenomegaly
- ► Gaseous distention of the stomach
- ► Gaseous distention of the splenic flexure of the colon (left)
- ► Ascites
- ► Subphrenic abscess

► Hematoma
► Other abdominal mass

Thoracic causes
► Atelectasis
► Acute pleuritis
► Pulmonary embolism
► Pulmonary infarction
► Pulmonary fibrosis
► Surgery
  • Lobectomy
  • Pneumectomy
► Diaphragm hernia
► Trauma
  • Thorax trauma
  • Traumatic rupture of diaphragm

Phrenic nerve paralysis
► Retrosternal goiter
► Surgery (thyroid)
► Trauma
► Aortic aneurysm
► Neoplasm in the mediastinum
  • Bronchial carcinoma
  • Malignant lymphoma
  • Metastases
► Poliomyelitis
► Peripheral neuritis
► Hemiplegia
► Guillain-Barré syndrome/Polyradiculitis

DDx
► Subpulmonic pleural fluid
► Complete diaphragmatic eventration

Diarrhea

Abnormally frequent (> 3x/day) discharge of semisolid or fluid feces from the bowel and/or a fecal volume > 250 g/24h. Very common symptom that can be acute, chronic, self-limiting or life-threatening. Main causes are infections, bacterial toxins and drugs. Acute **gastroenteritis** with viral or bacterial cause is typical, but usually no agent is traceable. Frequently self-limiting progression within 5 days. Dysentery is acute diarrhea with muco- purulent-bloody feces accompanied by fever. Pseudodiarrhea is an increased number of bowel movements without an increase in fecal volume (in irritable colon or proctitis).

Risk factors
► Recent travel to endemic area
► High-risk sexual behavior (sexually transmitted disease)
► Antibiotic use within 6 months (clostridium difficile)
► Immunosuppression

Acute diarrhea
► Infection
  • Bacterial infection
    ○ E. coli
      - *ETEC (enterotoxic E. coli)*
      - *EHEC (enterohemorrhagic E. coli)*
      - *EPEC (enteropathogenic E. coli)*
    ○ Salmonella
    ○ Campylobacter jejuni
    ○ Vibrio cholerae
    ○ Klebsiella
    ○ Enterobacter
    ○ Staphylococcus aureus
    ○ Shigella
    ○ Clostridium difficile (after antibiotic therapy!)
    ○ Yersinia enterocolitica
    ○ Chlamydia
    ○ Neisseria gonorrhoeae
    ○ Aeromonas
    ○ Plesiomonas
  • Viral infection
    ○ Norwalk virus
    ○ Rotavirus
    ○ Adenovirus
    ○ CMV
    ○ Influenza virus
    ○ Coxsackie virus
    ○ Poliovirus
    ○ ECHO viruses
  • Food toxins (not killed through cooking)
    ○ Staphylococcus aureus

- Bacillus cereus
- Clostridium perfringens
- Parasites
  - Entamoeba histolytica
  - Giardia intestinalis
  - Cryptosporidium
▶ Noninfectious causes
- Ischemic-hemorrhagic colitis
- Endocrine
  - Hyperthyroidism
  - Addison's disease
  - C-cell carcinoma
  - Other hormone-producing tumors
- Colon cancer
- Graft-host reaction after allogenic bone marrow transplantation
- Food allergy
- First manifestation of chronic inflammatory bowel disease
- Heavy metal intoxication
- Runners' diarrhea
▶ Drug-induced
- Alcohol
- Antibiotics (Clostridium difficile)
- Biguanides
- Chemotherapy
- Cholestyramin
- Chemotherapeutics
- Digitalis
- Diuretics
- Ergotamine
- Heavy metal poisoning
- Hydralazine
- Laxatives (abuse)
- Mushroom poisoning
- Opiate withdrawal
- Parasympathomimetics
- Quinidine
- Reserpine
- Uremia
- Warfarin
▶ Diseases associated with acute diarrhea
- Mono- and oligoarthritis (HLA-B27-positiv)
  - Yersinia

  - Shigella
  - Campylobacter
  - Salmonellas
- Erythema nodosum
  - Yersinia
- Guillain-Barré syndrome/Polyradiculitis
  - Campylobacter jejuni

Frequent germs of travelers' diarrhea
▶ Enterotoxic E. coli
▶ Shigella
▶ Campylobacter jejuni
▶ Salmonella
▶ Aeromonas
▶ Rotavirus
▶ Protozoa

Chronic diarrhea
▶ Types
- Osmotic diarrhea
- Motility diarrhea
- Secretory diarrhea
- Exudative diarrhea
▶ Causes
- Malassimilation (→ 233)
  - Maldigestion
  - Malabsorption
- Chronic inflammatory bowel disease
  - Crohn's disease
  - Ulcerative colitis
- Food allergy
- Sprue
- Motility disorders of the GI tract
- Irritable colon
- Diverticular disease
- Exudative diarrhea
- Infection
  - Bacterial toxins (e.g. cholera)
  - Tuberculosis
  - Enteropathogenic viruses
  - HIV
    - *Cryptosporidiosis*
    - *Amebiasis*
    - *Giardia*
  - Parasites
    - *Ascariasis*

- – *Whipworm*
- – *Hookworms*
- Neoplastic
  - ○ Carcinoma of the pancreas
  - ○ Carcinoid syndrome
  - ○ Gastrinoma
  - ○ Villous adenoma
  - ○ Villous carcinoma
  - ○ Colon cancer
  - ○ Medullary thyroid carcinoma
  - ○ Lymphomas
- Dietary
  - ○ Excess tea, coffee, cola
- Incontinence
  - ○ Diabetes mellitus
  - ○ Rectal surgery
  - ○ Radiation proctitis
- Endocrine, metabolic
  - ○ Diabetic enteropathy
  - ○ Autonomous neuropathy
  - ○ Neuroendocrine tumors
    - – *VIPoma*
    - – *Carcinoid*
  - ○ Verner-Morrison syndrome
  - ○ Zollinger-Ellison syndrome
  - ○ Prostaglandins
  - ○ Hyperthyroidism
  - ○ Medullary thyroid carcinoma
  - ○ Pellagra
  - ○ Addison's disease
- Postoperative
  - ○ Short bowel syndrome
  - ○ Dumping syndrome
  - ○ Postvagotomy
  - ○ Gastric surgery/Billroth operation
- Psychogenic
  - ○ Anxiety
  - ○ Vegetative lability
- Drugs
  - ○ Antacids
  - ○ Antiphlogistics
  - ○ Anthraquinones
  - ○ Castor oil
  - ○ Lactulose
  - ○ Mannitol

- ○ Prostaglandins
- ○ Sorbitol
- Miscellaneous
  - ○ Intestinal atrophy
    - – *After radiation therapy*
  - ○ Microscopic colitis
    - – *Collagenous colitis*
    - – *Lymphocytic colitis*
  - ○ Colitis after radiation therapy
  - ○ Unabsorbed dietary fat (steatorrhea)
  - ○ Chologenic diarrhea (bile acids, eg, after ileal resection)
  - ○ Amyloidosis
  - ○ Whipple's disease
  - ○ Idiopathic lymphangiectasis
  - ○ Obstructive jaundice
  - ○ Biliary fistula
  - ○ Fecal impaction
  - ○ Proctitis
  - ○ Polyposis
  - ○ Polyarteritis nodosa
  - ○ Mesenteric ischemia (ischemic colitis)
  - ○ Gastrocolic fistula
  - ○ Achylia

Diarrhea with FUO
See Fever of Unknown Origin → 143

Diplopia

Double vision
Binocular diplopia
Double vision only if both eyes are open
- ▶ Cranial nerves palsy
  - • Abducent nerve palsy
  - • Trochlear nerve palsy
  - • Oculomotor nerve palsy
- ▶ Giant cell arteritis
- ▶ Myasthenia gravis
- ▶ Endocrine ophthalmopathy (Grave's disease)
- ▶ Chronic progressive external ophthalmoplegia
- ▶ Orbital tumors, pseudotumors

- ▶ Orbital trauma, blow out fracture of orbit
- ▶ Myositis of the eye muscles
- ▶ Vascular disorders
- ▶ Meningitis, encephalitis
- ▶ Polyneuropathy
- ▶ Eclampsia
- ▶ Multiple sclerosis
- ▶ Wernicke's encephalopathy
- ▶ Anisocoria
- ▶ Polio
- ▶ Syphilis
- ▶ Subarachnoid hemorrhage
- ▶ Cerebrovascular disease
- ▶ Insulinoma

Monocular diplopia
Double vision even if one eye is covered
- ▶ Error of refraction
- ▶ Lens or corneal opacities

Disseminated Intravascular Coagulation

DIC
A hemorrhagic syndrome following uncontrolled activation of clotting factors and fibrinolytic enzymes throughout small blood vessels. Fibrin is deposited, platelets and clotting factors are consumed, and fibrin degradation products inhibit fibrin polymerization, resulting in tissue necrosis and bleeding.

Causes
- ▶ Infection
  - (Gram negative) sepsis
  - Meningococcemia
  - Rocky Mountain spotted fever
- ▶ Neoplasm
  - Mucin-secreting adenocarcinoma
  - Promyelocytic leukemia
  - Prostate cancer
  - Lung cancer
- ▶ Tissue damage
  - Trauma
  - Surgery
- Heat stroke
- Burn injury
- Dissecting aneurysm
- ▶ Obstetrical complication
  - Abruptio placentae
  - Amniotic fluid embolism
  - Retained fetal products
  - Eclampsia
- ▶ Autoimmune
  - Immune complex disorders
  - Allograph rejection
  - Incompatible blood transfusion
  - Anaphylaxis
- ▶ Metabolic
  - Diabetic ketoacidosis
- ▶ Miscellaneous
  - Shock
  - Snake bite
  - Cyanotic congenital heart disease
  - Fat embolism
  - Severe liver disease
  - Cavernous hemangioma

Double Stranded DNA Antibody
See Autoantibodies in Connective Tissue Diseases → 47
Positive in
- ▶ Systemic lupus erythematosus
  - Associated with lupus nephritis
  - Associated with lupus CNS Involvement
- ▶ Sjögren's syndrome
- ▶ Rheumatoid arthritis
- ▶ Chronic active hepatitis
- ▶ Biliary cirrhosis
- ▶ Epstein-Barr virus
- ▶ Cytomegalovirus

Double vision, See Diplopia → 103

Drowsiness, See Hypersomnia → 194

Drug Eruptions

Drug-induced reactions with lesions on the skin.

Drugs commonly causing serious reactions
- Allopurinol
- Anticonvulsants
- Bumetanide
- Captopril
- Furosemide
- NSAIDs
- Penicillamine
- Piroxicam
- Sulfonamides
- Thiazide diuretics

Acneiform eruptions
- Amoxapine
- Corticosteroids
- Halogens
- Haloperidol
- Isoniazid
- Lithium
- Phenytoin
- Trazodone

Acute generalized exanthematous pustulosis
- Acetaminophen
- Allopurinol
- Beta-lactam antibiotics
- Bufexamac
- Buphenine
- Carbamazepine
- Carbutamide
- Chloramphenicol
- Clobazam
- Cotrimoxazole
- Diltiazem
- Furosemide
- Hydroxychloroquine
- Imipenem
- Isoniazid
- Macrolides
- Mercury
- Nadoxolol
- Nifedipine
- Phenytoin
- Piperazine
- Pyrimethamine
- Quinidine
- Salbutiamine
- Streptomycin
- Tetracycline
- Vancomycin

Alopecia
- Allopurinol
- Anticoagulants
- Azathioprine
- Beta-blockers
- Bromocriptine
- Cyclophosphamide
- Hormones
- Lithium
- Methotrexate (MTX)
- NSAIDs
- Phenytoin
- Valproate

Bullous pemphigoid
- D-penicillamine
- Furosemide
- Neuroleptics
- Penicillins
- Phenacetin
- Psoralen plus UV-A
- Salicylazosulfapyridine
- Sulfasalazine

Erythema nodosum
- Halogens
- Oral contraceptives
- Penicillin
- Sulfonamides
- Tetracycline

Erythroderma
- Allopurinol
- Anticonvulsants
- Barbiturates
- Captopril
- Carbamazepine

- Cefoxitin
- Chloroquine
- Chlorpromazine
- Cimetidine
- Diltiazem
- Griseofulvin
- Lithium
- Nitrofurantoin
- Sulfonamides

Fixed drug eruptions
- Acetaminophen
- Anticonvulsants
- Aspirin
- Barbiturates
- Benzodiazepines
- Butalbital
- Dapsone
- Metronidazole
- NSAID
- Oral contraceptives
- Penicillins
- Phenacetin
- Phenolphthalein
- Sulfonamides
- Tetracyclines
- Tolmetin

Hypersensitivity syndrome
- Allopurinol
- Carbamazepine
- Dapsone
- Lamotrigine
- Minocycline
- NSAIDs
- Phenobarbital
- Phenytoin
- Sulfonamides

Lichenoid
- Antimalarials
- Beta-blockers
- Captopril
- Diflunisal
- Furosemide
- Gold
- Levamisole
- Penicillamine

- Phenothiazine
- Tetracycline
- Thiazides

Linear IgA dermatosis
- Captopril
- Diclofenac
- Glibenclamide
- Lithium
- Vancomycin

Lupus erythematosus
- Beta-blockers
- Chlorpromazine
- Cimetidine
- Clonidine
- Hydralazine
- Isoniazid
- Lithium
- Lovastatin
- Methyldopa
- Minocycline
- Oral contraceptives
- Procainamide
- Sulfonamides
- Tetracyclines

Maculopapular
- ACE inhibitors
- Allopurinol
- Amoxicillin
- Ampicillin
- Anticonvulsants
- Aprazolam
- Barbiturates
- Barbiturates
- Bupropion
- Carbamazepine
- Carbamazepine
- Chlorpromazine
- Desipramine
- Fluoxetine
- Isoniazid
- Lithium
- Maprotiline
- Nefazodone
- NSAIDs
- Phenothiazine

- Phenytoin
- Quinolones
- Risperidone
- Sulfonamides
- Thiazides
- Trazodone
- Trimethoprim-sulfamethoxazole

Pemphigus
- Aminophenazone
- Aminopyrine
- Azapropazone
- Captopril
- Cephalosporins
- D-penicillamine
- Gold
- Heroin
- Hydantoin
- Levodopa
- Lysine acetylsalicylate
- Oxyphenbutazone
- Penicillins
- Phenobarbital
- Phenylbutazone
- Piroxicam
- Progesterone
- Propranolol
- Pyritinol
- Rifampicin
- Thiamazole
- Thiopronine

Photosensitivity (→ 284)

Pigmentation
- Amitriptyline
- Chlorpromazine
- Clozapine
- Haloperidol
- Perphenazine
- Thioridazine

Stevens-Johnson syndrome
- Allopurinol
- Anticonvulsants
- Aspirin
- NSAIDS
- Barbiturates

- Carbamazepine
- Cimetidine
- Codeine
- Diltiazem
- Furosemide
- Griseofulvin
- Hydantoin
- Penicillin
- Phenothiazine
- Phenylbutazone
- Phenytoin
- Rifampicin
- Sulfonamides
- Tetracyclines
- Trimethoprim-sulfamethoxazole

Toxic epidermal necrosis
- Allopurinol
- Anticonvulsants
- Aspirin
- NSAIDs
- Isoniazid
- Penicillins
- Phenytoin
- Prazosin
- Sulfonamides
- Tetracyclines
- Trimethoprim-sulfamethoxazole
- Vancomycin

Urticaria
- ACE inhibitors
- Aspirin
- Cephalosporins
- Chlordiazepoxide
- Dextran
- Fluoxetine
- Imipramine
- Lithium
- NSAIDs
- Opiates
- Penicillin
- Polymixin
- Radiocontrast media
- Ranitidine
- Trazodone

Vasculitis
▶ Allopurinol
▶ Aspirin
▶ Cimetidine
▶ Gold
▶ Hydralazine
▶ NSAIDs
▶ Penicillin
▶ Phenytoin
▶ Propylthiouracil
▶ Quinolones
▶ Sulfonamide
▶ Tetracycline
▶ Thiazides

Vesiculobullous
▶ Aspirin
▶ Barbiturates
▶ Captopril
▶ Cephalosporins
▶ Furosemide
▶ Griseofulvin
▶ NSAIDs
▶ Penicillamine
▶ Penicillins
▶ Sulfonamides
▶ Thiazides

Drug fever
See Fever of Unknown Origin → 143

Dry Eyes

Keratitis sicca, Keratoconjunctivitis sicca

Aqueous tear deficiency
▶ Idiopathic
▶ Congenital alacrima
▶ Systemic vitamin A deficiency (xerophthalmia)
▶ Lacrimal gland ablation
▶ Sensory denervation
▶ Collagen vascular diseases
  • Rheumatoid arthritis
  • Wegener granulomatosis
  • Systemic lupus erythematosus

▶ Sjögren syndrome
▶ Autoimmune disorders associated with Sjögren syndrome
  • Rheumatoid arthritis
  • Scleroderma
  • Polymyositis
  • Polyarteritis nodosa
  • Hashimoto thyroiditis
  • Chronic hepatobiliary cirrhosis
  • Lymphocytic interstitial pneumonitis
  • Thrombocytopenic purpura
  • Hypergammaglobulinemia
  • Waldenström's macroglobulinemia
  • Progressive systemic sclerosis
  • Dermatomyositis
  • Interstitial nephritis
▶ Secondary conjunctival scarring
  • Ocular pemphigoid
  • Stevens-Johnson syndrome
  • Trachoma
  • Chemical burns
  • Thermal burns
  • Atopic disease
▶ Drugs
  • Antihistamines
  • Atropine
  • Betablockers
  • Oral contraceptives
  • Phenothiazines
▶ Infiltration of the lacrimal glands
  • Sarcoidosis
  • Tumors
▶ Postradiation fibrosis of lacrimal glands

Lipid tear layer disorders
▶ Blepharitis
▶ Rosacea

Mucin tear layer disorders
▶ Vitamin A deficiency
▶ Trachoma
▶ Diphtheric keratoconjunctivitis
▶ Mucocutaneous disorders
▶ Topical drugs

Dry mouth, See Xerostomia → 384

Dysacusis. See Hearing Loss, Hearing Impairment → 165

Dysarthria See Aphasia → 39

Dysmenorrhea
Painful menstruation
See Amenorrhea → 21
See Polymenorrhea → 289
Secondary dysmenorrhea
▶ Uterine deformation
▶ Gynatresia
▶ Uterine hypoplasia
▶ Membranous dysmenorrhea
▶ Retroflexion of uterus
▶ Stenosis of the uterine cervix
▶ Endometriosis
▶ Hysteromyoma
  • Submucous myoma
▶ Uterine polyps
▶ PID (→ 279)
▶ Adnexitis
▶ Cervical stenosis
▶ Parametritis
▶ Pelvic congestion
▶ IUD
▶ Tumor

Dysopias
See Vision Loss, Acute → 376
See Vision Loss, Chronic → 377
See Scotoma → 327
See Diplopia → 103
Transient worsening of vision
▶ Microthrombembolism
▶ Idiopathic amaurosis fugax
▶ Hypotension
▶ Heart failure
▶ Migraine
▶ Hypertension
▶ Giant cell arteritis

Persistent worsening of vision
▶ Without pain and without redness of the eye
  • Acute retinal artery occlusion
  • Hypertension
  • Retinopathy eclamptica
  • Giant cell arteritis
  • Vitreous hemorrhage
  • Retinal vein occlusion
  • Retinal detachment
  • Mycotic endophthalmitis
  • Cytomegalic virus retinitis
  • Neuropapillitis
  • Hysteric vision impairment
▶ With pain and redness of the eye
  • Glaucoma attack
  • Iritis
  • Panophthalmitis
  • Conjunctivitis
Acute color sensation impairment
▶ Drugs
  • Amylnitrite
  • Barbiturate
  • Chlorothiazine
  • Digitalis intoxication
  • Santonin
  • Streptomycin
  • Sulfonamides

Dyspareunia
Painful Intercourse
Localized pain
▶ Infection, inflammation
  • Human papillomavirus
  • Herpes simplex virus
  • Vulvar vestibulitis
  • Vaginitis
  • Cystitis
  • Urethritis
▶ Atrophic vaginitis
▶ Vaginismus
▶ Postpartum
Deep pain
▶ Chronic cervicitis

- Endometriosis
- Uterine fibroids
- Pelvic congestion
- Pelvic adhesions
- Retroverted uterus

Dyspepsia

Impaired gastric function due to some disorder of the stomach with epigastric pain, sometimes burning, nausea, and gaseous eructation.

Gastrointestinal
- Functional dyspepsia (!)
- Peptic ulcer disease
- Gastroesophageal reflux
- Gastroparesis
- Stomach infiltrative disease
- Ischemic bowel disease
- Crohn's disease
- Biliary tract disorder
- Pancreatitis

Malabsorption
- Lactose intolerance
- Fructose intolerance
- Sorbitol intolerance
- Mannitol intolerance

Tumor
- Esophageal cancer
- Gastric cancer
- Pancreatic cancer
- Hepatoma
- Abdominal malignancy
- Abdominal mass

Endocrine, metabolic
- Diabetes mellitus
- Thyroid disease
- Parathyroid disease
- Hypercalcemia
- Hyperkalemia

Infection (parasites)
- Giardia
- Strongyloides

Miscellaneous
- Connective tissue diseases

- Sarcoidosis

Drugs, toxins
- Acarbose
- Alcohol
- Alendronate
- Aspirin
- Cigarette smoking
- Cisapride
- Codeine
- Coffee
- Corticosteroids
- Erythromycin
- Iron
- Metformin
- Orlistat
- Potassium
- Theophylline

Herbals
- Chaste tree berry
- Feverfew
- Garlic
- Gingko
- Saw palmetto
- White willow

Dysphagia

Difficulty in swallowing due to problems in nerve or muscle control.

Disorders of the oral cavity
- Angina tonsillaris
- Tonsil abscess
- Vincent's angina
- Lateral funiculus angina
- Herpangina
- Typhoid fever angina
- Mumps
- Scarlet fever
- Diphtheria
- Mononucleosis
- Oral candidiasis
- Stomatitis
- Pharyngitis
- Ludwig's angina
- Lymph granulomatosis

- Agranulocytosis
- Stevens-Johnson syndrome

Disorders of the larynx
- Laryngeal cancer
- Aspiration of foreign body

Bolus/foreign body

Stenosis
- Neoplastic
  - Esophageal cancer
  - Leiomyoma
- Esophagitis
  - Reflux
  - Radiation
- Esophageal Crohn´s disease
- Esophageal sarcoidosis
- Graft-versus-host reaction
- Behçet's syndrome
- Allergic swelling
- Angina tonsillaris
- Peptic stenoses
- Postoperative stenoses
- Chemical burns
- Mucosal rings
  - Pharyngeal (Plummer-Vinson syndrome)
  - Lower esophageal ring (Schatzki ring)

External compression
- Goiter
- Diverticulum
- Abscesses
- Neoplastic
- Fibrosis
- Aortic aneurysm
- Enlarged left atrium
- Osteophytes
- Pleural and pericardial causes
- Extreme spinal curvature

Motoric dysphagia
- Nutcracker esophagus
- Reflux esophagitis
- Achalasia
- Poliomyelitis
- Scleroderma
- Myasthenia gravis

- Multiple sclerosis
- Rabies
- Tetanus

Functional dysphagia
- Globus hystericus

Disorders of the esophagus
- Achalasia
- Zenker's diverticulum
- Scleroderma
- Barret's syndrome
- Endobrachyesophagus
- Peptic stenosis
- Esophageal diverticulum
- Esophagotracheal fistula
- Esophageal spasm
- Intramural pseudodiverticulosis
- Presbyesophagus
- Esophagitis
  - Reflux
  - Radiation
  - Medication-induced esophagitis (Biphosphonates)
- Esophageal trauma
- Eeophageal infection
  - CMV
  - HSV
  - Idiopathic human immunodeficiency virus ulcers
  - Esophageal moniliasis
- Esophageal Crohn´s disease
- Esophageal sarcoidosis

Collagen vascular disease
- Scleroderma
  - CREST syndrome
- Dermatomyositis
- Systemic lupus erythematosus
- Rheumatoid arthritis

Neurologic
- Palatoplegia after damage to the vagal nerve or the accessory nerve
- Impaired sensitivity in the larynx
- Peripheral tongue paralysis with lesions of the hypoglossal nerve
- Pseudobulbar paralysis

▶ Syringobulbia
▶ Central vagal nucleus lesion
▶ Central hypoglossal nerve paralysis
▶ Poliomyelitis
▶ Peripheral neuropathy
▶ Myasthenia gravis
▶ Botulism
▶ Poliomyositis/ dermatomyositis
▶ Diabetic neuropathy
▶ Muscular dystrophy
▶ Huntington's chorea
▶ Multiple sclerosis
▶ Cerebrovascular insult
▶ Parkinson's disease
▶ Guillain-Barré syndrome/Polyradiculitis
▶ ALS

Disorders of the stomach
▶ Gastric tumors
▶ Gastroparesis
▶ Gastritis
▶ Pyloric stenosis
▶ Cascade stomach

Miscellaneous, secondary
▶ Amyloidosis
▶ Hyperthyroidism
▶ Hypothyroidism
▶ Chagas'disease
▶ Pseudoachalasia
▶ Alcoholism
▶ Paraneoplasia
▶ Hiatal hernia
▶ Hypokalemia
▶ Aortic arch aneurysm
▶ Aerophagia
▶ Globus syndrome
▶ Vascular abnormality

Dyspnea
Shortness of breath, a subjective difficulty or distress in breathing, usually associated with disease of the heart or lungs. Occurs physiologically during heavy exercise or at high altitude. Frequently characterized by an increase in the pCO_2 in the blood. If the pH value is still in the reference range (pH > 7.35 to < 7.45), it is called compensated respiratory acidosis. Compensation through the "metabolic" organs (liver and kidneys). See Alkalosis, Respiratory → 19 See Acidosis, Respiratory → 12 See Respiratory Failure → 319

Parenchymal lung disease
▶ Restriction
  • Pneumonia
  • ARDS
  • Parenchyma loss
  • Pulmonary fibrosis
  • Pleural fibrosis
  • Lymphangitic metastases
  • Kyphoscoliosis
▶ Reduced lung elasticity or pulmonary gas exchange area
  • Pneumothorax
  • Aspiration
  • Pulmonary edema
  • Atelectasis
  • Pulmonary embolism
  • Pleural effusion
  • Chylothorax
  • Miliary tuberculosis
  • Radiation pneumonitis
  • Pulmonary fibrosis
  • Lymphangitic metastases
  • Fibrosing alveolitis
    ◦ Idiopathic
    ◦ Exogenic-allergic alveolitis
    ◦ Medicamentous damage
    ◦ After inhalation of toxic gases
▶ Altitude sickness
▶ Sarcoidosis
▶ Histiocytosis X
▶ Pneumoconiosis
▶ Shock lung
▶ Weakened respiratory pump
  • Neuromuscular diseases
  • Pulmonary emphysema
    ◦ Asthma
    ◦ Pulmonary emphysema
  • Pleural effusion

- Pneumothorax
- Respiratory muscle fatigue with severely lowered cardiac output

Obstructive disease of the airways
▶ Chronic bronchitis
▶ COPD
▶ Asthma
▶ Acute tracheobronchitis
▶ Glottal edema
▶ Laryngostenosis
▶ Pulmonary emphysema
▶ Laryngeal/bronchospasm
▶ Pulmonary edema
▶ Mediastinal tumors
▶ Bronchial tumors
▶ Tracheal stenosis
▶ Foreign body aspiration
▶ Abnormality of thoracic vessels
▶ Esophageal diseases with tracheal compression
▶ Goiter, substernal goiter
▶ Tracheobronchial collapse
▶ Tracheomalacia
▶ Tracheal tumors
▶ Croup
▶ Laryngospasm

Cardiac disease
▶ Cardiac dysrhythmia
  • Atrial fibrillation
▶ Left ventricular failure
  • Cardiac valve defect
    ○ Mitral regurgitation
    ○ Aortic regurgitation
    ○ Aortic stenosis
    ○ Mitral stenosis
    ○ Stenosis of aortic isthmus
  • Coronary heart disease
    ○ Myocardial infarction
    ○ Angina pectoris
  • Perimyocarditis
  • Cardiomyopathy
  • Hypertension
  • Pericardial effusion/pericardial constriction
  • Complex cyanotic defect

- Intracardial masses
  ○ Tumors of the myocardium
▶ Left–right shunt (increased blood flow to lungs)
  • Atrioseptal defect
  • Patent ductus arteriosus
  • Ventricular septal defect
  • Complex defects
▶ Right ventricular failure
▶ Cor pulmonale
  • Primary pulmonary hypertension
  • Secondary pulmonary hypertension in obstructive and/or restrictive lung desease
▶ Biventricular heart failure
▶ Endocardial changes
  • Endocarditis
  • Endomyocardial fibrosis
  • Loeffler's endocarditis

Pulmonary vascular disease
▶ Decreased lung flow
  • Perimyocarditis
  • Pericardial effusion
  • Pulmonary stenosis
  • Tricuspid stenosis
  • Tetralogy of Fallot
  • Complex cyanotic defect
▶ Pulmonary edema

Disease of the chest wall or respiratory muscles
▶ Pleural and thoracic causes
  • Limited thoracic flexibility
    ○ Multiple rib fractures
  • Trauma
  • Deformity of the chest
    ○ Kyphoscoliosis
  • Pneumo-, hemato-, hydro-, chylothorax
  • Pleural effusion
  • Decreased thoracic or diaphragmatic excursions
    ○ Pleural callosity
    ○ Kyphoscoliosis
    ○ Obesity
    ○ Abdominal masses

Miscellaneous
► Physiologic dyspnea
► Psychogenic
  • Hyperventilation syndrome
    ○ Hysteria
    ○ Anxiety
► Impaired oxygen transport
  • Anemia
  • Intoxication
    ○ CO
    ○ HCN
► Metabolic acidosis
  • Shock
  • Diabetic coma
  • Uremia
► Increased respiratory drive
  • Hypoxemia
  • Metabolic acidosis
  • Heart failure
  • Intrapulmonary receptor stimulation
► Allergic
  • Asthma attack
  • Quincke's edema
► Neuromuscular/impairment of the respiratory center:
  • Myasthenia gravis
  • Guillain-Barré syndrome/ Polyradiculitis
  • Poliomyelitis
  • ALS
  • Phrenic nerve paresis
  • Brain stem infarction
  • Trauma
  • Encephalitis
► Drugs
  • Barbiturates
  • Methanol
  • Opiates
  • Progesterone
  • Salicylates
► Other
  • Gram-negative sepsis (!)
  • Cirrhosis

Time and position–dependent
► Intermittent dyspnea

  • Bronchial asthma
  • Aspiration
  • Pulmonary embolism
► Persistent dyspnea
  • Chronic obstructive bronchitis
  • Pulmonary emphysema
  • Cardiac diseases
  • Neuromuscular diseases
► Nocturnal dyspnea
  • Bronchial asthma
  • Heart failure
  • Gastroesophageal reflux
  • Sleep apnea syndrome
► Position-dependent dyspnea
  • Heart failure
  • Phrenic nerve paralysis
  • Pulmonary arteriovenous malformation

Dysproteinemia
Abnormality in plasma proteins, normally immunoglobulins.
See Protein in the Serum → 296

Dysrhythmias
See Cardiac Dysrhythmias → 62

Dyssomnia, See Insomnia → 212,
See Hypersomnia → 194

Dysuria
Painful urination; difficulty or pain in urination.

Urinary tract infection (UTI)
► Urethritis
  • Gonorrhea
  • Chlamydia
► Cystitis
  • Bacterial
    ○ Tuberculosis
    ○ E. coli
    ○ Proteus
    ○ Enterobacter

- ◦ Pseudomonas
- ◦ Klebsiella
- ◦ Enterococcus
- ◦ Streptococcus
- ◦ Mycobacteria
- • Viral
  - ◦ Herpes viruses
  - ◦ Adenoviruses
- • Mycotic
  - ◦ Candida
- • Parasitic
  - ◦ Bilharziosis
  - ◦ Schistosomiasis
- ▶ Pyelonephritis
  - • Enterobacteriaceae
- ▶ Prostatitis
  - • Enterobacteriaceae
- ▶ Epididymitis, orchitis
  - • Enterobacteriaceae
  - • Mumps
- ▶ Meatitis, urethritis
  - • HSV II
- ▶ Vaginitis
  - • Candidal vaginitis (dermatitis)
  - • Trichomonas vaginitis
  - • Atrophic vaginitis
- ▶ Genital herpes (HSV II)
- ▶ Gonorrhea
- ▶ Trichomoniasis
- ▶ Candida albicans

Obstructive uropathy
- ▶ Benign prostatic hypertrophy
- ▶ Urethral stricture

Contact dermatitis or vulvitis (women)
- ▶ Contraceptive foams, sponges
- ▶ Perfumed soap
- ▶ Spermicidal gel
- ▶ Tampons
- ▶ Toilet paper, napkins
- ▶ Vaginal douche, lubricant

Tumor
- ▶ Bladder cancer
- ▶ Infiltration
  - • Cervical cancer
  - • Rectal cancer

Rheumatologic
- ▶ Behçet's syndrome
- ▶ Reiter's syndrome

Drugs
- ▶ Beta blockers
- ▶ Busulphan
- ▶ Cantharidin
- ▶ Cyclophosphamide
- ▶ Dopamine
- ▶ Ifosfamide
- ▶ Isoniazide
- ▶ Phenothiazine

Miscellaneous
- ▶ Nephrolithiasis
- ▶ Ureter stone
- ▶ Urinary catheter
- ▶ Vesical calculus
- ▶ Bladder diverticulum
- ▶ Foreign body in the bladder
- ▶ Trauma
- ▶ After radiation therapy
- ▶ Psychogenic
- ▶ Diabetes mellitus
- ▶ Prolapsed uterus

Earaches

Otalgia, otodynia
Pain in the ear.

Ear disorders
- ▶ Outer ear
  - • Otitis externa
    - ◦ Acute otitis externa (Swimmer's ear)
    - ◦ Chronic otitis externa
    - ◦ Malignant otitis externa
  - • Obstruction of the outer ear
    - ◦ Ear canal foreign body
    - ◦ Cerumen impaction (ear wax)
  - • Auricle
    - ◦ Auricular perichondritis
    - ◦ Auricular erysipelas
  - • Tumor
- ▶ Middle ear
  - • Acute otitis media
  - • Chronic otitis media

- Cholesteatoma
- Sterile middle ear effusion
- Tumor
► Barotrauma
- High altitude exposure
- Other acute barotrauma
► Ruptured or perforated eardrum
► Eustachion tube
- Dysfunction
- Syringitis
► Herpes zoster oticus
► Acoustic nerve tumor

Referred pain
► Teeth
- Teeth infection
- Dental caries
► Arthritis of temporomandibular joint
► Sinusitis
► Parotitis
► Mastoiditis
► Sore throat
- Pharyngitis
- Tonsillitis
► Neck
- Lymphadenitis
- Metastatic tumor
► Other tumor
► Neurologic
- Cervical spine affection
- Trigeminal neuralgia
- Syphilitic meningitis

ECG, Cardiac Axis

Normal axis – horizontal range
(III negative, greatest amplitude in I)
► Physiologic in age > 50 years
► Left heart hypertrophy
► Arterial hypertension
► Obesity

Normal axis – vertical range (II > III > I)
► Right ventricular hypertrophy
► Obesity

Left axis deviation (I > II)
► Normal variation

► Mechanical shifts
- Expiration
- Ascites
- High diaphragm (pregnancy)
► Left ventricular hypertrophy
► Left atrial hypertrophy
► Left anterior hemiblock
► Left bundle branch block
► Congenital lesions
- Tricuspid atresia
- Ostium primum ASD
► Wolff-Parkinson-White syndrome
► Hyperkalemia
► Right ventricular ectopic rhythms
► Inferior myocardial infarction
► Emphysema
► Chronic obstructive pulmonary disease (COPD)
► Artificial cardiac pacing

Right axis deviation (III > II)
► Normal variation
- Children
- Tall thin adults
► Mechanical shifts
- Inspiration
- Emphysema
► Right bundle branch block
► Right ventricular hypertrophy
► Left ventricular failure with right ventricular strain
► Left posterior hemiblock
► Dextrocardia
► Left ventricular ectopic rhythms
► Some right ventricular ectopic rhythms
► Wolff-Parkinson-White syndrome
► Switched electrodes (of the two arms)
► Pulmonary hypertension
► Pulmonary embolus
► Chronic obstructive pulmonary disease (COPD)
► Congenital heart diseases
- Atrial septal defect
- Ventricular septal defect
► Anterolateral myocardial infarction

Extreme axis deviation
- Emphysema
- Hyperkalemia
- Lead transposition
- Artificial cardiac pacing
- Ventricular tachycardia

Sagittal type (RS in I, II and III tilted around the horizontal axis)
- Strain on right ventricle
- Cor pulmonale
- Pulmonary embolism
- Obesity

ECG, Hypokalemia and Hyperkalemia

See Hypokalemia → 202
See Hyperkalemia → 192

Hypokalemia
▶ ST depression
▶ Prominent U waves
▶ May merge into TU waves
▶ Repolarization disorders
▶ Dysrhythmias

Hyperkalemia
▶ T wave tenting (tall, peaked T waves)
▶ Prolongation of PR interval
▶ Shortening of QT interval
▶ Diminution of P wave height
▶ Broad QRS complex (Bundle-branch block-like changes)
▶ Finally ventricular tachycardia and asystole

ECG, P Wave

P wave inversion
▶ Ectopic atrial focus
▶ AV nodal rhythm
▶ In normal axis - horizontal range

High amplitude P
▶ Cor pulmonale
▶ Hypertension
▶ Congenital heart disease
▶ Pulmonary stenosis

▶ Tricuspid stenosis
▶ Tricuspid insufficiency
▶ Mitral valve disease
▶ Atrial septal defect
▶ Emphysema
▶ Chronic bronchitis
▶ Young individuals

Biphasic P wave
▶ Mitral stenosis
▶ Constrictive pericarditis
▶ Mitral regurgitation
▶ Aortic stenosis
▶ Hypertension
▶ Myocardial fibrosis
▶ Patent ductus arteriosus
▶ Aortic regurgitation

Ectopic P wave
▶ Wandering atrial pacemaker
▶ Premature atrial contractions
▶ (Non-)paroxysmal atrial tachycardia
▶ Premature junctional contractions
▶ Junctional escape rhythm
▶ (Non-)paroxysmal junctional tachycardia
▶ Premature ventricular contractions

Wide P wave (> 0.12 sec)
▶ Left atrial enlargement
  - Mitral stenosis
  - Mitral regurgitation

P wave absent
▶ Sinoatrial node block
▶ AV nodal rhythm

ECG, PR Interval

PR-interval: 0.12-0.21s

Long PR interval
▶ First degree AV block
  - Intra-atrial conduction delay
  - Slowed conduction in AV node
  - Slowed conduction in His bundle
  - Slowed conduction in bundle branch
▶ Second degree AV block
  - Type I (Wenckebach)
  - Type II (Mobitz)

- ► III° AV block
  - Acute posterior myocardial infarction
  - Bacterial endocarditis
- ► High vagal tone
- ► Drugs
  - Adenosine
  - Antiarrhythmics
  - Betablockers
  - Calcium channel blockers (verapamil)
  - Digitalis (overdose)
  - Propafenone
- ► Myocardial ischemia
- ► Hypothyroidism
- ► Atrial enlargement
- ► Atrio-septal defect
- ► Endocarditis
- ► Myocarditis
- ► Sarcoidosis with heart involvement
- ► Infections (toxic)
- ► Supraventricular extrasystoles

Short PR interval
- ► WPW syndrome
- ► Lown-Ganong-Levine syndrome
- ► Hyperthyroidism
- ► Tachycardia
- ► Cardiac pacemaker
- ► AV junctional rhythms (retrograde atrial activation)
- ► Ectopic atrial rhythms (originating near the AV node)
- ► Normal variant

ECG, Q Wave

Enlarged (Q wave > 25 % of the amplitude of the R wave)
- ► Normal variant
- ► Abnormally placed ECG-leads
- ► Myocardial damage
  - Myocardial infarction
  - Myocardial ischemia (transient)
  - Myocarditis
  - Hypertrophic cardiomyopathy
  - Neoplasm
  - Amyloidosis

- Sarcoidosis
- Dermatosclerosis
- Chagas' disease
- Echinococcus-cyst
- ► Ventricular hypertrophy
  - Cor pulmonale
  - Left heart hypertrophy
  - Left bundle-branch block with left heart hypertrophy
- ► Ventricular enlargement
- ► Acute and chronic cor pulmonale
  - Pulmonary embolism
  - Chronic obstructive pulmonary disease
- ► Wolff-Parkinson-White syndrome
- ► Tachycardia
- ► Ventricular extrasystoles
- ► Hyperkalemia
- ► Dextrocardia
- ► Cardiac surgery
- ► Spontaneous pneumothorax (especially left)
- ► Funnel chest
- ► Severe disease (shock, pancreatitis)

ECG, QRS Complex

Usually < 100ms with 0.6 mV-1.6 mV
High QRS amplitude
- ► Left ventricular hypertrophy (Sokolow's index: S in V_2 + the R in V_5 > 3.5 mV)
- ► Right ventricular hypertrophy (R in V_2 + S in V_5 > 1.05 mV)
  - Cor pulmonale
  - Pulmonary stenosis
  - Left to right shunt
  - Eisenmenger's syndrome
  - Pulmonary embolism
- ► Hyperthyroidism
- ► Fever
- ► Anemia
- ► Sympathicotonia

QRS complex lowered (low voltage)
- ► Artifact
- ► Norm variant
  - Pregnancy

- Obesity
▶ Pericardial effusion
▶ Pericard adhesion
▶ Myocardial fibrosis
▶ Ischemia
▶ Myocarditis
▶ Extensive myocardial infarction
▶ Hypothyroidism, mostly associated with sinus bradycardia
▶ Cardial infiltration
  - Amyloidosis
▶ Cardiomyopathy
▶ Dermatosclerosis
▶ Addison's disease
▶ Pleural effusion
▶ Chronic obstructive lung disease
▶ Left-sided pneumothorax

Wide QRS
▶ Incomplete (< 0.11 s) and complete (> 0.11 s) left bundle-branch block
  - Congestive cardiomyopathy
  - Hypertension
  - Coronary cardiac disease
  - Myocardial infarction
  - Myocarditis
  - Hyperkalemia
  - Class-I-Antidysrhythmic drugs
  - Wolff-Parkinson-White syndrome
  - Unintentional ECG-tracing with fast rate (50 or 100 mm/s)
  - Incomplete block pictures frequently also in cardiovascular healthy persons
▶ Incomplete (< 0.11 s) and complete (> 0.11 s) right bundle-branch block
  - Congenital cardiac disease with right ventricular load (atrio-septal defect, Fallot's tetralogy)
  - Cor pulmonale
  - Left to right shunt
  - Eisenmenger's syndrome
  - Acute pulmonary embolism
  - Myocardial infarction
  - Myocarditis
  - Class-I-Antidysrhythmic drugs
  - Hyperkalemia

  - Unintentional ECG-tracing with fast rate (50 or 100 mm/s)
  - Incomplete block pictures frequently also in cardiovascular healthy persons
▶ Focal block with "knotting" in the QRS complex (e.g. myocardial scar)
▶ Atypical heart position with not visible P
▶ Ventricular tachycardia with wide QRS complex (Caution: potentially life-threatening)
  - Ventricular tachycardia
  - Supraventricular tachycardia in preexisting bundle-branch block
    ◦ Sinus tachycardia
    ◦ Atrial tachycardia
    ◦ Atrioventricular reentry tachycardia
  - Supraventricular tachycardia in patients who receive anti-arrhythmics (especially class IA and IC)
  - Supraventricular tachycardia with preexcitiation (Wolff-Parkinson-White syndrome)
    ◦ Sinus tachycardia
    ◦ Atrial tachycardia
    ◦ Atrial fibrillation

Thin QRS complex
▶ Sinus rhythm
▶ Ectopic atrial rhythm
▶ Absolute arrhythmia in atrial fibrillation
▶ Atrial flutter
▶ Polytope atrial ectopias
▶ Supraventricular extrasystoles

Changing QRS complex
▶ Intermittent preexcitation complex
▶ Intermittent bundle-branch block
▶ Premature ventricular contractions
▶ Supraventricular extrasystoles

ECG, QT Interval
Duration depends on heart rate. Normally 0.25-0.45s
Short QT interval
▶ Sinus tachycardia
▶ Hyperkalemia

- ► Hypercalcemia
- ► Hypermagnesemia
- ► Acidosis
- ► Digitalis medication
- ► Coronary heart disease
- ► Hyperthyroidism

Long QT interval
- ► Congenital causes
  - Jervell and Lange-Nielsen syndrome
  - Ward-Romano syndrome
- ► Metabolic/ endocrinologic causes
  - Hypocalcemia
  - Hypokalemia
  - Extreme hyperkalemia
  - Alkalosis
  - Hypothyroidism
- ► Myocardial infarction and ischemia
- ► Ventricular enlargement
- ► Cardiomyopathy
- ► Myocarditis
- ► Complete heart block
- ► Bundle-branch block
- ► Mitral valve prolaps
- ► Sick sinus syndrome
- ► Drugs, toxins
  - Anti-arrhythmics
    - ○ Quinidine
    - ○ Procainamide
    - ○ Dysopyramid
    - ○ Amiodarone
    - ○ Sotalol
  - Antibiotics
    - ○ Erythromycin
    - ○ Clarythromycin
    - ○ Ketoconazole
    - ○ Ampicillin
    - ○ Pentamidine
    - ○ Amantidin
    - ○ Trimethoprim/sulfamethoxazole
  - Antihistaminics
    - ○ Terfenadine
    - ○ Astemizole
  - Thiazides
  - Furosemide
  - Serotonine antagonists
  - Cisapride
  - Quinine
  - Novocamid
  - Tricyclic antidepressants
  - Phenothiazines
  - Butyrophenone
  - Insecticides
  - Cocaine
  - Papavarin
  - Chronic alcoholism
- ► Hypothermia
- ► HIV infection
- ► Dysproteinemia
- ► Diabetic coma
- ► Hepatic coma
- ► Chronic hepatopathy
- ► Hemochromatosis
- ► Nephrosis
- ► Celiac sprue
- ► Amyloidosis
- ► Glycogen storage diseases
- ► Cerebrovascular brain damage

ECG, ST Segment

An isoelectric ST segment is normal.

ST segment depression
- ► Normal variants, artifacts
  - Pseudo-ST-depression (poor skin-electrode contact)
  - Sinus tachycardia (physiologic J-junctional depression)
  - Hyperventilation
- ► Ischemic heart disease
  - Subendocardial ischemia
    - ○ Exercise induced
    - ○ Angina attack
  - Non Q-wave MI
  - Acute Q-wave MI (reciprocal changes)
- ► Nonischemic causes
  - Right ventricular hypertrophy
  - Left ventricular hypertrophy
  - Mitral valve prolapse
  - Myocarditis
  - IV blocks

- o Right bundle-branch block
- o Left bundle-branch block
- o WPW syndrome
- Drugs, toxins
  - o Antiarrhythmics
  - o Barbiturates
  - o Carbon monoxide
  - o Digitalis
  - o Mushroom toxins
  - o Narcotics
  - o Nicotine
  - o Quinine
  - o Thallium
- Hypokalemia
- CNS disease
- Systemic diseases with myocardial involvement
  - o Systemic lupus erythematosus
  - o Dermatomyositis
  - o Rheumatoid arthritis
- Relative coronary insufficiency
  - o Hyperthyroidism
  - o Pheochromocytoma

ST segment elevation
- ▶ Normal variant ("early repolarization")
- ▶ Ischemic heart disease
  - Acute transmural injury
  - Ventricular aneurysm
  - Prinzmetal's (variant) angina
  - In exercise testing: extremely tight coronary artery stenosis or spasm
- ▶ Acute pericarditis
- ▶ Miscellaneous
  - Left ventricular hypertrophy
  - Left bundle branch block
  - Advanced hypokalemia
  - Hypothermia
  - Pulmonary embolism (SI-QIII)
  - Vagotonia

ECG, T Wave

Negative T wave (T inversion)
- ▶ Norm variant
  - Juvenile T wave pattern

- Hyperventilation
- ▶ Myocardial ischemia
- ▶ Myocardial infarction
- ▶ Pericarditis
- ▶ Myocarditis
- ▶ Myocardial contusion (trauma)
- ▶ Left/right ventricular hypertrophy with strain
- ▶ Digoxin effect
- ▶ Brain damage causing long QT interval
  - Subarrachnoid hemorrhage
- ▶ Mitral valve prolapse
- ▶ Idiopathic apical hypertrophy (a form of hypertrophic cardiomyopathy)
- ▶ Post-tachycardia T inversion
- ▶ Post-pacemaker T inversion
- ▶ Dilatative cardiomyopathy
- ▶ Intermittent left bundle-branch block

Flattened and/or low T
- ▶ Hypokalemia
- ▶ Hypocorticism
- ▶ Addison's disease
- ▶ Hypothyroidism
- ▶ Myocarditis
- ▶ CHD
- ▶ Myocardial ischemia
- ▶ Sympathicotonia
- ▶ Beginning left heart hypertrophy
- ▶ Anterior myocardial infarction
- ▶ Pericardial effusion
- ▶ Cardiomyopathy

Pre-terminal negative T
- ▶ Normal in lead III, in adolescents also in V3-4
- ▶ CHD
- ▶ Left heart hypertrophy
- ▶ Digitalis
- ▶ Pericarditis (scarring stadium)

Terminally negative T (exterior layer ischemia)
- ▶ Peri-/myocarditis
- ▶ Rheumatic/neoplastic infiltration
- ▶ Intoxication

High T
▸ Initial stadium of myocardial infarction (suffocation-T)
  • Fresh anterior myocardial infarction (V2-V4)
▸ Stadium II of posterior myocardial infarction (V2-V4)
▸ Acute and severe cardiac ischemia
  • Prinzmetal's angina
▸ Chronic phase of myocardial infarction (T wave inversion of formerly negative T waves before the infarction)
▸ Non-ischemic causes
  • Norm variant
  • Vagotonia
  • Acute hemopericard
  • Hyperkalemia
  • Damage to the left heart due to increased left ventricular strain and hypertrophy
  • Complete left bundle-branch block
  • Acute perimyocarditis

ECG, U−, Delta Wave

High U wave
▸ Hypokalemia
▸ Cardiomyopathy
▸ Left ventricular hypertrophy
▸ Diabetes mellitus
▸ Hyperthyroidism
▸ High vagal tone
▸ Bradycardia
▸ Drugs
  • Digitalis
  • Procainamide
  • Quinidine

Negative U wave
▸ Ischemic heart disease
  • Myocardial infarction
  • Angina, exercise-induced ischemia
  • Coronary heart disease (post extrasystolic)
  • Prinzmetal's angina
▸ Nonischemic causes
  • Left/right ventricular hypertrophy
  • Long QT syndrome
  • Pulmonary embolism

Delta wave
  • Wolff-Parkinson-White syndrome (ventricular preexcitation)

Edema
Painless, non-reddened swelling due to an accumulation of an excessive amount of watery fluid in cells, tissues, or serous cavities. Fluid accumulation in preformed body cavities is called hydrops; when generalized in the skin, it is called anasarca.

Pathophysiology
▸ Increased hydrostatic pressure
  • Heart failure
  • Venous thrombosis
▸ Reduced oncotic pressure
  • Protein deficiency
▸ Increased capillary permeability
  • Inflammatory capillary wall damage
  • Metabolic capillary wall damage

Generalized edema
▸ Heart failure
  • Left heart failure (pulmonary edema)
  • Right heart failure (generalized edema)
▸ Gastrointestinal, nutritional
  • Malabsorption, maldigestion (See Malassimilation → 233)
  • Exudative enteropathy
  • Liver failure
  • Malnutrition
  • Cachexia
  • Starvation edema
  • Anorexia nervosa
  • Bulimia nervosa
  • Hypoalbuminemia
  • Beriberi
▸ Endocrine
  • Premenstrual edema
  • Cushing's syndrome

- Addison's disease
- Hypothyroidism
- Hyperthyroidism
► Renal
  - Nephrotic syndrome
  - Acute glomerulonephritis
► Systemic
  - Anemia
  - Bartter's syndrome
  - Scleroderma
► Drugs
  - α-methyldopa
  - Diuretics
  - Estrogens
  - Glucocorticoids
  - Laxatives
  - Mineralocorticoids
  - Minoxidil)
  - Nifedipine
  - NSAIDs
  - Oral contraceptives
  - Progestogens
  - Sympathicolytics
► Idiopathic edema

Localized edema
► Infection
  - Carbuncle
  - Cellulitis
  - Boils
  - Abscess
  - Erysipelas
  - Gas gangrene
  - Osteomyelitis
► Venous obstruction
  - Thrombophlebitis
  - Thrombosis
  - Varicose veins
  - AV fistula
  - Aneurysm
  - Neoplasm
  - Lymph node mass
  - Tight clothing
► Lymphatic obstruction
  - Neoplasm
  - Surgical excision

  - Filariasis
  - Cellulitis
► Local trauma
  - Bruise
  - Contusion
  - Fracture
  - Ligamentous sprain
  - Tendonous strain
  - Insect bite
  - Snake bite
  - Irritant
  - Frostbite
  - Burn
  - Sunburn
► Congenital
  - AV fistula
  - Amniotic band
► Miscellaneous
  - Gout
  - Angioneurotic edema
  - Milroy's disease

Localized edema in the facial region and above diaphragma
See Face, Swollen → 138
► Quincke's edema (angioneurotic edema)
  - Physical stimuli
    ○ Sun
    ○ Cold
    ○ Trauma
  - Food
    ○ Nuts
    ○ Tomatoes
    ○ Fresh fruit
  - Drugs
    ○ ACE inhibitors
    ○ Cephalosporins
► Hereditary angioneurotic edema (C1-esterase inhibitor deficiency)
► Acquired C1-esterase inhibitor deficiency
► Melkersson-Rosenthal syndrome (triad of relapsing unilateral facial swelling, relapsing facial nerve paralysis, fissured tongue)
► Contact dermatitis

▶ Scleroderma
▶ Erysipelas
▶ Cellulitis
▶ Thoracic aneurysm
▶ Mediastinal cancer
▶ Trichinosis

Localized edema of extremities
See Leg Swelling → 220
▶ Phleboedema
 • Thrombophlebitis
 • Deep vein varicosis
 • Leg thrombosis
▶ Lymphedema (→ 231)
 • Congenital malformation of the
   lymph vessels
   ○ Aplasia
   ○ Hypoplasia
   ○ Dilation
 • Trauma
 • Infection
   ○ Erysipelas
   ○ Filariasis
 • Tumors
▶ Sudeck's atrophy
 • Musculoskeletal trauma
 • Peripheral nerve lesion
 • Myocardial infarction
 • Cerebral circulation impairment

Effluvium, See Alopecia → 19

Effusions, hemorrhagic
See Pleural Effusion → 286

Elastase in Blood Serum
Serine proteinase hydrolyzing elastin
occurring in granulocytes, macrophages
and endothelial cells. Released e.g. in
inflammatory and necrotic tissues.

Reference range	
In plasma	60–110 ng/ml
In pleural effusion	480–2900 ng/ml

Increase
▶ Sepsis
▶ Shock
▶ Shock lung in gestosis
▶ Multiple trauma
▶ Chronic joint disorders
▶ Hemodialysis

Electrophoresis, serum protein
See Protein in the Serum → 296

Empty-Sella Syndrome
Causes
▶ Familial
▶ Congenital absence of the diaphragma
  sellae
▶ Primary in middle-aged obese women
▶ Post-partum pituitary necrosis
  (Sheehan's syndrome)
▶ Pituitary infarction
 • Vascular diseases
 • Diabetes mellitus
 • Increased intracranial pressure
 • Head trauma
 • Meningitis
 • Cavernous sinus thrombosis
▶ Pituitary adenoma
▶ Surgery
▶ Irradiation
▶ Communicating hydrocephalus
▶ Rupture of intrasellar or parasellar cyst
▶ Autoimmune factors

Encephalopathy, Metabolic
Vertigo, memory loss, and generalized
weakness, due to metabolic brain disease
or secondary to other organ failure.
Metabolic, endocrine
▶ Hypoglycemia
▶ Diabetic ketoacidosis
▶ Hyperosmolar coma
▶ Hypothyroidism
▶ Hyperadrenocorticism

► Hyperparathyroidism
Cofactor deficiency
► Thiamine (in alcoholism, Wernicke's encephalopathy)
► Vitamin B_{12}
► Pyridoxine
Electrolyte disorder
► Hyponatremia
► Hypercalcemia
Systemic (endogenous toxins)
► Dialysis
► Liver disease
► Uremia
► Porphyria
► Sepsis
Drugs, toxins
► Carbon dioxide narcosis
► Carbon monoxide
► Drug withdrawal
► Ethanol
► Heavy metals
► Hypnotics
► Lead
► Narcotics
► Organophosphates
► Salicylates
► Sedatives
► Tricyclic antidepressants
Cerebrvascular
► Hypoxia
► Ischemia
Miscellaneous
► Heat stroke
► Epilepsy

Encopresis

Repeated, generally involuntary passage of feces. Considered a **mental disorder** if occurring in a child more than 4 years old.
DDx retentive encopresis
► Functional constipation
► Anal disorder
  • Anal fissure
  • Anal stenosis
  • Anal atresia
  • Anal fistula
  • Displacement of anus
  • Anal trauma
  • Postoperative
► Neurogenic causes
  • Hirschprung's disease
  • Chronic intestinal pseudo-obstruction
  • Pelvic mass
  • Spinal cord disorders
  • Cerebral palsy
► Neuromuscular disease
► Endocrine, metabolic
  • Hypercalcemia
  • Hypothyroidism
► Drugs, toxins
  • Antacids
  • Codeine
  • Lead intoxication
  • Narcotics
DDx functional encopresis
► Ulcerative colitis
► Acquired spinal cord disease
  • Sacral lipoma
  • Spinal cord tumor
► Rectoperineal fistula (with imperforate anus)
► Postoperative (damage to anal sphincter)

Endocarditis, Bacterial

Microbial infection of the endothelial surface of the heart
Risk factors
► Disorders
  • Prosthetic heart valve
  • Rheumatic heart disease
  • Congenital heart disease
    ○ Septal defects
    ○ Valve disease
  • Mitral valve prolapse
  • Calcific aortic stenosis
  • Asymmetric septal hypertrophy

- Marfan's syndrome
- IV drug use
- Previous bacterial endocarditis
- Surgical systemic-pulmonary shunts and conduits
- Central venous catheters
▶ Procedures
- Dental
  ◦ Extractions
  ◦ Implants
  ◦ Root canals
- Respiratory tract
- Tonsillectomy
- Adenoidectomy
- Surgical
  ◦ Sclerotherapy
  ◦ Biliary tract surgery
  ◦ Endoscopic retrograde cholangiopancreatography
  ◦ Prostatic surgery
  ◦ Cystoscopy
  ◦ Urethral dilation
  ◦ Cardiac surgery
  ◦ Cardiac catheterization
- Childbirth

Infectious source
▶ IV procedure (drug abuse, catheter)
- Staphylococcus aureus
- Group A streptococcus
- Gram negative rods
- Candida
▶ Dental procedure
- Viridans Streptococci
▶ Genitourinary procedure
- Enterococcus
- Gram negative rods
▶ Prosthetic valve
- Staphylococcus epidermidis
- Staphylococcus aureus
- Gram negative rods
- Enterococcus
- Diphtheroids
- Candida
▶ Colonic neoplasm, adenoma, polyp
- Streptococcus bovis

▶ Skin infection
▶ Respiratory infection

Enophthalmos
Recession of the eyeball within the orbit.
Causes
▶ Horner's syndrome
▶ Pancoast tumor
▶ Goiter with neck vein distension
▶ Hypothyroidism
▶ Esophagus carcinoma
▶ Mediastinal carcinoma
▶ Malnutrition
▶ Water loss
▶ Takayasu's syndrome
▶ Congenital enophthalmos
▶ Progressive hemiatrophy
▶ Syringomyelia
▶ After eye operation

Enteropathy, Protein-loosing
Multiplicity of abnormalities that result in the loss of plasma proteins from the gastrointestinal tract.
Gastrointestinal mucosal disorder
▶ Erosions, ulcerations of
- Esophagus
- Stomach
- Duodenum
▶ Inflammatory bowel diseases
- Crohn's disease
- Ulcerative colitis
▶ Graft versus host disease
▶ Pseudomembranous colitis (Clostridium difficile)
▶ Mucosal-based neoplasm
▶ Carcinoid syndrome
▶ Amyloidosis
▶ Idiopathic ulcerative jejunoileitis
▶ Kaposi sarcoma
▶ Neurofibromatosis
▶ Protein dyscrasia

Increased interstitial pressure,

lymphatic obstruction
- Tuberculosis
- Sarcoidosis
- Retroperitoneal fibrosis
- Lymphoma
- Lymphoenteric fistula
- Intestinal endometriosis
- Whipple disease
- Cardiac disease
  - Constrictive pericarditis
  - Congestive heart failure

Nonerosive upper GI disorder
- Whipple disease
- Connective tissue disorders
- AIDS
- Angioedema
- Henoch-Schönlein purpura
- Celiac sprue
- Tropical sprue
- Gastroenteritis
  - Allergic gastroenteritis
  - Acute gastroenteritis
  - Eosinophilic gastroenteritis
- Ménétrier disease
- Intestinal parasites
- Bacterial overgrowth
- Microscopic colitis

Eosinophilia

Series of allergic, infectious, neoplastic and idiopathic illnesses associated with an increase in the absolute number of the eosinophil granulocytes in the serum and/or tissue.

Reference range

Adult	0–450/µl

Allergic illnesses
- Asthma
- Urticaria
- Hay fever
- Contact dermatitis
- Angioneurotic syndrome/Quincke's edema
- Allergic vasculitis

- Food allergy
- Serum sickness
- Drug exanthema
- Mastocytosis
- Muscular spasms

Infection
- Parasitosis
  - Trichinosis
  - Ascariasis
  - Echinococcosis
  - Oxyuriasis
  - Filariasis
    - Tropical pulmonary eosinophilia
    - Onchocercosis
    - Mansonelliasis
  - Schistosomiasis
  - Toxakariasis
  - Ancylostomiasis
  - Scabies
- Miscellaneous infections
  - Scarlet fever
  - Tuberculosis
  - Measles
  - Erythema infectiosum
  - Gonorrhea
  - Lepra
  - Dysentery

Skin
- Dermatitis herpetiformis
- Erythema multiforme
- Pemphigus
- Scabies
- Neurodermatitis
- Contact dermatitis
- Exfoliative dermatitis
- Pityriasis rosea
- Ichthyosis
- Pemphigus vulgaris
- Facial granuloma
- Psoriasis

Malignant, hematologic
- Hodgkin's lymphoma
- Myeloproliferative disorder
- CML
- Generalized carcinoma

- Eosinophilic leukemia
- Mycosis fungoides
- Polycythemia
- Ovarial carcinoma
- Necrosis near tumors
- Hypereosinophilic syndrome
- Mastocytosis
- Advanced solid tumors

Collagen vascular diseases
- Rheumatoid arthritis
- Dermatomyositis
- Polyarteritis nodosa
- Vasculitis
- Felty's syndrome (splenomegaly with rheumatoid arthritis and leukopenia)
- Loeffler's endocarditis

Gastrointestinal
- Ulcerative colitis
- Regional enteritis
- Eosinophilic gastroenteritis

Endocrine
- Thyrotoxicosis
- Addison's disease
- Myxedema
- Hypopituitarism

Drugs
- Chlorpromazine
- Penicillin
- Streptomycin

Miscellaneous
- Chronic renal disease
- Radiation therapy
- Familial eosinophilia
- Graft-vs.-host disease
- Pernicious anemia
- Fibroblastic endocarditis
- Sarcoidosis
- Tropical eosinophilia
- Churg-Strauss syndrome
- Waterhouse-Friderichsen syndrome
- Henoch-Schönlein purpura
- Erythema nodosum
- Liver damage in cholestasis
- Eosinophilic pulmonary infiltrate

- After splenectomy
- Artheroembolic diseases

Epilepsy
Seizures
Chronic disorder characterized by paroxysmal brain dysfunction caused by excessive neuronal discharge, and usually associated with some alteration of consciousness. Differences are made between focal epilepsy (motoric, sensitive-sensory, autonomic, psychic, psychomotoric and twilight states), and generalized epilepsy (absence, myoclonic attacks, clonic attacks, tonic attacks, tonic-clonic attacks, atonic attacks). All diseases and damages of the CNS can cause a symptomatic epilepsy.

Cerebrovascular
- Thrombosis
- Embolism
- Intracranial hemorrhage and trauma
- Vasculitis
  - Lupus erythematosus
  - Polyarteritis nodosa
- Thrombophlebitis

Neoplasms
- Metastasis
- Meningeoma
- Astrocytoma

Infections
- Encephalitis
- Meningitis
- Brain abscess
- Neurosyphilis
- Creutzfeldt-Jakob disease
- HIV
- Cysticercosis

Metabolic, endocrine disorders
- Fever
- Hypoglycemia (and hyperglycemia)
  - Non-ketotic hyperglycemia
- Hypernatremia and hyponatremia
- Hypocalcemia

▶ Hypomagnesemia
▶ Phenylketonuria
▶ Hyperthyroidism
▶ Hypothyroidism

Other organic disorders
▶ Chronic renal failure
▶ Pellagra
▶ Pyridoxine deficiency
▶ Alkalosis
▶ Hepatic failure
▶ Huntington's chorea
▶ Reye's syndrome

Drugs, toxins
▶ Acyclovir
▶ Alcohol (withdrawal)
▶ Amphetamine (withdrawal)
▶ Analgesics
▶ Anesthetics
▶ Antidepressants
▶ Antipsychotics
▶ Barbiturates (withdrawal)
▶ Benzodiazepines (withdrawal)
▶ Betalactam antibiotics
▶ Cocaine (withdrawal)
▶ Cyclosporine
▶ Ganciclovir
▶ Heroine (withdrawal)
▶ Interferones
▶ Isoniazid
▶ Lithium
▶ Local anesthetics
▶ Meperidine
▶ Methylphenidate (withdrawal)
▶ Nalidixic acid
▶ Quinolones
▶ Radiocontrast drugs
▶ Salicylates
▶ Sedatives (withdrawal)
▶ Tacrolimus
▶ Theophylline
▶ Tramadol

Congenital diseases
▶ Infections
  • Toxoplasmosis
  • CMV

  • Syphilis
  • German measles
▶ Perinatal hypoxia or trauma
▶ Kernicterus
▶ Down syndrome
▶ Lipid storage diseases
  • Gaucher's disease
▶ Tuberous sclerosis
▶ Sturge-Weber syndrome
▶ Von Hippel-Lindau syndrome
▶ Phenylketonuria
▶ Acute intermittent porphyria

Miscellaneous
▶ Head trauma
▶ Hypoxic encephalopathy
▶ CNS hypoxia, ischemia
  • Hypotension
  • Stokes-Adams syndrome
  • Carotid sinus syndrome
▶ Hypertensive encephalopathy
▶ Eclampsia
▶ Alzheimer's disease
▶ Presenile dementia
▶ Pick's disease

Causes for occasional attacks
▶ Hypoglycemia
▶ Hyperglycemia
▶ Heat stroke
▶ Fever
▶ Uremia
▶ Alcohol withdrawal
▶ Drug withdrawal
▶ Intoxication
▶ Hypovolemia
▶ Tetany
▶ Hypoparathyroidism

DDx of seizures
▶ Syncopes
  • Vasovagal syncope
  • Arrhythmias
  • Valvular heart disease
  • Cardiac failure
  • Orthostatic hypotension
▶ Psychologic
  • Hyperventilation

E

- Panic attack
► Metabolic
  - Hypoglycemia
  - Hypoxia
► Migraine
► Transient ischemic attack (TIA)
► Sleep disorders
► Movement disorders (Tics)
► Pediatric
  - Apnea
  - Night terrors
  - Sleepwalking
  - Breath-holding spells
  - Migraine

Epiphora
Tearing, lacrimation
Increased tear secretion
Causes
► Emotion
► Foreign body irritation
► Corneal ulcer
► Conjunctivitis
► Keratoconjunctivitis sicca
► Measles
► Allergic
  - Hay fever
  - Coryza (allergic rhinitis)
► Lid abnormality
  - Acquired ectropion
  - Entropion
  - Floppy eyelid syndrome
► Lacrimal disorders
  - Acquired punctal stenosis
  - Canalicular stenosis
  - Canaliculitis
  - Dacryocystitis
  - Lacrimal sac tumors
  - Large hordeolum
  - Chalazion
► Neurologic
  - Cluster headache (unilateral tearing)
  - Cranial nerve VII compression
    (parasympathetic lacrimal fibers)

- Postraumatic state
► Toxins
  - Arsenic
  - Bromide (Bromism)
  - Iodine
  - Pilocarpine
► Caustic burn

Epistaxis
Nasal hemorrhage, nosebleed
Bleeding from the nose.
Local causes
► Trauma
  - Nose picking
  - Nasal foreign body
  - Forceful blowing
  - Hemorrhage of Kiesselbach's area
  - Nasal fractures
  - Sinus fracture
  - Other trauma to the face
  - Postoperative
► Air
  - Dry air
    ○ Dry climate
    ○ Winter months
  - Irritants
    ○ Vapors
    ○ Dust
► Repeated cocaine use
► Tumor
  - Juvenile nasopharyngeal fibroma
  - Bleeding septal polyp
  - Neoplasm
► Infection/inflammation
  - Nasal diphtheria
  - Nasal syphilis
  - Rhinitis sicca
  - Allergic rhinitis
Predisposing factors (systemic causes)
► Drugs
  - Anticoagulant therapy
  - Aspirin
  - NSAIDs
► Immune disorders

- ► (Febrile) infections
  - Influenza
  - Measles
  - Diphtheria
  - Typhoid fever
  - Psittacosis
  - Streptococcal infection
- ► Cardiovascular disorders
  - Hypertension
  - Arteriosclerosis
  - Aortic isthmus stenosis
- ► Hemorrhagic diathesis
  - Hemophilia
  - Thrombocytopenic purpura (Werlhof's disease)
  - Pancytopenia
  - Vasculopathies
    - ○ Osler's disease
    - ○ Wegener's granulomatosis
  - Coagulopathies
- ► Blood disorders
  - Thrombocytopathy
  - Leukemia
  - Erythrocythemia
  - Waldenström's macroglobulinemia
- ► Miscellaneous
  - Multiple myeloma
  - Vitamin deficiencies
    - ○ Vitamin K deficiency
    - ○ Avitaminosis C
  - Liver diseases
    - ○ Chronic hepatitis
    - ○ Cirrhosis
  - Alcoholism
  - Uremia

Erection impairment, See Priapism → 292, See Impotence → 208

Erythema Nodosum

Symptom complex characterized by painful nodes on the extensor surfaces of the lower extremities, initially red, later blue-green-yellow. The lesions suddenly occur and are associated with arthralgia and fever. The erythema usually lasts more than 6 weeks and can recur. Women are more frequently affected.

Infections
- ► Bacterial
  - Brucella
  - Campylobacter
  - Cat-scratch fever
  - Chlamydia
  - Corynebacterium diphtheriae
  - Francisella tularensis
  - Leptospira
  - Mycobacteria (Tuberculosis, leprosy)
  - Mycoplasma pneumoniae
  - Neisseria meningitidis
  - Salmonella
  - Streptococci
  - Yersinia
- ► Fungal
  - Coccidioidomycosis
  - Dermatophytosis
  - Histoplasmosis
  - North American blastomycosis
  - Sporotrichosis
- ► Protozoa
  - Hookworm infection
  - Toxoplasmosis
- ► Viral
  - Hepatitis
  - Herpes simplex
  - Infectious mononucleosis
  - Milker's nodule

Drugs
- ► Antimony compounds
- ► Bromides
- ► Estrogens
- ► Iodides
- ► Oral contraceptives
- ► Penicillins
- ► Phenacetin
- ► Salicylates
- ► Sulfonamides
- ► Vaccines

Malignant tumors
► Hodgkin's lymphoma
► Leukemia
► Postradiated pelvic cancer

Miscellaneous
► Behçet's syndrome
► Inflammatory bowel diseases
  • Crohn's disease
  • Ulcerative colitis
► Pregnancy
► Sarcoidosis
► Reiter's disease
► Radiation therapy

Erythrocyte, increase
See Polycythemia → 288

Erythrocyte, Morphology

Red blood cell morphology on peripheral smear. Variations of erythrocytes concerning color, size, shape and contents.

Acanthocytes
Spherical cells with blunt-tipped or club-shaped spicules of different lengths projecting from their surface at irregular intervals. Also called **spur cells.**
► Abetalipoproteinemia
► Chronic liver disease
  • Cirrhosis
  • Hepatic necrosis
► Hemolytic anemia
► Pyruvate kinase deficiency
► Uremia
► Acanthocytosis
► Infantile pyknocytosis

Anisocytosis (variation in the size), poikilocytosis (irregular shape)
► Possible in all anemia forms
  • Iron deficiency anemia
  • Pernicious anemia
  • Folic acid deficiency anemia
  • Sideroachrestic anemia
  • Tumor anemia

► Myelopathy
  • Spherocytosis
  • Elliptocytosis
  • Thalassemia
  • Paroxysmal nightly hemoglobinuria

Basophilic stippling (aggregated ribosomes)
► Lead poisoning
► Arsenic poisoning
► Thalassemia
► Sideroblastic anemia
► Hemolytic anemia
► Severe anemia
► Unstable hemoglobin
► Pyrimidine 5'-nucleotidase deficiency

Cabot's ring bodies (nuclear remnants)
► Lead toxicity
► Pernicious anemia
► Hemolytic anemia

Dacrocytes (Teardrop)
► Extramedullary hemopoiesis
► Myelofibrosis
► Severe hemolytic anemia
► Polycythemia vera
► Thalassemia

Eliptocytes
Oval erythrocytes, ovalocytes
► Various anemias
  • Megaloblastic anemia
  • Iron deficiency anemia
  • Refractory normoblastic anemia
  • Microcytic anemia
► Hereditary elliptocytosis
► Myelofibrosis
► Thalassemia

Heinz bodies
Small irregular, deep purple granules in erythrocytes due to damage of hemoglobin molecules.
► Hereditary hemolytic anemia
► Glucose-6-phosphate dehydrogenase deficiency
► Thalassemia
► Methemoglobinemia

- Premature infants
- Oxidant drugs
  - Primaquin
- Drug sensitivities

Howell–Jolly bodies
Nuclear fragments of condensed DNA in the erythrocyte.
- Asplenia (congenital absence of the spleen)
- Functional hyposplenism
- Postsplenectomy
- Hemolytic anemia
- Megaloblastic anemia
- Pernicious anemia
- Thalassemia
- Leukemia

Hypochromic microcytes: Defective Hemoglobin synthesis
- See microcytic anemia (→ 28)
- Iron deficiency anemia
- Thalassemia
- Sickle cell anemia
- Hemoglobinopathy

Intraerythrocytic parasites
- Malaria
- Bartonellosis
- Babesiosis

Macrocytes
- See macrocytic anemia (→ 28)
- Reticulocytosis
- Liver disease

Microcytes
- See hypochromic anemia (→ 28)
- See: hemolytic anemia (→ 28)

Schistocytes
Fragmented erythrocytes, like triangles or half-moons
- Microangiopathic hemolytic anemia
- Macroangiopathic hemolytic anemia
- Hemolytic anemia after burns
- Mechanical hemolysis (prosthetic heart valve)
- Disseminated intravascular coagulation (DIC)

- Thrombotic thrombocytopenic purpura
- Hemolytic uremic syndrome (HUS)
- Giant hemangioma
- Metastatic carcinoma
- Malignant hypertension
- Eclampsia (in pregnancy)
- Vasculitis
- Rejection of transplant (e.g. kidney)

Sickle cells
- Sickle cell anemia

Sideroblasts
- See sideroblastic anemia
- Nucleated erythrocytes

Spherocytes
Erythrocytes that are almost spherical in shape.
- Hereditary spherocytosis
- Autoimmune hemolytic anemia
- Hemolytic transfusion reactions
- Alcoholism
- Hemoglobin C disease
- After severe burns
- Severe hypophosphatemia
- Acute oxidant damage

Stomatocytes (slit or mouth–shaped pallor)
- Acute alcohol intoxication
- Drugs
  - Phenothiazines
- Neoplasm
- Cardiovascular disease
- Hepatobiliary disease
- Hereditary

Target Cells (codocytes)
Erythrocytes with a central color spot in the area of pallor, resembling a target.
- Hemolytic anemias
- Hemoglobin C disease
- Sickle cell anemia
- Iron deficiency anemia
- Thalassemia minor
- Postsplenectomy
- Liver disease

Erythrocyte, Osmotic Fragility

Osmotic fragility measures red blood cell resistance to hemolysis when exposed to a series of increasingly dilute saline solutions. The sooner hemolysis occurs, the greater the osmotic fragility of the cells.

High osmotic fragility
▸ Hereditary spherocytosis
▸ Autoimmune hemolytic anemia
▸ Severe burns
▸ Toxins
  • Alcoholism
  • Benzol intoxication
  • Acute oxidant damage
▸ Hemolytic disease of the newborn (erythroblastosis fetalis)

Low osmotic fragility
▸ Thalassemia
▸ Iron deficiency anemia
▸ Pernicious anemia
▸ Sickle cell anemia
▸ Hemolytic anemias
▸ Postsplenectomy
▸ Drugs
  • Sulfonamides
▸ Newborns (physiologic)

Erythrocyte Sedimentation Rate
ESR

Rate of settling of red blood cells in anticoagulated blood;
Normal ESR is relatively low, since the erythrocytes repel each other through their negative surface potential and thus hold themselves in suspension. After reduction of this potential, particularly after an increase in fibrinogens or globulins, also in acute-phase proteins, the formation of cell aggregates becomes possible, primarily in the form of rolls that sediment faster than individual cells. Also, erythrocyte size influences the ESR. Macrocytes sediment faster than normocytes.

Reference range	
Women	3–10 mm/h
(Probably higher because of lower hematocrit)	
Men	3–8 mm/h

Increased
▸ Falsely increased
  • Poikilocytosis
  • Acanthocytosis
  • Iron deficiency anemia
▸ Infections
  • Systemic fungal infection
  • Bacterial infection
  • Viral infection
  • Infectious hepatitis
  • Cat scratch disease
  • Primary atypical pneumonia
  • Secondary syphilis
  • Tuberculosis
  • Leptospirosis
▸ Hematologic, neoplastic
  • Severe anemia
    ○ Hemolytic anemia
    ○ Iron deficiency anemia
    ○ Vitamin B_{12} deficiency anemia
    ○ Sickle cell anemia
  • Multiple myeloma
  • Leukemia
  • Lymphoma
    ○ Hodgkin's lymphoma
    ○ Non-Hodgkin's lymphoma
  • Metastases
  • Chronic granulomatous disease
  • Macroglobulinemia
  • Hyperfibrinogenemia
▸ Renal disease
  • Acute glomerulonephritis
  • Chronic glomerulonephritis with renal failure
  • Pyelonephritis
  • Nephrosis
  • Hemolytic uremic syndrome (HUS)

- Gastrointestinal disease
  - Inflammatory bowel disease
  - Acute pancreatitis
  - Cholecystitis
  - Lupoid hepatitis
  - Acute liver failure
  - Peritonitis
- Collagen vascular, rheumatic disease
  - Rheumatic
    - Arteritis temporalis (!)
    - Polymyalgia rheumatica
  - Rheumatic fever
  - Rheumatoid arthritis
  - Systemic lupus erythematosus
  - Scleroderma
  - Dermatomyositis
  - Systemic vasculitis
  - Henoch-Schonlein purpura
  - Mediterranean fever
- Drugs
  - Anabolics
  - Drug hypersensitivity reaction
  - Oral contraceptives
  - Plasma expander
- Miscellaneous
  - Hypothyroidism
  - Thyroiditis
  - Sarcoidosis
  - Infantile cortical hyperostosis
  - Trauma
    - Surgery
    - Burn injury
  - Pregnancy
  - Myocardial infarction
  - Heart failure

Decreased
- Hematologic
  - Polycythemia vera
  - Sickle cell anemia
  - Hypofibrinogenemia
  - Afibrinogenemia
  - Cryoglobulinemia
  - Macroglobulinemia (e.g. hyperviscosity syndrome)
  - Spherocytosis

- Drugs
  - Corticosteroids
  - Salicylates

Erythrocythemia, See Polycythemia → 288

Erythropoietin

Protein enhancing erythropoiesis by stimulation of the formation of proerythroblasts and release of reticulocytes from bone marrow. Secreted by the kidney.

Increased
- See anemia (→ 28)
- Kidney diseases
  - Hydronephrosis
  - Polycystic kidneys
  - Renal tumors
  - Adenomas
- Secondary polycythemia
  - COPD
  - Pulmonary fibrosis
  - High altitude exposure
- Pregnancy
- Bone marrow insufficiency
  - Aplastic
  - Iron deficiency
- Hypoxia
- Doping with EPO
- Paraneoplasia
  - Ovarial carcinoma
  - Cerebellar tumors, hepatomas
- Familiar erythrocytosis

Decreased
- Renal failure
- Chronic kidney disease
- Polycythemia
- Chronic anemia
- Inflammation

Erythruria, See Hematuria → 172

Esophagitis

Infection
- Bacteria
- Viruses
  - Herpes
  - Cytomegalovirus
- Fungi
- Yeast (Candida)

Irritation
- Gastroesophageal reflux
- Vomiting
- Drugs, toxins
  - Alcohol
  - Nicotine
- Hernias
- Caustic burn
- Iatrogenic
  - Radiation
  - Gastric tube
  - Gastroscopy
  - Surgery
- Tumor
- Metastasis
- Crohn's disease

ESR. See Erythrocyte Sedimentation Rate
→ 134

Estradiol

Estradiol (E2) is the most effective ovarian estrogen and is mostly formed in the ripening follicle under the influence of FSH. Main effects: proliferation of the endometrium, effects on vagina and breasts, prevention of osteoporosis and regulating effects on pituitary and hypothalamus. Symptoms of estrogen deficiency include small, atrophic breasts, sparse pubic hair, atrophic vulva and vagina, dry vagina, dyspareunia, small, atrophic uterus and tubes, eunuchoidism and osteoporosis.

Reference range

In sexually mature women, dependent on the ovarian cycle

Follicle phase	10–50 pg/ml
Ovulation phase	50–375 pg/ml
Luteal phase	15–260 pg/ml
Post-menopause	< 14 pg/m
Oral contraceptives	< 50 pg/ml
Adult men:	6–44 pg/ml
Prepubertal girls:	< 5–15 pg/ml
Prepubertal boys:	2–8 pg/ml

Increased
- Estrogen-producing tumors
  - Granuloma
  - Thecal cell tumor
- Hyperthyroidism
- Obesity
- Cirrhosis
- Around ovulation1
- Drug-induced multiple ovulations

Decreased
See secondary hypogonadism → 200
- Primary ovarian insufficiency
  - Menopause
- Secondary ovarian insufficiency
  - Oral contraceptives
  - Pituitary insufficiency
- Anovular ovarian cycle
- Corpus luteum deficiency
- Osteoporosis

Estriol

Main product of the feto-placental unit. See also estradiol (→ 136) and estrone (→ 137).

Reference range	
1st–20th wk of gestation	1.3–3.2 ng/ml
24th wk of gestation	1.5–5.0 ng/ml
28th wk of gestation	2.2–6.5 ng/ml
32th wk of gestation	2.9–8.4 ng/ml
36th wk of gestation	4.0–16.0 ng/ml
40th wk of gestation	7.7–24.0 ng/ml

Decreased
▶ Placental insufficiency
▶ Fetal diseases
  • Anencephaly
  • Down's syndrome
▶ Maternal
  • Corticosteroid therapy
  • Antibiotic therapy

Increased
▶ Multiple pregnancy

Estrogens

There are three main types of estrogens important in hormone balancing: Estradiol (→ 136), Estriol (→ 137) and Estrone (→ 137).

Estrone

Essential estrogen in the postmenopausal woman. Synthesis mainly through conversion of androstenedione and DHEA in the fatty tissue. See also estradiol (→ 136), estriol (→ 137).

Reference range	50–80 pg/ml

Increased
▶ Estrone-containing drugs
▶ Severe post-menopausal obesity

Decreased
▶ Advanced age

Exanthema with fever
See Fever with Rash → 144

Exophthalmos, See Proptosis → 294

Expectoration, See Sputum → 339

Exsiccation, See Dehydration → 93

Extradural hemorrhage
See Bleeding, Intracranial → 56

Extrasystoles
See Cardiac Dysrhythmias → 62

Exudate, See Pleural Effusion → 286

Eye Discharge

Serous
▶ Viral conjunctivitis
▶ Allergic conjunctivitis
▶ Toxic conjunctivitis
Purulent
▶ Bacterial conjunctivitis
Mucoid
▶ Allergic conjunctivitis
▶ Keratoconjunctivitis sicca (→ 108)
▶ Toxic conjunctivitis
▶ Chlamydia conjunctivitis
Mucopurulent
▶ Chlamydia conjunctivitis
▶ Bacterial conjunctivitis
▶ Toxic conjunctivitis

Eye, dry, See Dry Eyes → 108

Eye Movement Disorders
See Strabismus → 340
See Heterophoria → 181
See Nystagmus → 260

Eye pain

Ophthalmalgia

With visible lesions
- ► Ocular foreign body
- ► Entropion conjunctivitis
- ► Hordeolum
- ► Chalazion
- ► Corneal ulcer
- ► Interstitial keratitis
- ► Iritis
- ► Iridocyclitis
- ► Glaucoma
- ► Ocular herpetic infection
- ► Conjunctiva calcification
- ► Band keratopathy

With blindness, but no visible lesions
- ► Retrobulbar neuritis

Without blindness or visible lesion
- ► Eye strain

Miscellaneous
- ► Febrile disease
- ► Sinusitis
  - • Ethmoid sinus
  - • Sphenoid sinus
  - • Frontal sinus
- ► Thyrotoxicosis

Eye, red, See Red Eye → 311

Face pain, See Facial pain → 140

Face, Red

Vascular
- ► Hypertension
- ► Facies mitralis
  - • Mitral stenosis
- ► Hyperkinetic heart syndrome
- ► Thrombophlebitis
- ► Lymphangitis

Infection
- ► Systemic
  - • Scarlet fever
  - • Measles
  - • German measles
  - • Typhus
- ► Localized
  - • Furuncle
  - • Herpes zoster
  - • Erysipelas
  - • Erysipeloid
  - • Erythema chronicum migrans (Lyme disease)

Metabolic, endocrine
- ► Cushing's disease
- ► Diabetes mellitus
- ► Carcinoid syndrome

Hematologic
- ► Polycythemia
- ► Hyperglobulia

Collagen vascular disease
- ► Lupus erythematosus
- ► Dermatomyositis

Dermatologic
- ► Rosacea
- ► Naevus flammeous
- ► Eczema

Drugs
- ► Allergic drug reaction
- ► Alcoholism
- ► Antabus reaction

Miscellaneous
- ► Sunburn
- ► Fever
- ► Emphysema (pink-puffer)
- ► Pickwickian syndrome
- ► Pellagra
- ► Familiar rubeosis
- ► Mastocytosis
- ► Boeck's disease

Face, Swollen

Renal disorder
- ► Glomerulonephritis
- ► Diabetic nephropathy

- Chronic kidney disease
- Nephrotic syndrome
- Nephritis of pregnancy
  - Preeclampsia

Endocrine
- Cushing's syndrome
- Pituitary insufficiency
- Exophthalmus
- Myxedema (Hypothyroidism)

Venous drainage obstruction
- Bronchial carcinoma
- Mediastinal sarcoma
- Hodgkin's lymphoma
- Superior vena cava syndrome (→ 344)
- Retrosternal goiter

Infections
- Measles
- Pertussis
- Mumps

Miscellaneous
- Quincke's edema
- Drug eruption
- Erysipelas
- Local swelling
  - Tooth inflammation
  - Sinusitis
- Drugs
  - Estrogens
  - Corticosteroids
- Dermatitis seborrhoica
- Parkinsonism
- Protein deficiency edema

Facial hair growth in women,
See Hirsutism → 182

Facial Nerve Paralysis

Bell's palsy

Loss of voluntary movement of the
muscles on one side of the face due to
abnormal function of the facial nerv

Trauma
- Cortical injury

- Temporal bone fracture
- Basal skull fracture
- Brain stem injury
- Penetrating middle ear injury
- Barotrauma
  - Altitude
  - Diving

Endocrine
- Diabetes mellitus
- Hyperthyroidism

Infection
- Tetanus
- Diphtheria
- Malignant otitis externa (osteomyelitis)
- Acute otitis media
- Chronic otitis media
  - Cholesteatoma
- Gradenigo's syndrome
- Mastoiditis
- Herpes viruses
  - Herpes zoster oticus
  - Herpetic vessicles (auricle, external canal)
- Lyme disease
- HIV infection
- Parotitis
- Meningoencephalitis
- Mumps
- Mononucleosis
- Leprosy
- Influenza
- Coxschievirus infection
- Syphilis
- Tuberculosis
- Botulism

Tumor
- Facial nerve neuroma
- Parotid tumor
- Glomus jugulare tumor
- Primary temporal bone tumors
- Meningiomas
- Hemangioma
- Hemangioblastoma
- Pontine glioma

Birth
▶ Birth trauma
  • Forceps delivery
▶ Molding
▶ Congenital facial palsy
  • Möbius' syndrome
  • Heerfordt's disease
  • Cardiofacial syndrome

Intoxication
▶ Alcoholism
▶ Thalidomide
▶ Lead
▶ Carbon monoxide

Iatrogenic
▶ Rabies vaccine
▶ Antitetanus serum
▶ Mandibular block anesthesia
▶ Surgery

Miscellaneous
▶ Pregnancy
▶ Hypertension
▶ Ischemic cerebral insult
▶ Sarcoidosis
▶ Myasthenia gravis
▶ Guillain-Barre syndrome (polyradiculitis)
▶ Familial Bell's palsy

Facial pain

Causes
▶ Trigeminal neuralgia
  • Posttraumatic neuralgia
  • Inflammation
  • Vascular processes
  • Tumors
  • Intoxication
▶ Glossopharyngeal neuralgia
▶ Geniculate neuralgia
▶ Neuralgia of the superior laryngeal nerve
▶ Postherpetic neuralgia
▶ Facial pain of central origin
▶ Myofacial pain syndrome
▶ Sjögren's syndrome
▶ Atypical facial pain

▶ Tic douloureux
▶ Cluster headache
▶ Bing-Horton syndrome
▶ Histamine neuralgia
▶ Acute sinusitis
▶ Rhinitis
▶ Hypotension in the nasal sinuses
▶ Otitis
▶ Abscess
▶ Teeth, mandibular joint
  • Costen's syndrome (pain in the mandibular joint area)
▶ Opthalmologic
  • Glaucoma
  • Conjunctivitis
  • Lid abscess
  • Iridocyclitis
  • Dacrocystitis
▶ Psychologic
  • Anxiety
  • Somatization syndrome

Fatigue

Lessened capacity for work and reduced efficiency of accomplishment with a feeling of weariness, sleepiness, or irritability.

Psychogenic, lifestyle (80%)
▶ Mood disorder
  • Anxiety disorder
  • Major depression
  • Bipolar disorder
▶ Eating
  • Anorexia nervosa
  • Bulimia nervosa
  • Malnutrition (proteins)
  • Overnutrition
  • Obesity
  • Pickwickian syndrome
▶ Sleep disorder (e.g. insomnia)
▶ Lifestyle
  • Work problems
  • Relationship problems

Organic causes (20%)
► Infections
  • Fever
  • Tuberculosis
  • HIV infection
  • AIDS
  • Lyme disease
  • Influenza
  • Chronic mononucleosis
  • Local infection (dental granuloma)
  • Chronic pyelonephritis
  • Infectious endocarditis
► Metabolic
  • Diabetes mellitus
  • Hypothyroidism
  • Hyperthyroidism
  • Hyperparathyroidism
  • Pituitary insufficiency
    ○ Hypopituitarism
    ○ Sheehan's syndrome
  • Addison's disease
  • Cushing's disease
  • Conn's syndrome
► Hematologic
  • Anemia
  • Leukemia
  • Lymphoma
  • Myelodysplastic syndrome
► Neoplasm
► Renal disease
  • Acute renal failure
  • Chronic renal failure
► Liver disease
  • Acute hepatitis
  • Chronic hepatitis
  • Chronic liver disease
  • Cirrhosis
► Gastrointestinal
  • GI bleeding
  • Chronic pancreatitis
  • Sprue
  • Crohn's disease
  • Ulcerative colitis
► Cardiovascular
  • Heart failure

  • Coronary artery disease
  • Hypotension
  • Infectious endocarditis
  • Cerebrovascular arteriosclerosis
► Pulmonary
  • Chronic obstructive pulmonary disease
  • Emphysema
  • Other chronic lung disease
  • Sleep apnea
► Rheumatologic
  • Fibromyalgia
  • Sjögren's syndrome
  • Polymyalgia rheumatica
  • Giant cell arteritis
  • Polymyositis
  • Dermatomyositis
  • Connective tissue disease
  • Inflammatory bowel disease
  • Sarcoidosis
► Neurologic
  • Multiple sclerosis
  • Parkinson's disease
  • Neuromuscular weakness
► Drugs, toxins
  • Alcohol abuse
  • Amitriptyline
  • Amphetamines
  • Antihistamines
  • Antihypertensives
  • Betablockers
  • Caffeine
  • Cigarette smoking
  • Clonidine
  • Chronic CO
  • Doxepin
  • Hypnotics
  • Illicit drug abuse
    ○ Opiates
    ○ Cannabis
  • Lead poisoning
  • Methyldopa
  • Psychotropics
  • Reserpine
  • Sedatives
  • Tranquilizers

F

- Trazodone

Fatty Liver

Yellow discoloration of the liver due to fatty degeneration of parenchymal cells. Common response of the liver to injury. See Liver diseases → 226

Endocrine, metabolic
▶ Diabetes mellitus
▶ Wilson's disease (early stage)
▶ Hereditary defects in
  • Glycogen metabolism
  • Galactose metabolism
  • Tyrosine metabolism
  • Homocystine metabolism
▶ Fructose intolerance
▶ Reye's syndrome
▶ Weber-Christian disease
▶ Refsum's disease
▶ Abetalipoproteinemia
▶ Aryl-dehydrogenase-deficiency
▶ Disorders of lipid metabolism

Nutrition
▶ Obesity
▶ Starvation, rapid weight loss
▶ Protein malnutrition, deficiency
▶ Parenteral nutrition
▶ Intestinal bypass surgery

Drugs, toxins
▶ Alcohol
▶ Amiodarone
▶ Carbon tetrachloride
▶ Corticosteroids
▶ Estrogens
▶ Methotrexate
▶ Phosphorus
▶ Salicylates
▶ Tetracycline
▶ Valproic acid
▶ Vitamin A

Miscellaneous
▶ Pregnancy
▶ Inflammatory bowel disease
▶ Cystic fibrosis

Feces Color

Bloody feces
See gastrointestinal bleeding (→ 152)
Light grey
▶ Bile duct occlusion
▶ Viral hepatitis
▶ Fatty stool
▶ After radiocontrast

Feces Consistency

Watery
▶ Acute gastroenteritis
▶ Cholera
▶ Intoxication
▶ Carcinoid syndrome
Slimy
▶ Gastroenteritis
▶ Chronic enterocolitis
▶ Amebic dysentery
▶ Colitis mucosa
▶ Allergic diarrhea
▶ Pellagra
Thin
▶ Rectal carcinoma
▶ Constipation

Ferritin

In healthy patients ferritin is an indicator of total body iron stores. It is also an acute phase reactant and is increased in inflammatory states. See Iron → 214

Reference range
m: 15–400 µg/l
f: 10–200 µg/l

Decreased
▶ Iron deficiency anemia
  • GI-hemorrhage
  • Hypermenorrhea
  • Hemoglobinuria
  • Hemorrhage
  • Coagulation defect

- Iron resorption impairment
  - Malabsorption
  - Celiac sprue
- Insufficient supply
  - Vegetarians
- Increased demand
  - Pregnancy

Increased
- Inflammatory states
- Iron overloading
  - Hemochromatosis
  - Hereditary hemolytic anemia
    ○ Glucose-6-phosphate dehydrogenase deficiency
    ○ Pyruvate kinase deficiency
    ○ Hereditary sideroblastic anemia
- Secondary iron overloading
  - Frequent blood transfusions
  - Ineffective erythropoiesis
  - Atransferrinemia
  - Sideroblastic anemia
  - Thalassemia major
  - Porphyria cutanea tarda
- Iron mobilization therapy in Iron overloading
  - Bloodletting
  - Chelating agents
- Liver disease
- Malignant diseases
  - Leukemia
  - Lymphoma
    ○ Hodgkin's lymphoma
    ○ Non-Hodgkin's lymphoma
  - Other tumors
    ○ Breast cancer
    ○ Bronchial carcinomas
    ○ Pancreas carcinoma
    ○ Neuroblastomas
- Miscellaneous
  - Hyperthyroidism
  - Rheumatoid arthritis
  - Inflammatory bowel disease

Fever of Unknown Origin
FUO

Temperature > 38.3°C (101°F) on several occasions, for > 3 weeks with failure to reach a diagnosis within one week of inpatient investigation.

Infection
- Bacterial
  - Abscesses
  - Tuberculosis
  - Urinary tract infection (UTI)
  - Pyelonephritis
  - Endocarditis
  - Meningitis
  - Pneumonia
  - Septicemia
  - Acute sinusitis
  - Otitis media
  - Hepatobiliary infections
    ○ Cholecystitis
    ○ Gallbladder empyema
  - Abdominal abscess
  - Diverticulitis
  - Osteomyelitis
  - Brucellosis
  - Salmonellosis
  - Neisseria
  - Borrelia
    ○ Relapsing fever
    ○ Rat-bite fever
    ○ Lyme disease
  - Treponema pallidum
  - Coxiella burnetii
  - Chlamydia
- Viral
  - HIV/AIDS
  - Herpes viruses
    ○ CMV
    ○ Epstein-Barr virus (EBV)
- Fungi
  - Candida albicans
  - Malassezia furfur
- Parasites

- Toxoplasmosis
- Malaria
- Trypanosoma
- Leishmania
- Amoeba

Neoplasm
▸ Lymphomas
  - Hodgkin
  - Non-Hodgkin lymphomas
▸ Leukemias
  - Acute leukemias
▸ Renal cell carcinoma
▸ Breast carcinoma
▸ Liver carcinoma
▸ Colon carcinoma
▸ Pancreas carcinoma
▸ Liver metastases
▸ Carcinomatosis
▸ Paraneoplasia
▸ Malignant histiocytosis

Collagen vascular, autoimmune disease
▸ Systemic lupus erythematosus
▸ Juvenile rheumatoid arthritis
▸ Polyarteritis nodosa (PAN)
▸ Rheumatoid arthritis
▸ Mixed connective tissue diseases
▸ Other vasculitides
  - Giant cell arteritis
  - Polymyalgia rheumatica
  - Wegener granulomatosis
  - Takayasu arteritis
  - Cryoglobulinemia

Granulomatous disease
▸ Sarcoidosis
▸ Inflammatory bowel disease
▸ Granulomatous hepatitis

Drug fever
▸ Alpha-methyldopa
▸ Amphetamines
▸ Antibiotics
▸ Antihistamines
▸ Aspirin
▸ Atropine
▸ Barbiturates

▸ Beta-lactam antibiotics
▸ Diphenylhydantoin
▸ Glucocorticoids
▸ Isoniazid
▸ Procainamide
▸ Quinidine
▸ Steroids

Inherited disease
▸ Familial Mediterranean fever
▸ Fabry's disease
▸ Lamellar ichtyosis
▸ Nephrogenic diabetes insipidus
▸ Anhydrotic ectodermal dysplasia
▸ Familial dysautonomia

Endocrine
▸ Hyperthyroidism
▸ Subacute thyroiditis
▸ Adrenal insufficiency

Miscellaneous
▸ Factitious fever (psychiatric problems, multiple hospitalizations)
▸ Acute gouty arthritis
▸ Dehydration
▸ Neurogenic fever
▸ Milk allergy
▸ Behçet's syndrome
▸ Anicteric hepatitis
▸ Cardiovascular
  - Pulmonary embolism
  - Thrombophlebitis
  - Myocardial infarction
▸ Necrotizing lymphadenitis (Kikuchi disease)
▸ Postoperative

Fever with Rash

Causes
▸ Drug hypersensitivity
  - Allopurinol
  - Anticonvulsants
  - Penicillin
  - Sulfonamides
  - Thiazides
▸ Viral infection

- Coxsackie viruses
- Dengue fever
- Ebola virus
- ECHO viruses
- Enterovirus infection
- Erythema infectiosum
- Herpes zoster (VZV)
- Lassa fever
- Measles
- Mononucleosis
- Roseola
- Rubella virus
- Varicella virus (VZV)
- Viral hepatitis
- Yellow fever
▶ Other infections
  - Babesiosis
  - Bacterial endocarditis
  - Brucellosis
  - Listeriosis
  - Lyme disease
  - Meningococcemia
  - Pseudomonas bacteremia
  - Rocky Mountain spotted fever
  - Secondary syphilis
  - Scarlet fever
  - Staphylococcemia
  - Typoid fever
▶ Miscellaneous
  - Serum sickness
  - Erythema multiforme
  - Erythema marginatum
  - Erythema nodosum
  - Systemic lupus erythematosus
  - Dermatomyositis
  - Allergic vasculitis
  - Pityriasis rosea

Fibrin Degradation Products

Fibrin degradation products are formed during the metabolism of fibrinogen and fibrin via plasmin. They are increased in activation of coagulation and hyperfibrinolysis (markedly increased fibrinolysis). See Disseminated Intravascular Coagulation → 104.

Reference range	
fibrin degradation products	< 1 mg/l
D-dimers	20-400 µg/l

Increased
▶ Primary hyperfibrinolysis
  - Contact with body-foreign surfaces
  - Postoperative
  - Release of plasmin from plasminogen-rich organs
    ○ Pancreas
    ○ Prostate
    ○ Lungs
  - Drugs
    ○ Catecholamines
    ○ Vasopressin
▶ Secondary hyperfibrinolysis
  - Disseminated intravascular coagulation
  - Thromboses
  - Venous and arterial thrombotic events
  - Subdural hematomas
  - Pulmonary embolism
  - Fibrinolytic therapy
▶ Miscellaneous
  - Bladder carcinoma
  - Tumor
  - Severe liver disease
  - False positive, if rheumatoid factor (RF) is present

Fibrinogen

Blood clotting factor and acute-phase protein that is formed in the liver. Serious liver parenchyma damage can result in a fibrinogen deficiency due to a synthesis disorder.

Reference range
180-350 mg/dl

Decreased
▶ Disseminated intravascular coagulation

- Loss coagulopathy
  - Ascites
  - Hemodilution
- Primary or secondary fibrinolysis
- Fibrinolytic therapy
  - Streptokinase
  - Urokinase
  - T-PA
- Asparaginase therapy
- Liver failure
- Tumor
  - Prostate carcinoma
  - Pancreas carcinoma
- Hematologic diseases
  - Multiple myeloma
- Hereditary afibrinogenemia or hypofibrinogenemia
- Severe infections
- Cachexia
- Shock
- Newborns
  - Congenital afibrinogenemia

Increased
- Acute infection
- Tissue inflammation or damage
  - Postoperative
- Myocardial infarction
- Drugs
  - Oral contraceptives
- Tumor
- Diabetes mellitus
- Pregnancy

Flank Pain

Side pain

Pain in the side of the trunk between the right or left upper abdomen and the back.. See Abdominal Pain, Acute → 7

Non-urologic
- Spinal arthritis
- Disk disease
- Muscle spasm
- Herpes zoster (shingles)
- Neuralgia

- Retroperitoneal processes
  - Abscess
  - Hematoma
- Appendicitis
- Peritonitis
- Inguinal hernia
- Adnexitis
- Extrauterine pregnancy
- Cholecystolithiasis
- Cholecystitis
- Splenomegaly
- Hepatitis
- Ileus (→ 206)
- Perforation

Urologic
- Infection, inflammation
  - Acute pyelonephritis
  - Kidney abscess
  - Urogenital tuberculosis
  - Echinococcosis
  - Bilharziosis
  - Ormond's disease
- Tumor
  - Renal carcinoma
  - Renal pelvis carcinoma
  - Ureter carcinoma
  - Tumor infiltration (stenosis)
- Injury
  - Renal trauma
  - Ureter ligature, rupture
- Vascular disorders
  - Renal artery embolism, thrombosis
  - Renal artery aneurysm
  - Renal vein stenosis
- Abnormal position
  - Nephroptosis
  - Renal dystopia
- Urolithisasis
  - Renal stone
    - Calculi
    - Nephrolithiasis
  - Nephrocalcinosis
- Miscellaneous
  - Urinary retention
  - Cystic kidneys

- Renal cysts
- Vesicourethral reflux
- Ureterocele
- Calix diverticulum
- Megaureter

Flatulence

Intestinal gas, bloating, belching, meteorism.

Presence of an excessive amount of gas in the stomach and intestines that is passed through the rectum. The sensation of being flatulent also occurs in people with normal amounts of intestinal gas.
Four main sources: swallowed air, CO_2 from H^+ (stomach) and HCO_3^- (pancreas), bacterial carbohydrate production in the colon and gaseous diffusion from the blood into the intestinal lumen.
Symptoms: pressure, fullness, anxiety, discomfort, colicky pains and angina-like symptoms.

Causes

▶ Swallowing air (aerophagia)
  - Improper swallowing while eating
  - Unconscious swallowing of air
  - Activities increasing aerophagia
    ○ Rapid drinking
    ○ Chewing gum
    ○ Cigarette smoking
    ○ Sucking on hard candy
    ○ Drinking carbonated beverages
    ○ Hyperventilation in anxious people
▶ Irritable bowel syndrome
▶ Food increasing bacterial gas production
  - Beans
  - Broccoli
  - Brussels sprouts
  - Cabbage
  - Cauliflower
  - Dark beer
  - Fiber (excessive amounts)
  - Fresh bread
  - Fructose

- Garlic
- Leek
- Onions
- Prunes
- Red wine
- Sorbitol (sugar-free sweetener)
▶ Inappropriate bacterial colonization
▶ Lactase deficiency
▶ Malabsorption
  - Pancreatic insufficiency (exocrine)
  - Gallbladder, bile duct dysfunction
  - Chronic gastritis
▶ Slowing down of gastrointestinal transit
  - Constipation
  - Poor dietary fiber
  - Parasites
  - Inflammatory bowel disease
  - Intestinal obstruction
    ○ Adhesive bands
    ○ Ileus (→ 206)
    ○ Pyloristenosis
    ○ Tumors
    ○ Colon cancer
    ○ Right ventricular failure
    ○ Portal hypertension
  - Diverticulosis, diverticulitis
  - Hypothyroidism
  - Hirschsprung disease
  - Celiac sprue
  - Scleroderma
▶ Drugs
  - Acarbose
  - Antibiotics
  - Chemotherapeutics
  - Narcotics

Flushing

Blushing, hot flashes
Transient erythema, redness of the skin.
Physiologic
▶ Menopausal flushing (drop in estrogens)
▶ Hot beverages
▶ Spicy foods
▶ Extremes of emotion

► Rapid changes in temperature
► High fever

Drugs
► Alcohol
  • Alcohol abuse
  • Alcohol intolerance (in Asians)
  • Alcohol while taking chlorpromazine or disulfiram
► Alpha-methyldopa (withdrawal)
► Aspirin
► Bromocriptine
► Calcitonin
► Clonidine (withdrawal)
► Diltiazem
► Disulfiram (alcohol withdrawal) reaction
  • Griseofulvin
  • Flagyl
  • Chlorpropamide
  • Chloral hydrate
► Hydralazine
► Isoniazid
► Levodopa
► Niacin
► Nifedipine
► Nitrates
► MAO inhibitor while taking tyramine (beer, cheese)

Miscellaneous disorders
► Carcinoid syndrome
► Mastocytosis
► Basophil chronic granulocytic leukemia
► Pheochromocytoma
► Medullary carcinoma of the thyroid
► VIPoma
► WDHA (diarrhea, hypokalemia, achlorhydria)
► Renal carcinoma
► Hypertonic crisis
► Thyrotoxicosis
► Quincke's edema
► Rosacea
► Trigeminal neuralgia
► Erythromelalgia
► Vegetative dystonia

Folic Acid Deficiency

Deficiency of pteroylglutaminic acid, vitamin M

Part of the vitamin B complex, necessary for normal production of red blood cells.

Reference range	
folic acid in serum/ plasma deficiency	3.6–15 mg/dl
adequate folic acid supply	> 4 µg/l
Erythrocyte folic acid	120–800 µg/l

Inadequate Folate intake
► Alcohol abuse
► Advanced age
► Vegetarians
► Malnutrition
► Malabsorption
► Ulcerative colitis
► Crohn's disease
► Celiac disease
► Postoperative (resection)

Increased Folate utilization
► Malignancy
  • Leukemias
  • Solid tumors
► Increased erythropoiesis
  • Chronic blood loss
  • Chronic hemolytic anemia
  • Macrocytic anemia
  • Other anemias
► Hyperthyroidism
► Pregnancy
► Lactation
► Childhood
► Psoriasis

Miscellaneous
► Hematological diseases
► Enzyme defects
► Congenital impairment of folic acid metabolism

Drugs
► Alcohol
► Chemotherapeutics

▶ Contraceptives
▶ Methotrexate
▶ Pentamidine
▶ Phenobarbitol
▶ Phenytoin
▶ Primidone
▶ Pyrimethamine
▶ Sulfamethoxazole
▶ Sulfasalazine
▶ Triamterene
▶ Trimethoprim

Follicle stimulating hormone
See Gonadotropins → 158

FSH, See Gonadotropins → 158

Fulminant hepatic failure
See Hepatic Failure, Fulminant → 179

FUO, See Fever of Unknown Origin → 143

Gait Abnormalities

Limp
Abnormalities in the manner of walking.
See Ataxia → 46
Neurologic
▶ Parkinsonism
▶ Infection
 • Tabes dorsalis
 • Poliomyelitis
 • Encephalitis
 • Meningitis
▶ Multiple sclerosis
▶ Ataxia
 • Friedreich's ataxia
 • Sensory ataxia
▶ Dystonia
▶ Neuromuscular disorders
▶ Cerebrovascular disease
▶ Cerebral palsy
▶ Cerebellar lesions
 • Tumor

 • Infarction
▶ Polyneuropathy
▶ Hydrocephalus
Skeletal disorder
▶ Joint infection
 • Septic arthritis
 • Osteomyelitis
 • Viral arthritis
▶ Degenerative joint disease
 • Hips
 • Back
 • Knees
 • Osteochondritis dissecans
 • Chondromalacia patellae
▶ Trauma to
 • Extremities
 • Hips
 • Vertebral disc
▶ Chondrodystrophia
▶ Damage of the symphysis
▶ Discitis
▶ Periostitis
▶ Epiphysial aseptic necrosis
 • Osgood-Schlatter disease
 • Legg-Calvé-Perthes disease
▶ Neoplasm
 • Local neoplasm
 • Metastases
▶ Foot pain
 • Foreign body in shoe
 • Poorly fitting shoes
 • Splinter in foot
 • Leg length discrepancy
Miscellaneous
▶ Metabolic
 • Osteomalacia
 • Rickets
▶ Hematologic
 • Sickle cell disease
 • Hemophilia
▶ Abdominal pain (→ 7)
 • Appendicitis
 • Hernias
 • Testicular torsion
▶ Drugs

G

- Alcoholism
- Benzodiazepines
▶ Psychologic
- Somatization syndrome

Galactorrhea

Spontaneous flow of milk from the nipple at a time other than during nursing, mostly due to hyperprolactinemia of different causes.

Causes

▶ Hyperprolactinemia ((→ 293))
▶ Normoprolactinemic galactorrhoea
- Local breast stimulation/irritation
  ○ Inflammation
  ○ Trauma
- Oral contraceptives
- Recently preceded pregnancy
- Idiopathic (with menses)
▶ Pseudogalactorrhea
- Intramammary lesion
  ○ Fibrocystic disease
  ○ Intraductal papilloma
  ○ Malignant neoplasm

Gamma globulins
See Protein in the Serum → 296

Gamma–Glutamyl Transpeptidase
GGTP, GTP, GGT

Enzyme that mainly occurs on the surface of membranes with high excretory or absorbent function (e.g. the bile duct epithelial tissues, the brush border membrane of small intestine cells, renal tubules or efferent ducts of the pancreas). The enzyme transfers glutamyl rests from glutathione onto amino acids and peptides. The organ with the greatest amount of the enzyme is the liver, which is mostly responsible for increases of the γ-GT. The γ-GT is one of the most sensitive indicators for liver and bile passage diseases. An increase in the γ-GT with a simultaneous increase of the liver specific enzymes like GPT or GLDH almost always indicates liver damage. Causes of an isolated increase of the γ-GT can be a fatty liver, subclinical stasis of the bile flow, chronic liver stasis with heart failure or alcohol abuse. The height of the quotient γ-GT /GPT can make differential diagnostic statements regarding the cause of a hepatopathy. Indication in liver diseases, cholestasis, differential diagnosis of hepatopathies and as progress assessment.

Reference range	
Women:	< 18 U/l
Men:	< 28 U/l
Children under 12 months	< 91 U/l

Increased

▶ Hepatic
- Cholestasis
- Jaundice
- Hepatic tumor or metastasis
- Fatty liver
- Cirrhosis
- Alcohol ingestion
- Hepatitis
- Hepatic necrosis
- Vascular
  ○ Right-ventricular failure with congested liver
  ○ Portal vein thrombosis
- Hepatotoxic drugs
  ○ Halothan
  ○ Phenothiazine
  ○ Steroids
  ○ Streptokinase
  ○ Sulfonyl ureas
  ○ Tetracycline
  ○ Thiazide diuretics
  ○ Thyroid depressants
  ○ Tuberculostatics (INH)
▶ Extrahepatic
- Inflammation

- Chronic inflammatory bowel diseases
- Pancreatitis
- Acute nephritis
- Endocrine, metabolic
  - Porphyria
  - Obesity
  - Diabetes mellitus
  - Disorders of the lipid metabolism
  - Hyperthyroidism
- Infection
  - Pneumonia
  - Infectious mononucleosis (EBV)
  - Cytomegalovirus infections
- Malignant disease
  - Cancer of the pancreas
  - Prostate carcinoma
  - Brain tumor
- Myocardial infarction

Gastric Emptying, Delayed

Gastric outlet obstruction (mechanical)
▶ Peptic ulcer disease
  - Pyloric channel ulcer
  - Ulcers in first portion of duodenum
▶ Gastric polyps
▶ Ingestion of caustics
▶ Pyloric stenosis (1:750 births)
▶ Congenital duodenal webs
▶ Gallstone obstruction (Bouveret syndrome)
▶ Pancreatic pseudocysts
▶ Bezoars
▶ Neoplasm
  - Pancreatic cancer
  - Ampullary cancer
  - Duodenal cancer
  - Cholangiocarcinomas
  - Gastric cancer
  - Metastases

Functional obstruction (gastroparesis)
▶ Drugs
  - Anticholinergics
  - Beta-adrenergics
  - Opiates
▶ Electrolyte disorder
  - Hypokalemia
  - Hypomagnesemia
▶ Metabolic
  - Diabetes mellitus
  - Hypoparathyroidism
  - Hypothyroidism
  - Pregnancy
  - Vagotomy
▶ Neuromuscular
  - Myotonic dystrophy
  - Autonomic neuropathy
  - Scleroderma
  - Polymyositis
▶ Psychiatric
  - Anorexia nervosa
  - Psychogenic vomiting
  - Idiopathic
▶ Viral infection
▶ Brainstem tumors
▶ GERD

Gastric ulcer
See Peptic Ulcer Disease → 279

Gastrin
Hormone secreted in the pyloric-antral mucosa of the stomach stimulating the secretion of HCl by parietal cells.

Reference range
40–200 pg/ml
Increased
▶ Zollinger-Ellison syndrome (gastrinoma)
▶ Hyperparathyroidism
▶ Pernicious anemia
▶ Retained gastric antrum
▶ Chronic atrophic gastritis
▶ Pyloric obstruction
▶ Gastric neoplasm
▶ Antral G cell hyperfunction
▶ Duodenal ulcer
▶ Vagotomy
▶ Helicobacter pylori gastritis

▸ Gastrinoma in MEN
▸ Chronic renal failure
▸ Drugs
  • Proton pump inhibitors
    ○ Omeprazole
    ○ Lansoprazole
  • H_2 blockers

Gastritis

Series of conditions that present with inflammation of the gastric mucosa or inner lining of the stomach. Symptoms: indigestion, heartburn, nausea, loss of appetite, abdominal pain (often worse after eating) and gastrointestinal bleeding.

Erosive/hemorrhagic gastritis
▸ Drugs, toxins
  • Alcohol
  • Aspirin
  • NSAIDs
▸ Severe stress
  • Burns
  • Sepsis
  • Trauma
  • Surgery
  • Shock
  • Respiratory failure
  • Liver failure
  • Renal failure

Chronic gastritis
▸ Gastritis in pernicious anemia (Type A gastritis, antibodies to parietal cells, body predominant)
▸ Helicobacter pylori associated (Type B gastritis, antral-predominant)

Uncommon specific gastritis syndromes
▸ Ménétrier's disease
▸ Eosinophilic gastritis
▸ Radiation
▸ Alcoholic gastropathy
▸ Granulomatous gastritis
  • Tuberculosis
  • Syphilis
  • Sarcoidosis
  • Crohn's disease
▸ Infection
  • CMV in HIV
  • Bacterial infections (submucosa)
  • Candida
▸ Lymphocytic gastritis
▸ Corrosive gastritis

Miscellaneous/DDx
▸ Peptic ulcer
▸ Gastroduodenal ulcer
▸ Perforated ulcer
▸ Gastric carcinoma
▸ Diseases of the biliary system
▸ Intoxications
▸ Functional dyspepsia
▸ Pancreatitis
▸ Pancreas carcinoma
▸ Reflux esophagitis
▸ (Ruptured) aortic aneurysm
▸ Volvulus
▸ Esophageal varices
▸ Mallory-Weiss tear
▸ Gastrinoma (Zollinger-Ellison syndrome)

Gastroenteritis, See Diarrhea → 101

Gastrointestinal Bleeding

Presence of blood or hemoglobin in the stool. Signs of a gastrointestinal bleeding can be vomiting of blood (hematemesis), tarry stools (melena) or red bloody stools (hematochezia). See Occult Blood → 262

Main causes
▸ Hemorrhoid bleeding
▸ Diverticula
▸ Tumors or polyps
▸ Ulcerative diseases
▸ Inflammatory colonic diseases
▸ Ischemic colonic diseases

Upper gastrointestinal bleeding
Hemorrhage above the duodenojejunal flexure
▸ Ulcer (50 %)

- Esophageal
- Gastrial
- Duodenal
- Stomal
- Erosion (20 %)
  - Lower esophagus
  - Stomach
  - Duodenum
- Vascular lesions
  - Varices (10 %)
    - Esophageal
    - Gastric
    - Duodenal
  - Ischemic enteritis
  - Angiodysplasia
  - Arteriovenous malformations
  - Vasculitis
    - Henoch-Schönlein purpura
    - Hemolytic uremic syndrome
    - Systemic lupus erythematosus
    - Polyarteritis nodosa
    - Rheumatoid vasculitis
- Mallory-Weiss tear (5 %)
- Neoplasms (3%)
  - Esophageal carcinoma
  - Gastric carcinoma
  - Small-bowel carcinoma
  - Upper gastrointestinal polypa
  - Lymphoma
  - Kaposi′s sarcoma
  - Carcinoid tumor
- Infection
  - Bacterial
    - Heliobacter pylori
  - Viral
    - CMV
    - Herpes
- Hemorrhagic diathesis
  - Coagulopathies
  - Anticoagulant therapie
- Rare causes
  - Epistaxis
  - Osler's disease
  - Metastatic tumor
  - Uremia

- Gastrointestinal foreign bodies
- Volvolus

Lower gastrointestinal bleeding
- Small bowel hemorrhages
  - Inflammatory bowel disease
  - Infections
    - Sallmonella
    - Shigella
    - Campylobacter
    - Vibrio
    - Ameba
    - Pseudomembranous colitis
  - Small bowel tumor
  - Vascular lesions
    - Angiodysplasia
    - Angioma
    - Teleangiectasia
    - Varices
    - Vasculitis′
    - Mesenteric infarction
  - Mechanical causes
    - Strangulation
    - Invagination
    - Meckel's diverticulum
    - Trauma
    - Foreign body
    - Postoperative stitching
- Colonorrhagies
  - Diverticulosis
  - Chronic inflammatory intestinal diseases
    - *Ulcerative colitis*
    - *Crohn′s disease*
    - *Radiation colitis*
    - *Behçet's syndrome*
  - Neoplasms
    - Colon polyps
    - Colorectal carcinoma
    - Juvenile polyposis
    - Familial adenomatous polyposis
    - Peutz-Jeghers syndrome
    - Gardner′s syndrom
    - Lymphomas
    - Carcinoid tumors
  - Vascular lesions

- Mechanical causes
- ▶ Colorectal hemorrhage
  - Hemorrhoids
  - Anal fissure
  - Anorectal injuries
  - Secondary bleeding after
    - ∘ Polypectomy
    - ∘ Biopsy
    - ∘ Hemorrhoidal sclerotherapy or ligature
  - Carcinoma
  - Proctitis
  - Radiation proctitis
  - Ulcer in the area of the rectum
    - ∘ Especially in advanced renal failure
  - Prolaps of the rectum

Genital hemorrhage
See Bleeding, Genital → 55

Genital Pain
Genital Sores
Pain in the area of vulva, vagina, scrotum, penis. See Dyspareunia → 109
See Vaginal Discharge → 372
See Vulvitis → 381
See Vulvar Pruritus → 380
See Scrotal Pain → 327
See Priapism → 292

Genital Ulcer
See Sexually Transmitted Diseases → 329
Common causes
- ▶ Syphilis (early stage)
- ◀ Chancroid (Haemophilus ducreyi)
- ▶ Herpes genitalis
- ▶ Pyoderma
Rare causes
- ▶ Cytomegalovirus infection
- ▶ Yeast
- ▶ Granuloma inguinale
- ▶ Lymphogranuloma venereum
- ▶ Scabies

- ▶ Genital trauma
- ▶ Fixed drug eruption
- ▶ Excoriations
- ▶ Langerhans cell histiocytosis
- ▶ Penis carcinoma

GGT, See Gamma-Glutamyl Transpeptidase → 150

GH, See Growth Hormone → 159

Glasgow Coma Scale
Classification of comatose states

Eye opening	spontaneous	4
	to verbal command	3
	to pain	2
	none	1
Best verbal response	oriented	5
	confused	4
	inappropriate words	3
	incompreh. sounds	2
	none	1
Best motor response	obeys commands	6
	localizes pain	5
	withdraws from pain	4
	flexion to pain	3
	extension to pain	2
	none	1
GCS-Score		**3–15**

GCS > 8 = Somnolent		
>12	mild	
12–9	moderate	
somnolence: sleepy, easy to wake		
stupor: hypnoid, hard to awake		
GCS < 8 = Unconscious		
8–7	coma grade I	light coma
6–5	coma grade II	
4	coma grade III	deep coma
3	coma grade IV	

Globulins, See Protein in the Serum → 296

Glaucoma

Increased intraocular pressure, with excavation and atrophy of the optic nerve and defects in the field of vision.

Primary glaucoma
▶ Open angle glaucoma (outflow blocked by microscopic outflow changes)
▶ Narrow angle glaucoma (outflow tract blocked by base of iris)

Secondary glaucoma
▶ Drugs that increase IOP in predisposed
  • Corticosteroids
  • Adrenergics, anticholinergics
    ○ Cold medications
    ○ Antidepressants
    ○ Antidiarrheals

Glomerulonephritis
See Nephrotic Syndrome → 256

Glossitis

Local causes
▶ Infections
  • Bacterial
  • Viral
    ○ Oral herpes simplex
▶ Mechanical irritation/injury
  • Burns
  • Rough edges of teeth
  • Dental caries
  • Dental prosthesis
  • Trauma
▶ Irritants
  • Cigarette smoking
  • Alcohol
  • Hot foods
  • Spices
▶ Allergic reaction
  • Toothpaste
  • Mouthwash

• Breath fresheners
• Others

Systemic causes
▶ Iron deficiency anemia
▶ Vitamin B_{12} deficiencies
  • Pernicious anemia
▶ Other vitamin B deficiencies
▶ Oral lichen planus
▶ Erythema multiform
▶ Aphthous ulcers
▶ Pemphigus vulgaris
▶ Syphilis
▶ Inherited glossitis

Atrophic glossitis
▶ Anemia
  • Folic acid deficiency
  • Vitamin B_{12} deficiency
  • Iron deficiency anemia
▶ Other vitamin deficiencies
  • Pyridoxine deficiency
  • Riboflavin deficiency
  • Niacin deficiency
▶ Chemotherapeutics

Glucose, See Hyperglycemia → 189
See Hypoglycemia → 199
See Glucosuria → 155
See HbA1, HbA1c → 162

Glucosuria

Urine sugar, urine glucose
Urinary excretion of glucose. The renal threshold for glucose is approximately 160 to 190mg/dl of blood. Physiologically glucose does not appear in the urine until the blood glucose rises above this level.
See Hyperglycemia → 189
See Hypoglycemia → 199
See HbA1, HbA1c → 162

Hyperglycemia
▶ Diabetes mellitus
▶ Excessive enteral sugar supply

Renal disorder
▶ Fanconi's syndrome
▶ Toxic nephropathy
  • Lead intoxication
  • Mercury intoxication
  • Tetracycline
▶ Inflammatory renal disease
  • Acute glomerulonephritis
  • Nephrosis
▶ Nephrotic syndrome
▶ Increased GFR without tubular damage

Drugs, toxins
▶ Benzothiazine
▶ Glucocorticoids/steroids
▶ Lead intoxication
▶ Mercury intoxication
▶ Thyroxin

Miscellaneous
▶ Pancreatitis
▶ Pregnancy glucosuria
▶ Hyperthyroidism
▶ Cushing's disease
▶ Severe hepatopathy
▶ Intracranial causes
  • Increased intracranial pressure
  • Brain tumor
  • Encephalitis
  • Trauma
▶ Benign glucosuria
▶ Pentosuria
▶ Fructosemia
▶ Galactosemia
▶ Starvation

False positive glucosuria
▶ Ascorbic acid
▶ Cephalosporins
▶ Nalidixic acid
▶ Probenacid

Glutamate-Oxalacetate-
aminotransferase
See Aminotransferases → 23

Glutamate-Pyruvate-aminotransferase
See Aminotransferases → 23

Goiter

Struma
Enlargement of the thyroid gland, not due to neoplasm, occurring endemically in certain regions. Often asymptomatic, sometimes thyroid sensitive to touch, dyspnea, dysphagia and/or cough. Epidemiology: Endemic in areas distant from sea (e.g. mountains). Goiter is related to deficient iodine intake. Often occurs before puberty. Sporadic form much more common in women (8:1); adolescent girls, pregnant, lactating or menopausal women.

Diffuse goiter (euthyroid or hypothyroid)
▶ Iodine deficiency (endemic goiter)
▶ Idiopathic (sporadic)
  • Puberty
  • Pregnancy
  • Menopause
▶ Exposure to thyroid growth factor/ Goitrogens
  • Excess TSH
  • Defects in thyroid hormone synthesis
  • Chemicals
    ◦ Cobalt
    ◦ Flavonoids
    ◦ Pyridines
    ◦ Biphenyls
    ◦ Phtalate esters and metabolites
    ◦ Phenol derivates
    ◦ Polycyclic aromatic hydrocarbons
  • Calcium and fluorides in water
  • Goitrogenic vegetable
    ◦ Bamboo shoots
    ◦ Broccoli
    ◦ Cabbage
    ◦ Cassava
    ◦ Cauliflower

- ○ Brussels sprouts
- ○ Turnips
- Drugs
  - ○ Amiodarone
  - ○ Antithyroid drugs
    - – *Carbimazole*
    - – *Methimazole*
    - – *Propylthiouracil*
  - ○ Iodide excess
  - ○ Aminoglutethimide
  - ○ Barbiturates
  - ○ Chloroquine
  - ○ Ethionamide
  - ○ Hydantoins
  - ○ Lithium
  - ○ Nitrates
  - ○ Paraaminobenzoic acid
  - ○ Phenylbutazone
  - ○ Sulfonamides
  - ○ Sulfonyl ureas
  - ○ Iopanoic acid
  - ○ Tumor necrosis factor alpha
- ▶ Goiter with malfunction
- Hypothyroidism
- Hyperthyroidism
  - ○ Thyroid gland autonomy
  - ○ Grave's disease
- Thyroiditis (acute, subacute, chronic)
- ▶ Immunogenic goiter
- Hashimoto's thyroiditis
- Grave's disease
- ▶ Cystic goiter
- ▶ Neoplastic
- Benign and malignant thyroid gland tumors
- Metastases of extrathyroidal tumors
- ▶ Uninodular/multinodular goiter
- Adenoma
- Tumoral tissue
  - ○ Parathyroid
  - ○ Thymic
- Focal thyroiditis
- Colloid nodule
- Neoplastic
  - ○ Medullary carcinoma

- ○ Papillary carcinoma
- ○ Mixed papillary-follicular carcinoma
- ○ Squamous cell carcinoma
- ○ Anaplstic carcinoma
- ○ Follicular carcinoma
- ○ Carcinosarcoma
- ○ Lymphoma
- ○ Sarcoma
- Different causes
  - ○ Cyst
  - ○ Hematoma
  - ○ Multiple adenomas
  - ○ Nontoxic nodular goiter
  - ○ Toxic multinodular goiter
  - ○ Compensatory hyperplasia after hemithyroidectomy
  - ○ Focal granulomatous disease
    - – *Sarcoidosis*
- ▶ Infiltration
- Amyloidosis
- Sarcoidosis
- Thyreoiditis
  - ○ Acute
  - ○ Hashimoto
  - ○ Silent (painless)
  - ○ Riedel
  - ○ DeQuervain
- ▶ Impairment of the thyroid hormone synthesis/enzyme defect
- ▶ Paraneoplastic production of TSH
- ▶ Acromegaly
- ▶ Resistance to thyroid hormone
- ▶ Extrathyroidal/ systemic disease
- Sarcoidosis
- Lymphoma
- Amyloidosis
- Parasite
- ▶ Neonatal
- Maternal iodine therapy
- Maternal antithyroid drug therapy
- ▶ Selenium deficiency
- ▶ Insulin-like growth factor
- ▶ Thyroid growth immunoglobulines

G

Hyperthyroid
▶ Neoplasic
  • Choriocarcinoma
  • Hydatiforme mole
  • Embrional cell carcinoma of the testis
▶ Gestational stimulation by human chorionic gonadotropin
▶ Grave´s disease
▶ Inappropriate TSH secretion
  • Pituitary resistence to thyroid hormone
  • TSH-secreting pituitary hormone
  • Thyreoiditis

Other lesions enlarging the thyroid gland
▶ Cystic hygroma
▶ Thyroglossal duct cyst
▶ Carotic aneurysm
▶ Dermoid
▶ Hemangioma
▶ Lipoma
▶ Lymph node
▶ Prarthyroid adenoma
▶ Teratoma

Gonadotropins

Hormone capable of promoting gonadal growth and function. FSH and LH are gonadotropins released by the anterior pituitary gland in response to pulsatile gonadotropin-releasing hormone stimulation. Gonadotropins are responsible in females for the early growth of ovarian follicles. In males, together with testosterone, they stimulate Sertoli cells to release the hormone inhibin and induces sperm production. Inhibin and testosterone reduce gonadotropin-releasing hormone (and hence gonadotropin) secretion via negative feedback.

Reference range in grown-up women:	
Follicle phase	
LH	1.8-13.4 mU/ml
FSH	3-12 mU/ml
Periovulatory phase	
LH	15.6-78.9 mU/ml
FSH	8-22 mU/ml
Luteal phase	
LH	0.7-19.4 mU/ml
FSH	2-12 mU/ml
Postmenopausal	
LH	> 50 mU/ml
FSH	12-30 mU/ml
Reference range in men	
LH	1.5-9.2 mU/ml
FSH	1-14 mU/ml

Increase of FSH and LH
▶ Primary hypogonadism
▶ Turner's syndrome
▶ Swyer-James syndrome
▶ Gonadal dysgenesis (45X0, 46XYMosaic)
▶ Climacterium praecox
▶ Chemotherapeutic therapy
▶ After radiation therapy
▶ During menopause or postmenopausal

Reduced FSH and LH
▶ Secondary hypergonadism
▶ Anorexia nervosa
▶ Traumatic or tumorous damage of the pituitary or the hypothalamus
▶ Hyperprolactinemia
▶ progestogen negative amenorrhea

Reduced FSH/LH quotient
▶ Polycystic ovary syndrome
▶ Hyperandrogenic ovarial insufficiency

Gout, See Uric Acid → 364

GPT, See Aminotransferases → 23

Granular casts, See Cylindruria → 92

Growth Failure

Microplasia, dwarfism, stunted growth
Slow growth velocity.
Causes
▶ Familial short stature
▶ Constitutional delay
▶ Malnutrition
▶ Systemic
  • Microcephaly
  • Cyanotic heart disease
  • Gluten enteropathy
  • Ulcerative colitis
  • Crohn disease
  • Renal tubular acidosis
  • Cystic fibrosis
  • Dermatomyositis
  • Psychosocial dwarfism
▶ Chromosomal abnormalities
  • Turner syndrome
  • Down syndrome (trisomy 21)
▶ Other congenital syndromes
  • Noonan syndrome
  • Russell-Silver syndrome
  • Prader-Willi syndrome.
▶ Intrauterine growth retardation
▶ Bone and cartilage disorders
  • Achondroplasia
  • Hypochondroplasia
▶ Endocrine causes
  • Hypothyroidism
  • Growth hormone deficiency
  • Growth hormone insensitivity (IGF-1 deficiency)
  • Glucocorticoid excess
    ∘ Cushing syndrome
    ∘ Cushing disease
  • Androgen excess
    ∘ Exogenous androgen
    ∘ Precocious puberty
    ∘ Congenital adrenal hyperplasia

Growth Hormone

Somatotropin, pituitary growth hormone, somatotropic hormone, STH, human growth hormone (hGH)
Protein hormone of the anterior lobe of the pituitary, produced by the acidophil cells, promoting body growth, fat mobilization, and inhibition of glucose utilization.

Reference range	
Prepuberty	0–8 ng/ml (fasting , 8 o'clock in the morning)
Postpuberty	< 5 ng/ml

Decreased
▶ Idiopathic
▶ Organic
  • Brain tumors
    ∘ Craniopharyngioma
  • CNS radiation
  • CNS surgery
  • Anatomical abnormalities
    ∘ Empty sella syndrome
    ∘ Septooptic dysplasia
▶ Genetic
Increased (gigantism, acromegaly)
▶ Primary pituitary GH excess
  • Benign pituitary tumor
▶ Secondary GH excess
  • Increased secretion of GHRH
    ∘ Intracranial source
    ∘ Ectopic source
  • Dysregulation of hypothalamic-pituitary-GH axis

Gums, Bleeding

Bleeding gingiva
Inflammation
▶ Gingivitis

- Poor oral hygiene
- Inadequate plaque removal
- Tartar
▶ Periodontitis

Oral trauma
▶ Toothbrush
▶ Flossing
▶ New dentures

Drugs
▶ Anticoagulants
▶ Aspirin

Hematologic
▶ Leukemia
▶ Coagulopathy
▶ Thrombocytopenia
▶ Hemorrhagic diathesis

Miscellaneous
▶ Epulis
▶ Infection
▶ Vitamin C deficiency
▶ Vitamin K deficiency
▶ Pregnancy (hormonal changes)

Gums, Hypertrophic
Hypertrophic gingiva
Causes
▶ Hormones
  • Puberty
  • Pregnancy
  • Menstruation
▶ Aphthous stomatitis
▶ Acute leukemia
▶ Drugs
  • Hydantoin

Gynecomastia
Breast swelling in men
Benign enlargement of the male breast resulting from proliferation of the glandular component of the breast.
Physiologic
▶ Gynecomastia in the newborn (estrogens of mother)

▶ Benign gynecomastia of adolescence
▶ Familial gynecomastia
▶ Gynecomastia of aging

Drugs
▶ Alcohol
▶ Anabolics
▶ Chemotherapeutics
▶ Chlorpromazine
▶ Cimetidine
▶ Clomiphene
▶ Diazepam
▶ Digitalis
▶ Estrogens (also topical estrogens)
▶ Etomidate
▶ Finasteride
▶ Flutamide
▶ HCG therapy
▶ Illicit drugs
  • Tamoxifen (bodybuilder)
  • Anabolic steroids (bodybuilder)
  • Heroin
  • Marijuana
▶ Isoniazid
▶ Ketoconazole
▶ Methadone
▶ Methyldopa
▶ Metoclopramid
▶ Metronidazole
▶ Nifedipine
▶ Omeprazole
▶ Penicillamine
▶ Phenothiazine
▶ Spironolactone
▶ Tricyclic antidepressants
▶ Verapamil

Decreased Testosterone
▶ Klinefelter syndrome
▶ Congenital anorchia
▶ Testicular trauma
▶ Torsion of testes
▶ Viral orchitis
▶ Kallman syndrome
▶ Hypopituitarism (pituitary tumors)
▶ Renal failure
▶ Androgen-insensitivity syndrome

▶ Five alpha-reductase deficiency syndrome

Increased Estrogens
▶ Testicular tumors
▶ Ectopic production of hCG
  • Lung carcinoma
  • Kidney carcinoma
  • Stomach cancer
  • Liver cancer
  • Other GI tract carcinoma
  • Extragonadal germ cell tumors
▶ Increased peripheral conversion
  • Chronic liver disease
  • Malnutrition
  • Hyperthyroidism
  • Adrenal tumors
  • Familial gynecomastia

Hyperprolactinemia (→ 293)

Hair loss, See Alopecia → 19

Halitosis
See Bad breath, fetor oris, halitosis, ozostomia, stomatodysodia. → 59

Hand Contracture
Finger contracture
Muscle shortening due to tonic spasm or fibrosis, or to loss of muscular balance.
Causes
▶ Injury (including burns)
▶ Immobilization
▶ Nerve damage, degeneration
▶ Inherited disorders (e.g. muscular dystrophy)
Types/DDx
▶ Dupuytren's contracture
▶ Alcoholic cirrhosis
▶ Claw hand
▶ Foot drop
▶ Wrist drop
▶ Volkmann's contracture
▶ Becker's muscular dystrophy
▶ Cerebral palsy
▶ Duchenne's muscular dystrophy
▶ Scleroderma
▶ Hand callosity
▶ Stenosing tendovaginitis
▶ Rheumatoid arthritis
▶ Acrosclerosis
▶ Ulnar lesion
▶ Gout
▶ Raynaud's disease
▶ Hurler's syndrome

Haptoglobin
Acute-phase reactant.

Reference range

50–220 mg/dl
See Hemopexin → 175

Increased
▶ Inflammation (acute-phase reactant)
▶ Infection (acute-phase reactant)
▶ Neoplasm
  • Malignant tumor
  • Hodgkin's lymphoma
  • Multiple myeloma
▶ Necroses
▶ Collagen-vascular disease
▶ Obstructive liver disease
▶ Drugs
  • Androgens
▶ Miscellaneous
  • Iron deficiency anemia
  • Nephrotic syndrome
  • Amyloidosis

Decreased
▶ Hemolysis
  • Intravascular
  • Extravascular
▶ Megaloblastic anemia
▶ Severe liver disease
▶ Large hematomas
▶ Infection
  • Epstein-Barr virus (EBV)
  • Cytomegalovirus
▶ Drugs

H

- Oral contraceptives
► Miscellaneous
  - Malabsorption
  - Congenital haptoglobin decrease

HbA1, HbA1c

Retrospective index of glucose control. Measurement of the number of glucose molecules, that were attached to hemoglobin by spontaneous, non-enzymatic and irreversible glycosylation (glycosylated hemoglobin). The extent depends on the duration of the blood sugar level increase and also on the lifecycle of hemoglobin. HbA1c (hemoglobin A1c or glycosylated hemoglobin) reveals average blood glucose over a period of two to three months. HbA1c test results are expressed as a percentage, with 4 to 6 % considered normal.

Reference range for diabetics
HbA1c levels of 7.0% or below

Increased
► Diabetes mellitus

HCG. See Human Chorionic Gonadotropin (HCG) → 185

HDL Cholesterol

See Cholesterol → 77 cholesterol
See Hypercholesterolemia → 188
See Cholesterol hyperlipidemia → 188
See Coronary Risk Factor → 66
See LDL Cholesterol → 218
Positive cardiac risk factor (atherogenic) if: HDL < 35 or total cholesterol to HDL ratio in men > 5.0, in women > 4.5.
Negative cardiac risk factor (protective) if: HDL > 60

Increased
► Drugs
  - Exogenous estrogens

  - Gemfibrozil
  - Niacin
► Moderate alcohol intake (1 oz/day)
► Regular aerobic exercise
► Weight loss (for obese patients)
  - HDL increases 2 mg/dl for each 4.5 kg of weight loss

Decreased
► Diabetes mellitus
► Menopause
► Obesity
► Puberty in males
► Uremia
► Apolipoprotein deficiency
► Liver disease
► Tangier disease
► Drugs, toxins
  - Anabolic steroids
  - Cigarette smoking
  - Probucol
  - Progestins

Headache
Prosopalgia

Most common pain symptom. Approximately every 10th patient consults a physician because of headaches. The majority of patients suffer from tension, vasomotoric or psychogenic headaches. Other common causes of headache include migraine, trigeminal neuralgia and cluster headaches.

Pain history
► Onset
► Constant
► Intermittent
► Increasing
► Decreasing
► Localization
► Associated autonomic symptoms
► Associated ocular symptoms
► Drugs/intoxication
► Family history

Neurologic and general medical

examination
- Tension headache
- Vasomotor headache
- Cervical spine syndrome
- Migraine
- Cluster headache
- Intracranial infections
  - Meningitis
  - Meningoencephalitis
  - Cerebral abscess
- Neuralgia
  - Trigeminal neuralgia
- Neuritis
- Hypertensive headache
- Headache with:
  - Hypotension
  - CHD
  - Heart failure
- Intracerebral hemorrhage/ cerebrovascular insult
- Arteritis temporalis
- Intracranial pressure
- Cerebrospinal pressure
- Spondylosis
- Cranial pain
  - Paget's disease
- Idiopathic headache

ENT examination
- Otologic headache
- Glossopharyngeal neuralgia
- Sinusitis
- Otitis
- Mastoiditis
- Abscess
- Tumor in the epipharyngeal and pharyngeal region
- Trigeminal neuralgia
- Herpes zoster
- Costen's syndrome

Eye examination
- Glaucoma
- Conjunctivitis
- Stye
- Tumor
- Abscess

- Herpes zoster
- Refractive abnormality

Dental examination
- Cavities
- Parodontitis
- Faulty jaw position
- Pulpitis
- Abscess
- Tumor

Laboratory chemical analysis
- Infection
- Intoxication
- Hematologic disease
- Uremia
- Arteritis temporalis
- Hyponatremia
- Hypoglycemia
- CSF puncture
  - Meningoencephalitis
  - Hemorrhage

Technical examinations
- CT/MRI
  - Cerebral infarction
  - Hemorrhage
  - Hematoma
  - Intracerebral aneurisms
  - Venous sinus thrombosis
  - Tumor
  - Abscess
  - Hydrocephalus
  - Changes in the nasal sinus region
- Doppler ultrasound examination
  - Vascular occlusion
  - Angiospasm
- Cervical spine x-ray
  - Fractures
  - Degenerative changes
  - Abnormality
- Skull x-ray
  - Fracture
  - Sinusitis
  - Calcification
  - Tumour
  - Deformations
- Angiography

- Angiostenosis
- Vascular abnormality
- Vascular spasm

Peracute, sudden headache
► Arteriovenous malformation
► Aneurysma (with or without hemorrhage)
► Subarachnoid hemorrhage
► Epidural hemorrhage
► Brain hemorrhage
► Impaired CSF drainage
► Acute glaucoma
► Meningitis
► Acute viral infection
► Hypertensive encephalopathy
► Sunstroke
► Cerebral trauma
► Hypoglycemia
► Acute sinusitis
► Initial manifestation of a persistent headache

Subacute, progredient headache
► Subdural hematoma
► Meningeal irritation
  • Infection
  • Carcinomatous infiltration
  • Intrathecal injection
► Meningoencephalitis
► Hypertensive crisis
► Brain abscess
► Sinus thrombosis
► Vasculitis
  • Temporal arteritis
  • Polyarteritis nodosa
  • Lupus
► Metabolic disorder
► Post-lumbar puncture
► Sunstroke
► Intracranial tumors

Subacute headache of several hours' duration
► Noise pollution
► Alcohol abuse
► Cigarette smoking
► Nitrite-containing drugs

Chronic progredient headache
► Intracranial tumors
► Pseudotumor cerebri
► Chronic subdural hematoma
► Meningitis
► Meningoencephalitis
► Ocular diseases
  • Inflammations
  • Trauma
  • Increased intraocular pressure
  • Poor refraction
► Dental diseases
  • Infections
  • Trauma
  • Temporomandibular joint malocclusion

Diffuse chronic headache
► Analgesic headache
► Depression
► Post-traumatic
► Uremia
► Lead intoxication
► Systemic diseases
  • Infectious mononucleosis
  • Inflammatory bowel disease
  • AIDS-related illness
  • Systemic lupus erythematosus
  • Hashimoto's thyroiditis
► Meningeal irritation
► Subarachnoid hemorrhage
► Intracranial pressure increase
► Intracranial masses
► Hydrocephalus
► Sinus thrombosis
► Cerebrospinal hypotension
  • After puncture
  • CSF fistula
  • Forced diuresis
  • Fever
  • CSF underproduction (postinfectious)
► Intracerebral vessel dilation
  • Nitrates
  • Hypertension
  • Post-traumatic

Relapsing headache
- ▶ Migraine
  - Simple migraine
  - Migraine with and without aura
  - Ophthalmoplegic migraine
  - After taking oral contraceptives
  - Complex migraine
  - Basilar migraine
- ▶ Nonmigrainous vascular headache
  - Effort (physical activity)
  - Vasomotor rhinitis
  - Cough
  - Fever
  - Hypotension
  - Hypertension
  - Hypoxia
  - Anemia
  - Endocrine
    - ○ Hypoglycemia
    - ○ Hypothyroidism
    - ○ Hyperthyroidsm
    - ○ Serotonin-secreting tumors
    - ○ Adrenal insufficiency
    - ○ Polycystic ovary syndrome
    - ○ Premenstrual syndrome
- ▶ Cluster (histamine) headache
- ▶ Hypertension
- ▶ Tension headache
- ▶ Vasomotor headache
- ▶ Sleep-induced headache
- ▶ Hypoglycemia
- ▶ Hypotension
- ▶ Muscle contraction (tension)
- ▶ Cervical spine
  - Trauma
  - Cervical spondylosis
  - Ankylosing spondylitis
  - Tumor
- ▶ Psychosomatic headache
- ▶ Psychogenic headache

Dietary/medicamentous/toxic or physical headache
- ▶ Drugs
  - Acetaminophen
  - Chloroquine
  - Ephedrine
  - Ergotamine
  - Isoniazide
  - MAO inhibitors
  - Nitrite-containing drugs
  - Oral contraceptives
  - Phenacetin
  - Reserpine
  - Theophylline
- ▶ Dietary headache
  - Alcohol
  - Dopamine (cheese, red wine)
  - Hydroxyphenylethylamine (cheese, red wine)
  - Glutamate
  - Cola
- ▶ Toxin-induced headache
  - Arsenic
  - Benzene
  - Carbon monoxide
  - Carbon tetrachloride
  - Dyes
  - Insecticides
  - Lead
  - Paints
  - Solvents
- ▶ Physical cause
  - Altitude sickness
  - Ionizing radiation
  - Sunstroke
- ▶ Substance withdrawal
  - Alcohol
  - Amphetamine
  - Caffeine
  - Ergotamine
  - Steroid

Hearing Loss, Hearing Impairment

Conductive
- ▶ Cerumen impaction
- ▶ Foreign bodies
  - Earwax
- ▶ Middle ear effusion

- Acute or chronic otitis media
- Eustachian tube dysfunction
▶ Otitis externa
▶ Cholesteatoma
▶ Otosclerosis
▶ Trauma
- Head trauma
- Barotrauma
  ◦ Rapid descent in air or water
  ◦ Physical straining
▶ Mastoiditis

Perceptive (sensitivity to sound)
▶ Noise induced hearing loss
- Acute
- Long term
▶ Presbycusis (aging process)
▶ Neoplasm
- Acoustic neuroma
- Metastases
▶ Infection
- CMV
- EBV
- Herpes simplex
- Herpes zoster
- Influenza
- Measles
- Mumps
- Tertiary syphilis
- Lyme disease
▶ Hematologic, vascular
- Sickle cell anemia
- Leukemia
- Polycythemia vera
- Berger's disease
- Ménière's disease
- Infarction
- Fat emboli
- Hyperlipoproteinemia
- Macroglobulinemia
- Hypercoagulable states
- Diabetes mellitus (microvascular)
▶ Ototoxic drugs, toxins
- Aminoglycosides
- CO
- Diuretics

- Hydrocarbons
- Lead
- Mercury
- Neomycin
- Quinine
- Salicylates
- Streptomycin
- Vancomycin
▶ Miscellaneous
- Trauma
- Multiple sclerosis
- Congenital deafness
- Hereditary conditions
- Diabetes mellitus
- Hypothyroidism
- Autoimmune disease
- Pregnancy

Heartburn
Pyrosis
Substantial pain or burning sensation associated with regurgitation of acid-peptic gastric juice into the esophagus. See Dysphagia → 110, See Achalasia → 10.

Reduced LES (lower esophageal sphincter) pressure
▶ Foods
- Alcohol
- Chocolate
- Coffee
- Fatty foods
- Peppermint
- Soft drinks with caffeine
- Tea
▶ Drugs
- Albuterol (inhaled)
- Anticholinergics
- Caffeine
- Calcium channel blockers
- Cigarette smoking
- Nitrates
- Theophylline
- Progesterone
▶ Medical

- Hiatal hernia
- Diabetes (neuropathy)
- Postoperative states
  - Vagotomy
  - Fundectomy
  - Gastrectomy
  - Cardiotomy
- Autoimmune diseases
  - CREST syndrome
  - Raynaud phenomenon
  - Scleroderma
▶ Idiopathic (primary reflux esophagitis)

Elevated internal stomach pressure
▶ Lifting
▶ Straining
▶ Coughing
▶ Clothes
▶ Obesity
▶ Ascites
▶ Constipation
▶ Pregnancy

Body position
▶ Lying down
▶ Bending over

Direct irritation of esophagus
▶ Aspirin
▶ Cigarette smoke
▶ Citrus fruits, juices
▶ Ibuprofen
▶ Spicy foods
▶ Tomatoes
▶ Tomato sauces

DDx
▶ Myocardial ischemia
▶ Peptic ulcer disease
▶ Cholelithiasis

Heart Failure, Acute

Acute inadequacy of the heart as a pump to maintain the circulation of blood, with congestion and edema in the tissues.

The patient complains of breathlessness (dyspnea) and exhaustion at rest. Dramatic presentation with dyspnea, edema, either pulmonary or peripheral organ underperfusion and tachycardia.

Common causes of left heart failure
▶ Myocardial ischemia
▶ Hypertension
▶ Aortic stenosis
▶ Aortic regurgitation
▶ Mitral regurgitation

Common causes of right heart failure
▶ Left heart failure
▶ Cor pulmonale (→ 85)
▶ Cardiomyopathy
▶ Diffuse myocarditis.
See Heart Failure, Chronic → 168

Causes
▶ Bradycardias
▶ Tachycardias
▶ Hypertensive crisis
▶ Myocardial disorder with left-ventricular failure
  • Myogenic pump failure
  • Drugs, toxins
    ○ Betablockers
    ○ Verapamil
  • Postoperative
  • Myocarditis
  • Septum rupture in myocardial infarction
  • Cardiomyopathy
    ○ Congestive cardiomyopathy
    ○ Constrictive cardiomyopathy
▶ Cardiac valve disorder
  • Prosthesis dysfunction
  • Decompensated aortic stenosis
  • Decompensated mitral stenosis
  • Valvular destruction in endocarditis
  • Rupture of the papillary muscles in infarction
▶ Pulmonary hypertension
  • Pulmonary embolism
▶ Pericardial tamponade
  • Aortic dissection

H

- (Constrictive) pericarditis
  - Idiopathic
  - Uremic
- Rupture of the free ventricular wall in infarction
▶ Miscellaneous
  - Circulatory shock
  - Pulmonary edema
  - Dyspnea of non-cardiac genesis
  - Cyanosis of non-cardiac genesis
  - Edema of non-cardiac genesis
  - Cervical vein stasis of non-cardiac genesis
  - Pleural effusion of non-cardiac genesis

Heart Failure, Chronic

Reduced physical endurance due to ventricular malfunction. Chronic inadequacy of the heart as a pump to maintain the circulation of blood, with congestion and edema in the tissues. Clinical syndrome with different etiology. Distinguish between acute and chronic heart failure as well as low-output heart failure (CHD, valvular stenoses, cardiomyopathy) and high-output failure (anemia, hyperthyroidism). The patient complains of symptoms of breathlessness and exhaustion.

See Heart Failure, Acute → 167

Right-ventricular failure
▶ Pulmonary hypertension, chronic lung disease
  - Bronchial asthma
  - Chronic bronchitis
  - Lung emphysema
  - Pulmonary fibrosis
  - Pneumoconiosis
  - Silicosis
  - Allergic alveolitis
  - Sarcoidosis
  - Dermatosclerosis involving the lungs
  - Kyphoscoliosis

- Pleural fibrosis
- Honeycomb lung
- Neck vein distension
- Tachycardia
- Hyperglobulia
▶ Pulmonary stenosis
▶ Pulmonary insufficiency
▶ Tricuspid insufficiency
▶ Mitral stenosis
▶ Pickwickian syndrome
▶ After pulmonary resection
▶ Severe relapsing pulmonary emboli
▶ Myocardial infarction of the right ventricle
▶ After left-ventricular failure

Left-ventricular failure
▶ Low-output heart failure
  - CHD
    - Myocardial infarction
    - Angina
  - Hypertensive cardiac disease
  - Arrhythmia
    - Absolute tachyarrhythmia in atrial fibrillation
  - Cardiac valve defect
    - Rupture of the papillary muscles
    - Aortic stenosis
    - Mitral regurgitation
    - Aortic regurgitation
  - Cardiac aneurysm
  - Perimyocarditis
  - Cardiomyopathy
  - Drugs, toxins
    - Adriblastin
    - Alcohol
    - Amytriptilin
    - Barbiturates
    - Catecholamines
    - Cobalt
    - Cocaine
    - Doxorubicin
    - Imipramine
    - Negative inotropic drugs
    - Phenothiazines
  - Sepsis

- Diastolic ventricle filling defect
  - Hypovolemia
  - Pericardial tamponade
  - Pericardial effusion
  - Constrictive pericarditis
  - Restrictive cardiomyopathy
  - Mediastinal tumors
  - Pancoast's tumor
  - Vena cava thrombosis
- Protein deficiency
- Alcohol abuse
▶ High-output failure
- Anemia
- Arteriovenous fistula
- Hypoxia
- Paget's disease
- Beriberi
- Hyperthyroidism

Other causes of ventricular failure
▶ Congenital heart disease (→ 82)
▶ Infiltrative disease
  - Cardiac amyloidosis
  - Hemochromatosis
▶ Metabolic
  - Carnitine deficiency
  - Thyroid disease
  - Diabetes mellitus
  - Thiamine deficiency
  - Ascorbic acid deficiency
▶ Pulmonary edema of non-cardiac genesis
▶ Dyspnea of non-cardiac genesis
▶ Cyanosis of non-cardiac genesis
▶ Edema of non-cardiac genesis
▶ Cervical vein stasis of non-cardiac genesis
▶ Pleural effusion of non-cardiac genesis

Heart, hypertrophy
See Hypertrophy of the Heart → 196

Heart Murmur, Continuous
Systolic-diastolic murmur
▶ Patent ductus arteriosus

▶ Arterio-venous fistula
  - Traumatic
  - Postoperative
▶ Postoperative aortopulmonary fistula
▶ Aortopulmonary window without severe pulmonary hypertension
▶ Pulmonary embolism
▶ Coronary arteriovenous fistula
▶ Coarctation of aorta
▶ Ruptured sinus of Valsalva aneurysm
▶ Lung angioma
▶ Abnormal origin of the left coronary artery from the pulmonary artery
▶ Lutembacher's syndrome
▶ Fallot's tetralogy
▶ Transposition of great vessels

Heart Murmur, Diastolic
Generally quieter than systolic murmurs. Aortic murmurs are best heard while the patient is sitting, mitral murmurs while lying on the left side.

Early diastolic
▶ Aortic valve regurgitation
  See Aortic Insufficiency → 38
▶ Pulmonic valve regurgitation
  - Pulmonary hypertension
  - Dilation of the right ventricle
  - Congenital or valvular disease

Mid-to-late diastolic
▶ Mitral stenosis
  - Endocarditis
▶ Mitral valve prosthesis
▶ Tricuspid valve stenosis
▶ Atrial myxoma
▶ Left atrial ball-valve thrombus
▶ Austin-Flint murmur
▶ Relative mitral stenosis due to high circulation volume
  - Anemia
  - Patent ductus arteriosus
  - Mitral regurgitation
  - Ventricular septal defect
▶ Relative tricuspid valve stenosis due to

high circulation volume
- Atrioseptal defect
- Tricuspid valve insufficiency
► Pulmonary insufficiency
- Graham-Steel murmur
► Coronary artery stenosis
► Dry pericarditis

Heart Murmur, Systolic

Cardiac sound during ventricular systole.

Early systolic
► Physiologic (innocent)
► Small ventricular septal defect
► Large ventricular septal defect with pulmonary hypertension
► Severe acute mitral regurgitation
► Severe acute tricuspid regurgitation
► Tricuspid regurgitation without pulmonary hypertension

Midsystolic
► Physiologic (innocent)
- Anemia
- Hyperthyroidism
- Hypothyroidism
- Pulmonary ejection murmur
- Aortic ejection murmur
► Pathologic
- Obstruction to left ventricular outflow
  ○ Valvular aortic stenosis
  ○ Supravalvular aortic stenosis
  ○ Hypertrophic cardiomyopathy
  ○ Aortic valve prosthesis
- Aortic dilation
- Coarctation of aorta
- Supraclavicular arterial bruit
- Obstruction to right ventricular outflow
  ○ Supravalvular pulmonic stenosis
  ○ Pulmonic valvular stenosis
  ○ Subpulmonic infundibular stenosis
- Flow murmur of atrial septal defect
- Idiopathic dilation of pulmonary artery
- Pulmonary hypertension

Holosystolic
► Mitral regurgitation
► Tricuspid regurgitation secondary to pulmonary hypertension
► Ventricular septal defect
► Patent ductus arteriosus
► Aortopulmonary window with pulmonary hypertension

Late systolic
► Mitral valve prolapse
► Tricuspid valve prolapse

Heart Sounds

HS, cardiac sounds

Noise made by muscle contraction and the closure of the heart valves during the cardiac cycle.
See Heart Murmur, Continuous → 169
See Heart Murmur, Diastolic → 169
See Heart Murmur, Systolic → 170

Loud S1 (1st HS accentuated)
► Mitral stenosis
► Short PR interval
► Hyperkinetic heart
- Hyperthyroidism
- Fever
- Anemia
- Heavy exercise
- Psychic stress
- Large AV fistula

Soft S1 (1st HS diminished)
► First-degree AV Block
► Long PR interval
► Mitral regurgitation
► Reduced left ventricular contractility
- Congestive heart failure
- Coronary artery disease
- Constrictive pericarditis
► Pulmonary emphysema
► Thick chest wall

Variable S1 (1st HS variable)
► Third degree AV Block
► Atrial fibrillation

Loud A2 (2nd HS in right 2nd interspace accentuated)
▶ Systemic hypertension
▶ Dilated aortic root

Soft A2 (2nd HS in right 2nd interspace diminished)
▶ Aortic stenosis (calcific)

Loud P2 (2nd HS in left 2nd interspace accentuated)
▶ Pulmonary arterial hypertension
▶ Dilated pulmonary artery
▶ Atrial septal defect

Soft P2 (2nd HS in left 2nd interspace diminished)
▶ Pulmonic stenosis
▶ Aging

Splitting of S2
▶ Physiologic
  • Normally A2 precedes P2, increased in inspiration, decreased in expiration
▶ Wide split
  • Right bundle branch block
  • Pulmonic stenosis
  • Mitral regurgitation
▶ Fixed split (no respiratory change in splitting)
  • Atrial septal defect
  • Right ventricular failure
▶ Narrow
  • Pulmonary hypertension
▶ Paradoxical split (splitting narrows with inspiration or appears on expiration)
  • Aortic stenosis
  • Left bundle branch block
  • Congestive heart failure

Third heart sound S3
▶ Physiologic
  • Children
  • Young adults
  • Pregnancy (third trimester)
▶ Left ventricular volume overload/failure
  • Mitral regurgitation
  • Tricuspid regurgitation
  • Congestive heart failure

Fourth heart sound S4
▶ Physiologic
  • Trained athletes
  • Advanced age
▶ Stiff left ventricle
  • Hypertension
  • Aortic stenosis
  • Hypertrophic cardiomyopathy
  • Coronary artery disease

Ejection click (sound)
▶ Dilated aorta
▶ Dilated pulmonary artery
▶ Aortic stenosis
▶ Pulmonic stenosis

Systolic click (midsystolic click)
▶ Mitral valve prolapse

Heinz bodies
See Erythrocyte, Morphology → 132

Hemarthrosis

Blood in a joint.

Causes
▶ Trauma
  • Fractures
▶ Hematologic
  • Anticoagulant therapy
  • Bleeding disorder
    ○ Von Willebrandd's disease
  • Thrombocytopenia
  • Thrombocytosis
▶ Charcot's joint (tabes dorsalis, neuropathic)
▶ Idiopathic
▶ Miscellaneous
  • Hemangioma
  • Synovioma
  • AV fistula
  • Ruptured aneurysm
  • Pigmented villonodular synovitis

Hematochezia

Blood in the feces
See Gastrointestinal Bleeding → 152
See Occult Blood → 262

Hematocrit

Packed cell volume (PCV, hct).
Proportion by volume, of the blood that consists of red blood cells, expressed as a percentage.

Reference range
Women: 35–47%
Men: 40–52%

Decreased
► Pregnancy
► Recovery stage after acute hemorrhage
► Hematocrit lags blood loss (not reliable)
► Physical training
► Increase of plasma volume with constant RBC mass
► Anemias
   See Anemia → 28

Increased
► Polycythemia vera
► Dehydration
   • Water loss
      ○ Polyuria
      ○ Diarrhea
      ○ Vomiting
   • Insufficient water intake
► Newborns
► Hyperglobulia
   • Spherocytosis
   • Thalassemia
► Hypoxia
► High altitude exposure
► Increase of erythropoietin
► Burn injury
► Smoking
► Trauma
► Shock

Hematoma, epidural
See Bleeding, Intracranial → 56

Hematoma, subdural
See Bleeding, Intracranial → 56

Hematothorax
See Pleural Effusion → 286

Hematuria

Blood in the urine
Urine contains blood or red blood cells. Up to 5 erythrocytes/visual field are normal. Microscopic hematuria: > 5 erythrocytes/visual field. In gross hematuria the urine is overtly bloody, smoky, or tea colored.

Main causes
► Prostate hyperplasia
► Cystitis
► Contamination during menstruation
► Prostatitis
► Bladder carcinoma
► Stones
► Glomerulonephritis
► Pyelonephritis
► Renal carcinoma

Renal causes
► Primary glomerulopathies
   • IgA-nephropathy
   • Glomerulonephritis
      ○ Crescentic glomerulonephritis
      ○ Postinfectious glomerulonephritis
      ○ Thin basement membrane disease
      ○ Membranoproliferative glomerulonephritis
      ○ Focal glomerulonephritis
   • Malignant hypertension
   • Diabetic glomerulosclerosis/ diabetic nephropathy
   • Kidney amyloidosis
► Tubulointerstitial nephropathies, nephritis

- Pyelonephritis
  - Kidney-tuberculosis
  - Streptococci
  - Staphylococci
  - Pneumococci
  - Pseudomonas
  - E. coli
  - Legionella
  - Salmonella
  - Mycoplasma
  - Plasmodium
  - Toxoplasma
  - Trichinella spiralis
  - Schistosoma
  - Filaria
  - Bilharziosis
  - Hepatitis B
  - Mononucleosis
  - Cytomegalovirus
  - Varicella
  - ECHO viruses
  - Adenoviruses
  - Influenza
- Necrotizing papillitis
  - Analgesic kidney
  - Diabetes mellitus
- Acute interstitial nephritis
- Nephrolithiasis
- Traumatic kidney lesion
- Neoplastic
  - Hypernephroma
  - Metastases (bronchial carcinomas, ovarial carcinoma, Hodgkin's lymphoma)
- Cystic kidneys
- Drugs:
  - Analgesic (Analgesic nephritis)
  - Captopril
  - D-penicillamine
  - Gold
  - Heroin
  - Lysergic acid
  - Mercury
  - Vaccines
- Hydronephrosis

- Nephropathy in systemic diseases
  - Diabetes mellitus
  - Goodpasture's syndrome
  - Hemolytic-uremic syndrome
  - Thrombotic thrombocytopenic purpura
  - Malignant hypertension
  - Fabry's disease
  - Nail-patella syndrome
  - Allergic granulomatosis
- Vascular
  - Renal infarct
  - Renal vein thrombosis
  - Renal artery aneurysms
- Collagen vascular disease
  - Polyarteritis nodosa
  - Lupus erythematosus
  - Wegener's granulomatosis
  - Schönlein-Henoch's disease
  - Dermatosclerosis
- After endocarditis
- Radiation nephropathy
- Urate nephropathy
- Balkan nephropathy
- Nephrocalcinosis
- Shunt nephritis
- Deformations
  - Polycystic kidney disease
  - Sponge kidney
  - Alport's syndrome
  - Benign familiar hematuria

Prenatal causes

▶ Hemorrhagic diathesis
  - Anticoagulants
    - Warfarin therapy (sign of overdose !)
  - Chemotherapeutics
  - Thrombocytopenia
  - Thrombocytopathies
  - Consumption coagulopathy
  - Hemophilia
  - Factor lack
▶ Hematopoietic system
  - Hemoglobinopathy
  - Sickle cell anemia
  - Thalassemia

- Polycythemia
- Neoplasm
- Multiple myeloma
► Hemolytic-uremic syndrome
► Heavy exercise
► Systemic
  - Amyloidosis
  - Sarcoidosis
► Osler's disease
► Cardiovascular
  - Arteriosclerosis
  - Heart failure
  - Hypertension
  - Shock
► Drugs, toxins, foods causing red coloration of the urine
  - α-methyldopa
  - Blackberries
  - Daunorubicin
  - Doxyrubicin
  - Food dyes
  - Phenothiazine
  - Porphyrines
  - Red beets
  - Rhodamine
  - Rifampicin
  - Urates

Postrenal/ urologic causes
► Cystitis
  - Bladder tuberculosis
► Urolithiasis
► Tumor
► Trauma
► Prostate hyperplasia
► Masturbation
► Calculi
  - Urolithiasis
  - Renal stones
  - Vesical calculi
  - Urethrolithiasis
► Inflammation
  - Bilharziosis
  - Urogenital tuberculosis
    ○ Kidney
    ○ Ureter

  ○ Bladder
  ○ Prostate
- Urethritis
- Acute/chronic cystitis
- Pyelonephritis
► Deformation
  - Cystic kidney
  - Renal cyst
  - Renal hypoplasia
  - Calyx diverticulum
  - Megaureter
  - Vesico-ureteral-renal reflux
  - Urethral valves
  - Meatus stenosis
► Tumor
  - Kidneys
    ○ Metastases
    ○ Wilms' tumor
    ○ Kidney call carcinoma
  - Carcinoma of the renal pelvis.
  - Carcinoma of the ureter
  - Prostate carcinoma
  - Urethra carcinoma

Gross hematuria
► Miction-independent hematuria
  - Tumor
  - Inflammation
  - Injury
► Initial hematuria
  Hemorrhage from urethra
  - Stone
  - Injury
  - Foreign body
  - Inflammation
  - Bladder carcinoma
  - Prostate carcinoma
► Total hematuria
  Hemorrhage from kidney, ureter, bladder)
  - Prostate adenoma /carcinoma
  - Cystitis
  - Bladder infiltration
  - Renal trauma
  - Urogenital tuberculosis
  - Renal vein thrombosis

- Renal vein infarct
- Pyelonephritis
- Hydronephrosis
- Renal cysts
- Cystic kidneys
- Urolithiasis
- Carcinoma of the kidney
- Urothelium carcinoma
▶ Terminal hematuria
Hemorrhage from bladder outlet
- Foreign body
- Endometriosis
- Bilharziosis
- Tuberculosis
- Stone
- Cystitis
- Bladder carcinoma
- Prostate adenoma / carcinoma

Hemoglobin

Oxygen-carrying pigment and major protein in erythrocytes. Hemoglobin forms an unstable, reversible bond with oxygen. Oxyhemoglobin (oxygenated state) transports oxygen from the lungs to the tissues where oxygen is released. Deoxyhemoglobin (reduced state).

Reference range
Women: 12-16 mg/dl
Men: 14-18 mg/dl
Increased
See Polycythemia → 288
Decreased
▶ Anemia
See Anemia → 28
▶ Hemorrhage
- Gastrointestinal (→ 152)
- Genotourinary (→ 55)

Hemoglobin cyanosis, See Cyanosis → 91

Hemoglobin, glycosylated
See HbA1, HbA1c → 162

Hemoglobinopathy
See Hemoglobin → 175

Hemoglobinuria, See Hematuria → 172

Hemolytic anemia, See Anemia → 28

Hemopexin

Acute-phase reactant.

Reference range
Hemopexin	50-115 mg/dl
See Haptoglobin → 161
Decreased
▶ Severe intravascular hemolysis
▶ Hemolytic anemia
▶ Chronic liver disease
▶ Malabsorption
▶ Porphyria cutanea tarda
Increased
▶ Rapidly growing melanomas

Hemoptysis

Bloody sputum, spitting up blood, coughing up blood
See Gastrointestinal Bleeding → 152
Infection, inflammation
▶ Bronchitis
▶ Bronchiectasis
▶ Pneumonia (e.g. Klebsiella)
▶ Laryngitis
▶ Pharyngitis
▶ Tracheitis
▶ Tuberculosis
▶ Lung abscess
▶ Echinococcal cyst
▶ Actinomycosis
▶ Aspergilloma
▶ Oral candidiasis
▶ Septic pulmonary emboli
Tumor
▶ Bronchogenic carcinoma

► Bronchial adenoma
► Metastases
► Mediastinal tumors
► Esophageal tumors
► Malignant lymphoma
► Endometriosis
► Pulmonary hemangioma

Cardiovascular
► Pulmonary infarction
► Mitral stenosis
► Heart failure
► Pulmonary congestion, alveolar edema
► Pulmonary embolism
► Ruptured aortic aneurysm
► Primary pulmonary hypertension
► Pulmonary arteriovenous fistula

Trauma
► Lung contusion
► Ruptured bronchi
► Violent coughing
► Aspiration, foreign body
  • Pulmonary aspiration
    ○ Bleeding gums (→ 159)
    ○ Nosebleed (epistaxis)
    ○ Tonsillectomy
  • Shrapnel

Other pulmonary disorders
► Broncholithiasis
► Cystic fibrosis
► Pulmonary hemosiderosis

Systemic disorders
► Vasculitis
  • Wegener's granulomatosis
  • Goodpasture syndrome
  • Polyarteritis nodosa
  • Behçet's syndrome
  • Systemic lupus erythematosus
► Sarcoidosis
► Pulmonary fibrosis
► Histiocytosis X
► Hemorrhagic diathesis
► Amyloidosis

Iatrogenic
► Biopsy

► Bronchoscopy
► Laryngoscopy
► Mediastinoscopy
► Spirometry

Hemorrhage, subarachnoid,
Hemorrhage, extradural,
Hemorrhage, subdural,
Hemorrhage, intracerebral,
See Bleeding, Intracranial → 56

Hemorrhagic Diathesis

Bleeding tendency, bleeding disorder
Pathologic bleeding tendency
(spontaneous hemorrhage or hemorrhage
without appropriate trauma) due to one or
several coagulation defects. This
impairment affects the vessels, the
plasmatic blood clotting factors or the
thrombocytes. The clinical picture contains
purpura (→ 309), muscle and intra-
articular bleeding, epistaxis and mucosal
hemorrhage (→ 243). Consider
thrombocyte count, bleeding time,
thrombin time, partial thromboplastin
time, D dimers and quantitative
determination of fibrinogen.
See Coagulation → 79, See Disseminated
Intravascular Coagulation → 104,
See Purpura → 309,
See Mucosa Hemorrhage → 243

Frequent causes
► Anticoagulation therapy
► Thrombocyte impairment
► Vascular impairment
► Hepatopathies
► Vitamin K deficiency
► Hereditary coagulopathies

Vascular impairment
► Schönlein-Henoch's purpura
► Purpura fulminans
► Senile-atrophic/ purpura senilis
► Chronic hypercortisolism
► Avitaminosis C

- Uremia
- Dysproteinemia
  - Paraproteinemia
  - Cryoglobulinemia
  - Hyperglobulinemia
- Infection (vascular allergic purpura)
  - Syphilis
  - Bacterial meningitis
  - Scarlet fever
  - Sepsis
  - Diphtheria
  - Bacterial endocarditis
  - Leptospirosis
  - Influenza
  - Measles
  - Pocks
  - Varicella
  - Rickettsia
  - Malaria
  - Toxoplasmosis
- Drugs (vascular allergic purpura)
  - Aspirin
  - Atropine
  - Barbiturates
  - Penicillins
  - Phenacetin
  - Sulfonamides
  - Warfarin
- Osler's disease
- Amyloidosis
- Hereditary hemorrhagic teleangiectasia
- Hereditary vessel, connective tissue defect
  - Ehlers-Danlos syndrome with increased vessel fragility
  - Osteogenesis imperfecta
  - Marfan syndrome
  - Pseudoxanthoma elasticum
- Pachymeningeosis haemorrhagica interna

Quantitative thrombocyte impairment
See Thrombocyte Count → 349

Thrombocyte dysfunction
- Aspirin-like-defect
- Anti-aggregation with aspirin

- Thrombopathic thrombopenia
- Fibrinolytic fission products (disseminated intravascular coagulation)
- Uremia
- Cirrhosis
- Paraproteinemia
- Myeloproliferative syndrome
- Hereditary
  - Von-Willebrand's disease
  - Thrombasthenia
  - Bernhard-Soulier syndrome (BSS)
- Glanzmann's thrombasthenia
- Pernicious anemia
- Myelodysplasia
- Miscellaneous heritable disorders of connective tissue
- Hegglin's anomaly
- Gray platelet syndrome

Acquired coagulopathies
- Drugs
  - Antibiotics
  - Cephalosporins
  - Cholestyramin
  - Heparin
  - L-asparaginase
  - Sulfonamides
  - Tetracyclines
  - Warfarin
- Fibrinolysis therapy
- Hepatopathies (hepatitis, cirrhosis)
  - Increased consumption of blood clotting factors
    - Diffuse intravascular coagulation
    - Fibrinolysis
    - Fibrinogenolysis
  - Thrombocyte malfunction
    - Alcoholism
    - Uremia
  - Thrombopenias
    - Splenomegaly with portal hypertension
    - Folic acid deficiency
    - Consumption coagulopathy
    - Alcoholism
  - Coagulation factor deficiency

- Factor-deficiencies: V, VII, IX, X, XI, XIII
- Antiplasmin
- Prothrombin
- Fibrinogen
- Reduced hepatic catabolism
  - Fibrinolytic fission products
  - Activated blood clotting factors
  - Plasminogen activators
▶ Vitamin K deficiency
- Warfarin
- Cephalosporins
- Vitamin K deficiency with newborns
- Dietary deficiencies
- Parenteral nutrition
- Biliary obstruction (reduced uptake of fat-soluble vitamins)
- Malabsorption (reduced uptake of fat-soluble vitamins)
- Faulty intestinal flora (reduced formation of vitamin K)
- Severe gastrointestinal bleeding
- Therapy with cholestyramin (binds fat-soluble vitamins)
▶ Malabsorption
▶ Dietary deficiencies
▶ Disseminated intravascular coagulation
- Severe bacterial, viral, mycotic and parasitic infections
- Severe trauma
  - Large operations
  - Acute pancreatitis
  - Burns
  - Myocardial infarction
  - Cranio cerebral trauma
- Neoplasm
  - Carcinomas
  - Metastases
  - Acute leukemias
- Obstetrical complications
  - Septic abortion
  - HELLP syndrome
  - Amniotic fluid embolism
  - Premature placenta ablation
  - Intrauterine embryo death

- Vasculopathies
  - Vasculitis
  - Cyanotic cardiac vitium
  - Large aneurysms
  - Large vascular prostheses
- Miscellaneous
  - Shock
  - State after circulatory arrest
  - Anaphylactic shock
  - Graft-vs.-host disease
  - Graft-versus-host-syndrome
  - Lactic acidosis
  - Hypothermia
  - Severe hepatopathy

Hereditary coagulopathies
▶ Hemophilia A, B
▶ Von Willebrand's disease
▶ Wiskott-Aldrich syndrome
▶ Dysfibrinogenemia
▶ Afibrinogenemia
▶ Deficiency of
- Factors: II, V, VII, X, XI, XII, XIII
- α_1-antitrypsin
- Protein C
- α2-macroglobulin
- C1-inhibitor
- α2-antiplasmin
▶ Bernard-Soulier syndrome (BSS)
▶ Thrombasthenia
▶ Hermansky-Pudlak syndrome
▶ Chediak -Higashi syndrome
▶ Osler's disease
▶ Ehlers-Danlos syndrome
▶ Nonthrombocytopenic purpura
▶ Gray platelet syndrome
▶ Teleangiectasia

Hemorrhagic effusions
See Pleural Effusion → 286

Hepatic Cysts

Congenital hepatic cysts
▶ Solitary cyst (biliary microhamartomas)
▶ Polycystic liver disease

Acquired hepatic cysts
- Inflammatory cyst
- Retention cyst
- Echinococcal cyst (Hydatid cyst)
- Amebic cyst
- Neoplastic cyst
- Peliosis hepatis (blood-filled cavities)

Hepatic abscess
- Amebiasis
- Bacterial infection
  - Aerobic gram negative bacteria
  - Streptococcus species
  - Staphylococcus aureus
  - Anaerobic bacteria (clostridium difficile)
  - Syphilis
  - Neisseria gonorrheae

Hepatic Failure, Fulminant

Liver damage that leads to a life-threatening impaired liver function within 8 weeks. See Liver diseases → 226

Infections
- Hepatitis A-G
- Herpes viruses
  - Herpes simplex virus 1/2
  - Cytomegalovirus
  - Epstein-Barr virus
  - Paramyxovirus
- Parainfluenza virus

Ischemic causes
- Hepatic arterial or venous occlusion
- Hypotension
- Shock
- Hyperthermia
- Primary graft nonfunction post liver transplantation

Drugs, toxins
- Acetaminophen
- Allopurinol
- Amanita phalloides mushroom poisoning
- Amiodarone
- Antidepressants
- Carbon tetrachloride
- Disulfiram
- Enflurane
- Gold
- Halothane
- Isoflurane
- Isoniazid
- Ketoconazole
- Methyldopa
- NSAIDs
- Phenytoin
- Propylthiouracil
- Rifampicin
- Sulfonamides
- Tetracycline
- Valproic acid

Metabolic
- Wilson's disease
- Acute fatty liver of pregnancy
- Reye's syndrome

Miscellaneous
- Autoimmune chronic active hepatitis
- Massive malignant infiltration of the liver
- Budd-Chiari syndrome (stenosis or occlusion of the hepatic vein)
- Heatstroke
- Sepsis

Hepatitis, See Liver diseases → 226

Hepatomegaly

Megalohepatia
Enlargement of the liver.
See Liver diseases → 226

Inflammation
- Hepatitis (→ 226)
  - Infectious hepatitis
    ○ Viral hepatitis
    ○ Schistosomiasis
  - Alcoholic hepatitis
  - Toxic hepatitis
  - Drug-induced

- Autoimmune
► Liver abscess
  - Pyogenic
  - Amebic
► Cholangitis
► Pericholangitis
► Other infection
  - Infectious mononucleosis
  - Miliary tuberculosis
  - Leishmania donovani (Kala-azar)
  - Amebiasis

Cirrhosis (→ 78)
► Alcoholic cirrhosis
► Posthepatitic
► Postnecrotic
► Biliary cirrhosis
► Hemochromatosis with cirrhosis

Neoplasm
► Malignant
  - Hepatocellular carcinoma
  - Cholangiocarcinoma
  - Angiosarcoma
  - Metastases
    ○ Pancreas carcinoma
    ○ Colon carcinoma
    ○ Lung carcinoma
    ○ Breast carcinoma
    ○ Stomach carcinoma
► Benign
  - Hepatic adenoma
  - Hemangioma
  - Focal nodular hyperplasia

Hematologic, lymphoproliferative
► Lymphoma
► Leukemia
► Myelofibrosis with myeloid metaplasia
► Multiple myeloma

Granulomatous
► Sarcoidosis
► Miliary tuberculosis

Metabolic
► Hemochromatosis
► Alpha1-antitrypsin deficiency
► Wilson's disease

► Cystic fibrosis
► Kwashiorkor (dietary protein deficiency)

Biliary obstruction (→ 75)
► Choledocholithiasis
► Pancreatitis
► Biliary stricture
► Carcinoma
► External compression

Hepatic congestion
► Congestive heart failure
► Constrictive pericarditis
► Budd-Chiari syndrome
► Thrombosis
► Tumor
► Inferior vena cava web

Storage, infiltrative disorders
► Alcoholic fatty infiltration
► Lipid storage disease
  - Gaucher's disease
  - Niemann-Pick disease
► Fatty liver (→ 142)
► Glycogen storage disease
► Amyloidosis
► Wilson's disease
► Hurler syndrome

Miscellaneous
► Cysts (See Renal Cysts → 314)
► Hydatid disease of liver

Hepatopathy, See Liver diseases → 226

Hepatosplenomegaly

Enlargement of liver and spleen.
See Hepatomegaly → 179
See Splenomegaly → 337
See Liver diseases → 226

Portal hypertension (→ 291)
► Cirrhosis
► Budd-Chiari syndrome (stenosis or occlusion of the hepatic vein)
► Banti's disease (idiopathic portal hypertension)
► Sarcoidosis

- Primary biliary cirrhosis
- Cystic liver
- Multiple liver metastases
- Congested liver
- Fatty liver
- Extrahepatic cholestasis
  - Tumors
  - Carbonic anhydrase inhibitors
- Stones
- Drug-induced jaundice

Infections
- Viral hepatitis
- Brucellosis (Bang's disease)
- Infectious mononucleosis
- Abdominal typhoid fever
- Amebiasis
- Malaria
- Leptospirosis
- Relapsing fever
- Echinococcosis
- Schistosomiasis
- Leishmaniasis
- Histoplasmosis
- Bilharziosis

Reticuloses
- Letterer-Siwe disease (reticulosis in children and adolescents)

Hematologic, myeloproliferative
- Idiopathic thrombocythemia
- Polycythemia
- Osteomyelosclerosis
- Chronic myelosis
- Hodgkin's lymphoma
- Leukemia
- Hemolytic anemia/hemoglobinopathy
  - Thalassemia
  - Sickle cell anemia
  - Glucose 6 phosphate deficiency
  - Immune-hemolytic anemia

Metabolic disorders
- Gaucher's disease
- Wilson's disease
- Niemann-Pick disease
- Hemochromatosis

- Galactosemia
- Amyloidosis
- Pfaundler-Hurler syndrome
- Type IV glycogenosis
- Familial hyperlipemia

Miscellaneous
- Cystic fibrosis
- Histiocytosis X
- Felty's syndrome (splenomegaly with rheumatoid arthritis and leukopenia)
- Morbus haemolyticus neonatorum
- Still's disease (juvenile form of rheumatoid arthritis)
- Osler's disease
- Sideroblastic anemia
- Moschcowitz microangiopathy
- Miliary tuberculosis
- Recurrent pulmonary embolism

Heterophoria

Latent tendency for deviation of the eyes from parallelism. Prevented by binocular vision.

Manifestation as strabismus (→ 340) in
- Severe fatigue
- Nervousness
- Fever
- Alcohol abuse
- Other origin of binocular vison disability

hGH, See Growth Hormone → 159

Hiccup
Singultus

Involuntary spasm of the diaphragm leading to a sudden inspiration that is stopped by an abrupt closure of the glottis, producing a sound.

Transient Hiccups (< 48 h, self limiting)
- Gastric distention
  - Overindulgence in food or alcohol
  - Excessive laughter
  - Cigarette smoking

- Carbonated beverages
- Aerophagia
- Air insufflation during gastroscopy
► Sudden change in gastric temperature
- Intake of very hot or very cold foods
- Movement into hot or cold environment
- Cold shower
► Psychologic
- Sudden excitement
- Emotional stress

Intractable Hiccups (> 48 h)
► Systemic-toxic causes
- Uremia
- Sepsis
- Alcohol abuse
- Drugs
  ○ Barbiturates
  ○ Chlordiazepoxide
  ○ Dexamethasone
  ○ Diazepam
► Neurologic disorders
- Encephalitis
- Meningitis
- Hydrocephalus
- Cerebrovascular insufficiency
  ○ Vertebrobasilar ischemia
- Intracranial hemorrhage
- Brain tumor
- Dementia
- Tabes dorsalis
- Postoperative states
- Cardiac pacemaker (stimulation of diaphragm)
► Mediastinal, thoracic disorders
- Trauma of the phrenic nerve
- Lung disorder
  ○ Tuberculosis
  ○ Sarcoidosis
  ○ Pulmonary fibrosis
  ○ Pneumonia (pleural irritation)
  ○ Pleuritis
  ○ Bronchial carcinoma
  ○ Bronchial obstruction
  ○ Bronchitis

- Heart disorder
  ○ Pericarditis
  ○ Adherent pericardium
  ○ Cardiomegaly
  ○ Myocardial infarction
- Esophagus disease
  ○ Reflux esophagitis
  ○ Esophageal obstruction
  ○ Esophagus carcinoma
- Miscellaneous
  ○ Aortic aneurysm
  ○ Mediastinitis
  ○ Mediastinal tumor
► Diseases of the neck area
- Goiter
- Lymphadenopathy
  ○ Inflammatory
  ○ Metastatic
► Abdominal disorders
- Diaphragmatic hernia of stomach
- Subphrenic abscess
- Subphrenic peritonitis
- Liver tumor or mass
- Liver abscess
- Cirrhosis
- Cholecystitis, cholelithiasis
- Gastric disease
- Ulcer disease
- Gastric carcinoma
- Acute gastrointestinal obstruction
- Splenic infarction
- Pancreatitis
- Pancreatic pseudocyst
- Pancreas carcinoma
- Peritoneal carcinomatosis
- After abdominal surgery
► Psychiatric diseases
- Anxiety disorder
- Anorexia nervosa

Hirsutism

Presence of excessive bodily and facial terminal hair, in a male pattern, especially in women. Distinguish between

hypertrichosis (growth of hair in excess of the normal on the whole body or on individual skin areas without increased facial- and pubic hair), **hirsutism** (hypertrichosis in a male pattern on the face and body: upper lip, beard, areolas, sternum, linea alba, lumbosacral, arms and legs) and **virilism** (hirsutism and masculinizing organic changes: clitoris hypertrophy, deep voice, breast atrophy, abnormal cessation of menses, masculine face and body hair, approximation to the masculine anatomy, effluvium, professor angles).

Causes
▶ Idiopathic hirsutism
▶ Ovarian hyperandrogenism
  • Tumors producing androgens
    ○ Sertoli-Leydig cell tumor
    ○ Granulosa-theka cell tumor
    ○ Hilus cell tumor
  • Stein-Leventhal syndrome (Polycystic ovary syndrome: PCO)
  • Arrhenoblastoma
▶ Adrenal hyperandrogenism
  • Tumors producing androgens
  • Cushing's syndrome
  • Adrenogenital syndrome (11-hydroxylase deficiency/ 17-hydroxylase deficiency)
▶ Combined adrenal and ovarian hyperandrogenism
▶ Pituitary tumor
  • Prolactin-secreting tumor
  • Cushing's disease
  • Acromegaly
▶ Neurologic
  • Multiple sclerosis
  • Encephalitis
  • Head trauma
▶ Drugs
  • ACTH
  • Anabolic steroids
  • Androgenic hormones
  • Acetazolamide

  • Corpus luteum hormones
  • Cyclosporine
  • Danazol
  • Diazoxid
  • Metopyron
  • Minoxidil
  • Oral contraceptives
  • Penicillamine
  • Phenytoin
  • Progestin
  • Spironolactone
  • Steroids
▶ Miscellaneous
  • Anorexia nervosa
  • Obesity
  • Postmenopausal
  • Hypothyroidism
  • Dermatomyositis
  • Increased sensitivity of end organs to androgenic hormones
  • Distinct insulin receptor insensitivity/ -resistance
  • Familial glucocorticoid resistance
  • Disturbance of sex differentiation
    ○ Gonadal dysgenesis
    ○ Male pseudo hermaphroditism
  • Cutaneous porphyria
  • Morgagni's syndrome
  • Gordan-Overstreet syndrome
  • Hurler's syndrome
  • Trisomy E

Hives, See Anaphylaxis → 27
See Urticaria → 371

HLA-B27
Humane Leukocyte Antigen B27
Conditions associated with HLA-B27
▶ Ankylosing spondylitis (Bechterew's disease)
▶ Reiter's syndrome
▶ Shigella arthritis
▶ Salmonella arthritis
▶ Yersinia arthritis

▶ Gonococci arthritis
▶ Rheumatoid arthritis
  • Still's disease
  • Felty's syndrome (splenomegaly with rheumatoid arthritis and leukopenia)
▶ Psoriatic arthritis
▶ Enteropathic spondylarthritis

Hoarseness

Organic
▶ Infection, inflammation
  • Acute viral laryngitis
  • Bacterial tracheitis/laryngitis
  • Laryngotracheobronchitis
▶ Non-infectious inflammation (chronic irritation with vocal edema, nodules, contact ulcers or chronic laryngitis)
  • Smoke irritation
  • Chronic cough, severe cold
  • Excessively dry and warm room combined with low water intake
  • Allergy
  • Chronic inhalation of chemical irritant agents usually caused by the professional activity
  • Gastro-esophageal reflux disease (GERD)
  • Overstress of vocal cords by crying, speaking, singing
▶ Trauma
▶ Neoplasm
  • Benign tumors
    ○ Vocal cord polyps
    ○ Papillomas
    ○ Chondromas
    ○ Lipomas
    ○ Neurofibromas
    ○ Hemangiomas
  • Malignant tumors
    ○ Squamous cell carcinoma
    ○ Larynx carcinoma
    ○ Bronchial carcinoma
▶ Cysts
  • Retention cysts

• Laryngocelesventricular prolapse
▶ Systemic
  • Hypothyroidism
  • Virilization
  • Rheumatoid arthritis
  • Systemic lupus erythematosus
  • Sarcoidosis
  • Wegener's granulotomosis
  • Amyloidosis
▶ Neurologic
  • Central lesions
    ○ CVA
    ○ Guillain-Barré syndrome
    ○ Head injury
    ○ Multiple sclerosis
    ○ Neural tumors)
  • Peripheral lesions
    ○ Tumors: glomus jugulare, thyroid, bronchogenic, esophageal, neural
    ○ Surgery
    ○ Cardiac
      - *Left atrial entargment*
      - *Aneurysm of aortic arch*
  • Neuromuscular
    ○ Myasthenia gravis
    ○ Spastic dysphonia

Functional
  • Psychogenic aphonia (hysterical aphonia)
  • Habitual aphonia
  • Ventricular dysphonias

Homocysteine

See Cardiac Risk Factor → 66
Homocysteine is elevated in 15-30% of patients with premature CAD.

Reference range
Optimal: 5-13.5µmol/l
Borderline : 13.5 µmol/l
Hyperhomocysteinemia: > 15 µmol/l

Hyperhomocysteinemia
▶ Vitamin deficiency
  • Folate deficiency
  • Vitamin B_6 deficiency

- Vitamin B$_{12}$ deficiency
► Chronic disease
  - Chronic renal failure
  - Hypothyroidism
  - Psoriasis
  - Cancer
  - Cigarette smoking
► Drugs
  - Anticonvulsants
  - Methotrexate
  - Nitrous Oxide
► Homocystinuria (inherited)

Homovanillic acid
See Urine Catecholamines → 368

Horner's syndrome
Ptosis, miosis, and anhidrosis (dryness) on the side of the paralysis of the superior cervical sympathetic nerve.
Causes
► Brainstem stroke
► Retroparotid mass
  - Parotid gland tumor
  - Carotid body tumor
  - Lymphoma
  - Metastasis
  - Tuberculous adenitis
► Mediastinal mass (→ 235)

Howell-Jolly bodies
See Erythrocyte, Morphology → 132

Human Chorionic Gonadotropin (HCG)
Choriogonadotropin, chorionic gonadotropic hormone, chorionic gonadotropic hormone.
Glycoprotein from the urine of pregnant women, produced by the placental trophoblastic cells, stimulating ovarian secretion of estrogen and progesterone during the first trimester, required for the integrity of conceptus. Important in the early diagnostic of a pregnancy and in the diagnostic of a miscarriage. Major clinical marker in women with gestational trophoblastic neoplasia (GTN)

Reference range
< 3 mU/l in serum
Increased
► Pregnancy
► Tumors
  - Testicular cancer (non-seminomas)
    ○ Choriocarcinoma
    ○ Embryonal cell carcinoma
  - Placental chorion carcinoma
  - Hydatidiform mole
  - Pancreas carcinoma
    ○ Adenocarcinoma
    ○ Islet-cell carcinoma
  - Seminoma
  - Colon carcinoma
  - Ovarial carcinoma
  - Breast carcinoma
  - Renal carcinoma
► Miscellaneous
  - Progress control in threatening miscarriage (decelerated HCG increase)
  - Delimitation of the EUP (decelerated HCG increase)
  - Postmenopausal females with kidney insufficiency dependent on dialysis
  - Chemotherapy (necrosis of malignant tumor)
  - Down syndrome

Human growth hormone
See Growth Hormone → 159

Hyaline casts, See Cylindruria → 92

Hydrocephalus

Excessive accumulation of fluid resulting in dilation of the cerebral ventricles and raised intracranial pressure.

Congenital
► Aqueductal stenosis (malformation)
► Incomplete development of the Magendie or Luschka foramina
► Dandy-Walker malformation
► Arnold-Chiari malformation
► Agenesis of the foramen of Monro
► Congenital toxoplasmosis
► Bickers-Adams syndrome

Acquired in infants and children
► Mass lesions
  • Tumors
    ○ Medulloblastoma
    ○ Astrocytoma
  • Cysts
  • Abscesses
  • Hematoma
► Intraventricular hemorrhage
  • Prematurity
  • Head injury
  • Rupture of a vascular malformation
► Infections
  • Meningitis
  • Cysticercosis
► Increased venous sinus pressure
  • Achondroplasia
  • Craniostenoses
  • Venous thrombosis
► Iatrogenic
  • Hypervitaminosis A
► Idiopathic

Acquired in adults
► Subarachnoid hemorrhage (SAH)
► Idiopathic hydrocephalus
► Head injury
► Tumors
  • Ependymoma
  • Ssubependymal giant cell astrocytoma
  • Choroid plexus papilloma
  • Craniopharyngioma
  • Pituitary adenoma
  • Hypothalamic glioma
  • Optic nerve glioma
  • Hamartoma
  • Metastatic tumors
► Prior posterior fossa surgery
► Congenital aqueductal stenosis
► Meningitis
► Nonobstructive (ex vacuo)
  • Alzheimer's disease
  • Pick's disease
  • Huntington's disease
  • Multiple cerebral infarctions
► See also acquired causes in infants and children

Causes of normal pressure hydrocephalus (NPH)
► Subarachnoid hemorrhage (SAH)
► Head trauma
► Meningitis
► Tumors
► Posterior fossa surgery
► Idiopathic

Hyperalbuminemia, See Albumin → 16

Hypoalbuminemia, See Albumin → 16

Hyperaldosteronism

Conn's syndrome, aldosteronism
Overproduction of aldosterone (→ 17), resulting in hypokalemia, alkalosis, muscle weakness, polydipsia, polyuria and hypertension.

Primary hyperaldosteronism (Conn's disease)
► Solitary adrenal adenomas (85%)
► Bilateral adrenal hyperplasia (15%)
► Adrenal carcinoma
► Unilateral adrenal hyperplasia

Secondary hyperaldosteronism
► Renin-producing tumors

- Chronic renal failure
- Renovascular hypertension
  - Renal artery stenosis
- Edema with reduced aldosterone metabolism
  - Cirrhosis
  - Nephrotic sndrome
  - Heart failure
- Pregnancy
- Bartter's syndrome
- Pseudo-Bartter's syndrome
- Mineralocorticoid excess
- Very low sodium diet
- Dexamethasone-sensitive hyperaldosteronism
- Cushing's syndrome
- Postoperative hyperaldosteronism
- Diuretics
- Laxatives
- Hyponatremia
- Hypovolemia

Hyperbilirubinemia, See Bilirubin → 51

Hypercalcemia

An increase in total plasma calcium concentration above 10.4 mg/dL (2.60 mmol/L). Hypercalcemia usually results from excessive bone resorption. Regulation of serum concentration occurs through PTH, vitamin D and calcitonin. Symptoms in hypercalcemia include headaches, weakness, confusion, depression, hallucinations, psychosis, coma, hyporeflexia, bradycardia, shortened QT interval, hypertension, digitalis hypersensitivity with arrhythmias, nausea, vomiting, constipation, gastroduodenal ulcer disease, pancreatitis, insulin resistance, glucose intolerance, polyuria, polydypsia, nephrolithiasis, muscle weakness, chondrocalcinosis and vascular calcification.

Main causes
- Primary hyperparathyroidism
- Secondary hyperparathyroidism
- Hypercalcemia
- Humoral hypercalcemia of malignancy
- Exogenous vitamin D
- Sarcoidosis
- Immobilization
- Drugs.

Increased uptake
- Milk-alkali syndrome
- Vitamin D intoxication

Endocrine impairment
- Primary hyperparathyroidism (approx. 20%)
  - Isolated or multinodal adenoma
  - Parathyroid hyperplasia
  - Carcinoma
  - Within the course of multiple endocrine neoplasms (MEN-I and MEN-II)
- Secondary/tertiary hyperparathyroidism
  - Acute and chronic renal failure
  - Autonomous hyperparathyroidism after long-term renal failure. Parathyroid hyperplasia no longer controllable due to calcemia.
    ○ Osteomalacia
- Hyperthyroidism
- Polyuric phase after acute renal failure:
  - Hyperparathyroidism in the preceding oliguric-anuric phase
- Cushing's syndrome
- Adrenal failure
- Acromegaly
- Pheochromocytoma
- VIPoma

Paraneoplasia (15%), secretion of osteolytic substances
- Tumors producing PTH
  - Ovarian cancer
  - Bronchial carcinomas
  - Kidney cancer
- Interleukin-1, TNF alpha, osteoclast-activating factor in:

▶ Myeloma/lymphoma
▶ Secretion of prostaglandins

Osteolyses in malignant processes/bone infiltration/bone destruction (55%)
▶ Paget's disease
▶ Acute osteoporosis
▶ Bone fracture
▶ Breast cancer
▶ Multiple myeloma
▶ Hodgkin's lymphoma
▶ Leukemia
▶ Polycythemia
▶ Hepatocellular carcinoma

Drugs
▶ Aluminum intoxication
▶ Estrogens/antiestrogens
▶ Lithium
▶ Steroids
▶ Tamoxifen
▶ Theophylline
▶ Thiazide diuretics
▶ Vitamin A/E
▶ Vitamin D/A.T.10 (calcinosis factor) intoxication

Ectopic 1,25-dihydroxycholecalciferol production
▶ Granulomatous diseases
  • Sarcoidosis
  • Tuberculosis
▶ Leprosy
▶ Histoplasmosis
▶ Coccidioidomycosis
▶ Berylliosis
▶ Oral candidiasis
▶ Silicone-induced granuloma
▶ Plasma cell granuloma

Reduced renal calcium excretion
▶ Familial hypocalcuric hypercalcemia
▶ Thiazide diuretics
▶ Dehydration

Miscellaneous
▶ Systemic diseases with kidney involvement
  • Multiple myeloma

• Sjögren's syndrome (drying up of the salivary, lacrimal and sebaceous glands)
• Sarcoidosis
▶ Immobilization
  • Paraplegia
▶ Hereditary diseases
  • Familial hypocalcuric hypercalcemia
  • Medullary spongy kidney
  • Bartter's syndrome
  • Gitelman's syndrome
  • Hypophosphatemia
▶ After kidney transplant (combination of existing secondary hyperparathyroidism with normal kidney function and vitamin D production after transplant; usually transient impairment)
▶ Hyperproteinemia
▶ Total parenteral nutrition
▶ Williams' syndrome
▶ Aspirin in large amounts
▶ Increased response to vitamin D
  • Idiopathic hypercalcemia in infants
▶ Rare causes
  • Coccidioidomycosis
  • Leprosy
  • Granulomatous diseases with tuberculosis
  • Vasoactive intestinal polypeptide-producing tumor

Hypercalcemia, See Calcium → 61

Hypercholesterolemia
Cholesterol hyperlipidemia
See Cardiac Risk Factor → 66
See LDL Cholesterol → 218
See HDL Cholesterol → 162
Reference values depend on existing CHD risk factors (pre-existing arteriosclerosis, familial hypercholesterolemia, smoking, obesity, diabetes, fibrinogen) and LDL/HDL ratio. Total cholesterol/HDL ratio has been proven to be effective in gauging the risk

of present or future coronary heart disease. High risk for CHD with a ratio over 11.5 (men) and 9.2 (women).

Cholesterol management
▶ With two or more cardiac risk factors
  • Goal LDL cholesterol < 130mg/dL:
    ○ Low fat diet if LDL cholesterol > 130mg/dL
    ○ Anti-hyperlipidemic therapy if LDL cholesterol > 160mg/dL.
▶ With CHD or diabetes mellitus
  • Goal LDL cholesterol < 100mg/dL:
    ○ Low fat diet if LDL cholesterol > 100mg/dL
    ○ Anti-hyperlipidemic if LDL cholesterol > 130mg/dL

Forms, causes
▶ Primary hypercholesterolemia
  • Familial hypercholesterolemia
    ○ Homozygous
    ○ Heterozygous
  • Familial dysbeta lipoproteinemia
  • Familial hypoalpha lipoproteinemia
  • Familial mixed hyperlipemia
  • Polygenetic hypercholesterolemia
  • Cholesterol storage disease
  • Apolipoprotein E polymorphism
  • Chylomicronemia
  • Lipoprotein(a) elevation
▶ Secondary hypercholesterolemia
  • Acute intermittent porphyria
  • Obesity
  • Prosperity syndrome = metabolic syndrome
  • Diabetes mellitus
  • Hypothyroidism
  • Nephrotic syndrome
  • Chronic renal failure
  • Chronic liver diseases
    ○ Cirrhosis
  • Cholestatic liver diseases
  • Malignant diseases
  • Cushing's syndrome
  • Drugs
    ○ Contraceptives
    ○ Diuretics
    ○ Beta blockers
    ○ Steroid therapy
  • Hemochromatosis
  • Acromegaly
  • Dysglobulinemia
    ○ Malnutrition
    ○ Malabsorption
    ○ Maldigestion
  • Malaria
▶ Reactive physiologic hypercholesterolemia
  • Hypercholesterolemia /hyperlipidemia e.g. after consumption of
    ○ Alcohol
    ○ Large meals
    ○ Fatty food

Hypercortisolism
See Cushing's Syndrome → 91

Hyperglobulia, See Polycythemia → 288

Hyperglycemia

Abnormally high concentration of glucose in the circulating blood, seen especially in patients with diabetes mellitus.
See Hypoglycemia → 199
See Glucosuria → 155,
See HbA1, HbA1c → 162

Primary
▶ Type I diabetes mellitus
  • Idiopathic
  • Immune mediated
    ○ Late onset autoimmune diabetes mellitus
▶ Type II diabetes mellitus
  ○ With and without obesity
▶ Gestational diabetes

Secondary
▶ Diseases of the exocrine pancreas
  • Pancreatitis
    ○ Acute

- ○ Chronic
- ○ Recurrent
- Pancreas tumor, neoplasm
- Trauma
- Pancreatectomy
- Idiopathic hemochromatosis
- Cystic fibrosis
- Fibrocalculous pancreatopathy
- Hemochromatosis
- Genetic defects of the β cell function
  - ○ Chromosome 20 (formerly MODY1)
  - ○ Chromosome 7 (formerly MODY2)
  - ○ Chromosome 12 (formerly MODY3)
  - ○ Mitochondrial DNA
▶ Endocrine
- Increased counterregulatory hormone production
  - ○ Cushing's disease
  - ○ Acromegaly
  - ○ Pheochromocytoma
  - ○ Glucagonoma
  - ○ Hyperthyroidism
  - ○ Somatostatinoma
  - ○ Conn's syndrome
  - ○ VIPoma
  - ○ Hyperaldosteronism
- Temporarily increased counterregulatory hormones (temporary hyperglycemia)
  - ○ Acute pancreatitis
  - ○ Stress
  - ○ Myocardial infarction
  - ○ Infection
  - ○ Stroke
  - ○ Renal insufficiency
  - ○ Surgery
  - ○ Trauma
  - ○ Hepatic disorder
  - ○ Status epilepticus
  - ○ Wernicke encephalopathy
  - ○ Subarachnoid hemorrhage
▶ Liver disease
- Cirrhosis
- Hemochromatosis
▶ Infections

- Congenital German measles
- Cytomegalovirus
- Other infections
▶ Insulin resistance
- Disorders of the insulin receptor
  - ○ Acanthosis nigricans
  - ○ Insulin resistance type A
  - ○ Rabson-Mendenhall syndrome
  - ○ Leprechaunism
  - ○ Lipatrophic diabetes
- Secondary insulin resistance
  - ○ Obesity
  - ○ Lack of exercise
  - ○ Stress
  - ○ Pregnancy
  - ○ Cirrhosis
  - ○ Endocrinopathies
▶ Drugs, toxins
- ACTH
- α-interferon
- Alcohol
- Anesthetics
- Benzodiazepines
- Cadmium
- Calcium-channel blockers
- Chlorpromazine
- Chlorthalidone
- Clonidine
- Contraceptives
- Corticosteroids
- Cyclophosphamide
- Danazol
- Dapsone
- Diazoxid
- Diphenylhydantoin
- Diuretics
- Epinephrine
- Estrogens
- Glucagon
- Glucocorticoids
- Haloperidol
- Imipramine
- Indomethacin
- L asparaginase
- Lithium

- Morphine
- Nicotinic acid
- Opiates
- Pentamidine
- Phenothiazines
- Phenytoin
- Prazosin
- Propranolol
- Rifampin
- Salicylates
- STH
- Sympathomimetics
- Thyroxine
- Tranquilizers
- Tricyclic antidepressants
- Miscellaneous
  - Decreased glucose tolerance
  - CNS disease
  - Muscle diseases
  - Lipodystrophy

Syndromes associated with diabetes
▶ Prader-Willi syndrome
▶ Porphyria
▶ Dystrophia myotonica
▶ Laurence-Moon-Biedel syndrome
▶ Huntington's chorea
▶ Friedreich's ataxia
▶ Wolfram syndrome
▶ Turner's syndrome
▶ Klinefelter's syndrome
▶ Down's syndrome

Hyperhidrosis
Polyhidrosis, sudorrhea.
Excessive or profuse sweating.
Endocrine
▶ Hyperthyroidism
▶ Pheochromocytoma
▶ Hypoglycemic shock
▶ Insulinoma
▶ Carcinoid syndrome
▶ Acromegaly
▶ Menopause
▶ Hypogonadism

▶ Castration
▶ Diabetes mellitus
▶ Diabetic neuropathy
▶ Hypoglycemia
▶ Mastocytosis
▶ Obesity
▶ Glycogenoses I, III, VI
▶ Fabry's disease
Infections
▶ Chronic infections
▶ Tuberculosis
  - Night sweat !
▶ Pneumonia
▶ Endocarditis lenta
▶ Acute rheumatic fever
▶ Brucellosis
▶ HIV infection
▶ Viral infections
Neoplasm
▶ Hodgkin's lymphoma
▶ Non Hodgkin's lymphoma
▶ Chronic myelocytic leukemia
▶ Sarcomas
▶ Hypernephroma
▶ Primary liver cell carcinoma
Cardiovascular
▶ Shock
▶ Heart attack
▶ Left heart failure
▶ Pulmonary embolism
▶ Acute hypertensive crisis
Drugs, toxins
▶ Acrylamide
▶ Arsenic
▶ Estrogen
▶ Mercury
▶ n-Hexane
▶ Nicotine
▶ Spironolactone
▶ Thyroxin
Neurologic
▶ Polyneuropathy
▶ Encephalitis
▶ Tabes dorsalis

H

- ▶ Syringomyelia
- ▶ Parkinson's disease
- ▶ CNS trauma

Miscellaneous

- ▶ Rheumatoid arthritis
- ▶ Collagen vascular disease
- ▶ Fever
- ▶ Obesity
- ▶ Menopause
- ▶ Autonomic dystonia
- ▶ Dumping syndrome
- ▶ Withdrawal in drug addicts
- ▶ Fructose intolerance
- ▶ Phenylketonuria
- ▶ Rickets

Hyperhydration

See Hypernatremia → 193

Hyperkalemia

A greater than normal concentration of potassium ions in the circulating blood. Indications for determination of potassium levels are cardiac dysrhythmias, acute or chronic renal failure, diarrhea, vomiting, known electrolyte imbalance, administration of diuretics and laxatives, and acid-base imbalance. ECG: tall, peaked T waves that later flatten, broad QRS complex. Finally, tachycardic arrhythmias can occur resulting in bradycardia and asystole.

Hyperkalemia

Serum potassium > 5.5 mmol/l

Pseudohyperkalemia

- ▶ Hemolysis of sampled blood
  - Stagnation
  - Rapid aspiration
  - Delayed centrifugation
  - Extravascular hemolysis
- ▶ Potassium release in sampled blood
  - Thrombocytosis
  - Leukocytosis

Increased intake

- ▶ Oral potassium intake:
  - Only in advanced renal failure
  - Replacement salts containing potassium
- ▶ Parenteral potassium supply
  - KCl (!)
  - Transfusion
  - Potassium containing drugs
    - K^+-Penicillin

Decreased renal potassium excretion

- ▶ Acute renal failure
- ▶ Chronic renal failure
- ▶ Drugs
  - ACE inhibitors
  - Angiotensin II receptor blockers
  - Co-trimoxazol
  - Cyclosporine
  - Heparin
  - NSAIDs
    - Indomethacin
    - Ibuprofen
  - Pentamidine
  - Potassium-sparing diuretics
    - Amiloride
    - Spironolactone
    - Triamterene
  - Tacrolimus
- ▶ Mineralocorticoid deficiency
  - Addison's disease
  - Bilateral adrenalectomy
  - Hypoaldosteronism
    - Hyporeninemic hypoaldosteronism
    - Specific enzyme defect
    - Tubular unresponsiveness
- ▶ Primary defect in potassium transport
- ▶ Congestive heart failure
- ▶ Graft-vs.-host disease of the kidney

Cellular shift of potassium

Intra- to extracellular shift

- ▶ Acidosis
  - Respiratory acidosis
  - Metabolic acidosis
    - Ketoacidotic coma (Hypoinsulinemia)

- Hyperosmolality (see hypertonic dehydration → 314)
  - Radiocontrast
  - Hypertonic dextrose
  - Mannitol
- Drugs
  - Alpha-adrenergic agonists
  - Arginine infusion
  - Betablockers
  - Digitalis overdose
  - Succinylcholine
  - Hyperkalemic periodic paralysis
- Release of potassium from cells:
  - Severe soft tissue injury
    ○ Crush syndrome
  - Rhabdomyolysis
  - Burns
  - Hemolytic crisis
  - Chemotherapeutic therapy
  - Heavy exercise
  - Hypoinsulinemia
  - Tourniquet syndrome (delayed opening of total arterial vascular occlusions)

Hyperlipidemia, hyperlipoproteinemia,
See Triglycerides → 360
See Hypercholesterolemia → 188
See Coronary Risk Factor → 66
See LDL Cholesterol → 218
See Protein in the Serum → 296

Hypernatremia
> 145 mmol/L
Causes
- Idiopathic hypernatremia
- Water loss
  - Inability to obtain enough water
    ○ Impaired thirst drive
      - *Hypothalamic lesion*
    ○ Coma
    ○ Dementia
- Excessive sodium intake
  - Sodium administration

  - ○ Sodium bicarbonate
  - Ingestion of large quantities of sodium (seawater)
- Endocrine disorders
  - ○ Ectopic ACTH production
  - ○ Cushing´s syndrome
  - ○ Hyperaldosteronism
- Loss of water in excess of sodium
  - Renal loss
    ○ Central diabetes insipidus
    ○ Impaired renal concentrating
      - *Osmotic diuresis (diabetic ketoacidosis; tube feedings, diuretic phase of acute renal failure)*
    ○ Use of diuretics
    ○ Hypokalemia
    ○ Hypercalcemia
    ○ Decreased protein intake
    ○ Multiple myeloma
    ○ Amyloidosis
    ○ Sarcoidosis
  - Peritoneal dialysis
  - Skin loss
    ○ Burns
    ○ Excessive sweating
- Drugs
  - Alcohol
  - Amphoterecin B
  - Colchicine
  - Diuretics
  - Foscarnet
  - Lithium
  - Phenytoin
  - Sulfonylureas
  - Vinblastine

Hypernatremia with normal total body sodium
- Diabetes insipidus
- Idiopathic hypernatremia

Hypernatremia with reduced total body sodium
- Water loss
  - Excessive sweating
  - Diabetes insipidus

H

► Hydropenia
► Lack of thirst

Pseudohyponatremia
► High plasma osmolality
  • Hyperglycemia
  • Mannitol
  • High urea levels with renal failure
► Normal plasma osmolality
  • Hyperlipidemia
  • Hyperproteinemia

Hyperoxaluria, See Nephrolithiasis → 255

Hyperphosphatemia
See Phosphate → 283

Hyperphosphaturia, See Phosphate → 283

Hyperprolactinemia, See Prolactin → 293

Hyperreflexia, See Reflexes → 313

Hypersomnia
Sleepiness, daytime tiredness, hypersomnolence
Excessive drowsiness at inappropriate times (hypersomnolence) and/or excessively long sleep periods (hypersomnia).
Causes
► Idiopathic daytime hypersomnolence
► Neurologic
  • Brain tumor
  • Brain abscess
  • Increased intracranial pressure
  • Epilepsy
  • Myoclonic movements
► Primary sleep disorders
  • Narcolepsy (→ 252)
  • Sleep apnea
  • Sleep deprivation
  • Circadian rhythm abnormalities (shift workers)
  • Sleep hygiene
► Systemic
  • Chronic obstructive pulmonary disease
  • Congestive heart failure
  • Coronary artery disease
  • Hypotension
  • Anemia
  • Hypothyroidism
  • Addison's disease
  • Precoma in metabolic encephalopathy
  • Post-hepatitis syndrome
► Head trauma
► Drugs
  • Alcohol
  • Antihistamines
  • Barbiturates
  • Benzodiazepines
► Depression
► Infection
  • Mononucleosis
  • Other viral syndromes
  • Encephalitis
  • Meningitis

Hypertension
High systemic arterial blood pressure.

Blood Pressure	Systolic (mm Hg)	Diastolic (mm Hg)
Optimal	< 120	< 80
Normal	< 130	< 85
High normal	130-139	85-89
Mild hypertension	140-159	90-99
Moderate hypertension	160-179	100-109
Severe hypertension	180-209	110-119
Very severe hypertension	> 210	> 120

Primary (idiopathic) hypertension
Secondary hypertension
► Endocrine
  • Pheochromocytoma
  • Primary hyperaldosteronism

- Conn's syndrome
- Cushing's syndrome
- Carcinoid syndrome
- Obesity
- Gestational hypertension
- Hyperthyroidism
- Acromegaly
- Renin producing tumors
- Primary hyperparathyroidism
- Endothelin producing tumor

▶ Renovascular
- Renal artery stenosis
- Arteriosclerosis
- Fibromuscular hyperplasia
- Aneurysm
- Thrombosis
- Embolism or thrombosis of the renal artery
- Trauma to the renal artery
- Arteriovenous fistula
- Arteriitis
- Dissection of the aorta
- Dissection of the renal arteries

▶ Other renal disorder
- Acute/chronic glomerulopathies
- Diabetic nephropathy
- Interstitial nephritis
- Kidney involvement in systemic diseases
- Hydronephrosis
- Acute renal failure
- Analgesic nephritis
- Liddle's syndrome
- After kidney transplantation
- Polycystic nephropathy
- Reflux nephropathy
- Hydronephrosis
- Perirenal hematoma
- Retroperitoneal fibrosis
- Malignant tumors
- Compression
  ○ Retroperitoneal fibrosis
  ○ Tumor

▶ Drugs, toxins, nutrition
- Anabolics

- Anesthetics
- Antirheumatics
- Appetite suppressants
- Bromocriptine
- Cadmium
- Carbeoxolon
- Cocaine
- Corticosteroids
- Cyclosporine
- Disulfiram
- Ergotamine
- Erythropoietin
- Fentanyl
- Heavy metals
- Ketamine
- Lead
- Licorice (mineralocorticoid effect)
- Lithium
- MAO inhibitors
- Metoclopramid
- Naloxone
- Oral contraceptives
- Pentazocine
- Scopolamine
- Serotonine antagonists
- Taramin (in red wine, older cheese)
- Thallium
- Thiazides
- Yohimbine

▶ Hypervolemia, hyperviscosity
- Polycythemia
- Dialysis
- Transfusions of larger blood volumes

▶ Neurogenic
- Elevated intracranial pressure (→ 213)
- Severe head trauma
- Meningitis
- Encephalitisis
- Quadriplegia
- Guillain-Barré syndrome/ Polyradiculitis

▶ Psychogenic
- Hyperventilation
- Anxiety

H

- Stress
▶ Cardiovascular
  - Aortic isthmus stenosis
  - Aortic regurgitation
  - Patent ductus arteriosus
  - Arteriovenous fistula
  - III° AV block
▶ Gestational hypertension
  - Eclampsia
  - Preeclampsia
  - Transient hypertension
  - Chronic hypertension
▶ Miscellaneous
  - Porphyria
  - Burns
  - Perioperative
  - Hypoglycemia
  - Alcohol withdrawal
  - Pancreatitis

Hypertension, pulmonary
See Pulmonary Hypertension → 306

Hyperthyroidism

Clinical term for a heterogeneous group of diseases that go along with an increase of thyroxin (T_4) and/or triiodothyronin (T_3). Symptoms: tachycardia, motorAgitation with small tremors, intolerance of heat, hyperhydrosis, warm sweaty skin, ravenous hunger, diarrhea, weight loss, hair loss, muscle weakness. Hyperthyroidism can manifest in older individuals only in the form of apathy, weight loss or atrial fibrillation.

Causes
▶ Grave's disease (imunogenic hyperthyroidism)
▶ Autonomous thyroid function
  - Toxic multinodular goiter
  - Toxic adenoma
  - Disseminated autonomy
▶ Thyroiditis (initial or progress stage)
  - Hashimoto's thyroiditis (chronic)
  - Subacute thyroiditis (De Quervain)
  - Silent thyroiditis (pregnancy related)
  - Suppurative thyroiditis (acute)
  - Riedel's thyroiditis (invasive fibrous)
  - Radiation thyroiditis
▶ Thyroid destruction by drugs
  - Amiodarone
▶ Exogenous hyperthyroidism
  - Iatrogenic, factitious
  - Iodine excess
▶ Ectopic hyperthyroidism
  - Struma ovarii
  - Metastatic differentiated thyroid cancer
  - Thyroid carcinoma
▶ Secondary hyperthyroidism
  - TSH-secreting pituitary adenoma
  - Thyxroid hormone resistance syndrome
  - HCG-secreting tumors
  - Gestational thyrotoxicosis

Hypertonic dehydration
See Dehydration → 93

Hypertrichosis, See Hirsutism → 182

Hypertriglyceridemia
See Triglycerides → 360

Hypertrophy of the Heart

(Left) ventricular hypertrophy
▶ Hypertension
▶ Valve disease
  - Aortic stenosis
  - Aortic regurgitation
  - Mitral regurgitation
▶ Congenital heart diseases
  - Patent ductus arteriosus
  - Aortic coarctation
▶ Primary cardiomyopathies
  - Familial dilated and hypertrophic cardiomyopathy (CM).

- Idiopathic dilated cardiomyopathy (DCM)
- Hypertrophic cardiomyopathy (HCM)
- Restrictive CM
▸ Secondary cardiomyopathies
  - Chronic renal failure
  - Acromegaly
  - Thalassemia
  - Alcoholic CM

Right ventricular hypertrophy
▸ Congenital heart diseases
  - Ventricular septal defect
  - Atrial septal defect
  - Transposition of great vessels
  - Tetralogy of Fallot
  - Eisenmenger's syndrome
▸ Valve disease
  - Pulmonic stenosis
  - Pulmonic regurgitation
  - Tricuspid regurgitation
  - Mitral stenosis
▸ Cor pulmonale
  - Chronic obstructive pulmonary diseases (COPD)
▸ Chronic alveolar hypoventilation (pickwickian syndrome)
▸ Left ventricular hypertrophy or dilation

Left atrial enlargement
▸ Ventricular septal defect
▸ Mitral stenosis
▸ Mitral regurgitation
▸ Mitral valve prolapse
▸ Patent ductus arteriosus
▸ Left heart failure
▸ Infectious endocarditis
▸ Atrial aneurysm
▸ Myxedema (in left atrium)

Right atrial enlargement
▸ Ebstein's anomaly
▸ Tricuspid regurgitation
▸ Tricuspid stenosis
▸ Atrial septal defect (with large left to right shunt)
▸ Pulmonic stenosis
▸ Right heart failure

▸ Atrial aneurysm
▸ Tumor (in right atrium)
▸ Right atrioventricular valve prolapse

Hyperuricacidemia, See Uric Acid → 364

Hyperuricuria, See Uric Acid → 364

Hyperventilation
Overventilation, overbreathing
Increased alveolar ventilation resulting in respiratory alkalosis (→ 19)
Causes
▸ Psychogenic
  - Anxiety (!)
  - Panic disorder
  - States of excitation
  - Pain
▸ Fever
▸ Hypoxemia
  - Anemia
  - High altitude exposure (> 10.000 ft)
  - CO
  - Left-ventricular failure
  - Cyanotic cardiac desease
▸ Hypercapnia
▸ Pulmonary
  - Pulmonary fibrosis
  - Pulmonary edema
  - Pulmonary embolism
  - Asthma
  - Pneumothorax
▸ Metabolic
  - Metabolic acidosis
  - Diabetes mellitus
  - Hypoglycemia
  - Uremia
  - Thyrotoxicosis
▸ Neurologic
  - Hepatic encephalopathy (→ 124)
  - Encephalitis
  - Tumor
  - Trauma

- Subarachnoid hemorrhage
- After epileptic attack
▸ Drugs
  - Adrenaline
  - Aminophylline
  - CO
  - Progesterone
  - Salicylates
▸ Sepsis
▸ Shock

Hypoaldosteronism

Primary hypoaldosteronism
▸ Adrenal cortical insufficiency [Addison's disease (→ 14)]
▸ Isolated aldosterone synthesis defects
▸ Adrenogenital syndrome (some forms)

Secondary hypoaldosteronism
▸ Hyporeninemia
▸ Pituitary insufficiency
▸ Cushing's syndrome with elevated ACTH secretion

Hypocalcemia

Hypocalcemia is a decrease in total plasma calcium concentration below 8.8 mg/dL (2.20 mmol/L) in the presence of normal plasma protein concentration. Clinical signs of hypocalcemia include tetany, Chvostek's and Trousseau's signs, dystonia, aphasia, confusion, chorea-like motions, QT elongation, decreased ST, heart failure, diarrhea, achlorhydria, malabsorption, muscle weakness, dry skin, hair loss and bilateral cataracts.

Main causes
▸ Hypoparathyroidism
▸ Pseudohypoparathyroidism
▸ Vitamin D deficiency
▸ Renal failure
▸ Magnesium depletion
▸ Acute pancreatitis
▸ Hypoproteinemia

▸ Enhanced bone formation
▸ Septic shock
▸ Hyperphosphatemia
▸ Drugs
▸ Excessive secretion of calcitonin,

Hypoalbuminemia
▸ Normal serum ionized calcium

Reduced uptake
▸ Malabsorption
▸ Maldigestion
▸ Short bowel syndrome
▸ Vitamin D deficiency

Increased loss
▸ Alcohol abuse
▸ Chronic renal failure
▸ Nephrotic syndrome
▸ Diuretic therapy

Endocrine
▸ Hypoparathyroidism
  - Congenital aplasia of the parathyroid gland
  - Idiopathic/autoimmune
  - Infiltrative
  - Postoperative after thyroidectomy
▸ Pseudohypoparathyroidism
  - Decreased PTH effect on end organs/endogenous resistance
▸ Calcitonin secretion in medullary thyroid carcinoma
▸ Adrenocortical hyperplasia
▸ Steroid therapy

Vitamin D deficiency in secondary hyperparathyroidism
▸ Decreased UV/sun
▸ Malabsorption
▸ Kidney diseases with reduced formation of activated vitamin D
▸ Anticonvulsants

Hypomagnesemia
▸ Therapy with cisplatin
▸ Therapy with aminoglycosides
▸ Alcohol

Paraneoplasia
▸ Breast cancer

- Bronchial cancer
- Thyroid cancer

Drugs
- Aminoglycosides
- Calcitonin
- Cis-platinum
- Colchicine
- Dilantin
- EDTA
- Ethylene glycol
- Gentamycin
- Loop diuretics
- Mithramicin
- Phenobarbital
- Phenytoin
- Protamine

Miscellaneous
- Sepsis
- Alkalosis
- Acute pancreatitis
- Chronic renal failure
- Nephrotic syndrome
  - Decreased total calcium with normal ionized calcium
- Hyperphosphatemia
  - Phosphate administration
    - Enemas, laxatives
    - Intravenous administration
  - Renal failure
  - Rhabdomyolysis
  - Tumor lysis syndrome
- Increased diuresis with physiologic saline solution
- Transfusion of citrated blood
- Cirrhosis
- Osteopetrosis
- Neonatal tetany

Hypocortisolism, See Cortisol → 87

Hypoglycemia

Abnormally small concentration of glucose in the blood. Usually a complication of diabetes. Distinguish between **fasting hypoglycemia** (subacute or chronic with apathy, seizures, paralysis, confusion) and **postprandial hypoglycemia** (acute/reactive with palpitations, cold sweat, agitation, tremor)

Reference range

blood sugar < 40 mg/dl (< 2.2 mmol/l)
See Hyperglycemia → 189
See Glucosuria → 155
See HbA1, HbA1c → 162

Fasting hypoglycemia
- Reduced gluconeogenesis
  - Endocrine
    - Adrenal insufficiency
    - Catecholamine deficiency
    - Glucagon deficiency
    - Hypopituitarism
    - Hypothyroidism
    - Multiple endocrine neoplasia (MEN)
  - Enzyme defect
    - Glucose 6 phosphate dehydrogenase deficiency (glycogenosis type I)
    - Glycogenosis type V
  - Substrate deficiency
    - Ketotic hypoglycemia of infancy
    - Severe malnutrition, wasting
    - Late pregnancy
  - Severe liver disease
    - Hepatic congestion
    - Severe hepatitis
    - Cirrhosis
    - Liver cell carcinoma
  - Renal disease
    - Renal hypoglycemia
    - Uremia
  - Hypothermia
  - Drugs
    - Alcohol
    - Propranolol
    - Salicylates
- Overutilization of glucose
  - Hyperinsulinism
    - Insulinoma
    - Insulin autoimmunity
    - Drugs

- *Disopyramide*
- *Exogenous insulin*
- *Pentamidine*
- *Quinine*
- *Sulfonylureas*
  ○ Endotoxic shock
- Appropriate insulin level
  ○ Extrapancreatic tumor
  ○ Systemic carnitine deficiency
  ○ Deficiency in enzymes of fat oxidation
  ○ Cachexia (fat depletion)

Postprandial/reactive hypoglycemia
▶ Beginning stages of diabetes (reactive late hypoglycemia)
▶ Gastric emptying disorder (dumping syndrome)
  • Autonomous neuropathy
  • Post-surgical conditions with rapid gastric emptying
    ○ Gastrectomy
    ○ Gastrojejunostomy
    ○ Pyloroplasty
    ○ Vagotomy
▶ Enzyme defects
  • Glucose-6-phosphatase
  • Fructose-1,6-diphosphatase
  • Liver phosphorylase
  • Glycogen synthase
▶ Fructose intolerance
▶ Galactosemia
▶ Leucine sensitivity
▶ Elevated vagal tone
▶ Idiopathic

Miscellaneous
▶ Malabsorption
▶ Maldigestion
▶ Benign glucosuria
▶ Whipple's disease
▶ Tumors
▶ Hypoglycemia in newborns
  • Gestational diabetic mother
  • Diabetic mother
▶ Idiopathic hypoglycemia McQuarrie
▶ Autonomic dystonia

▶ Heavy exercise

Drugs
▶ Alcohol
▶ Betablockers
▶ Biguanides
▶ Insulin
▶ MAO inhibitors
▶ NSAIDs
▶ Phenylbutazone
▶ Salicylates
▶ Sulfonyl ureas
▶ Warfarin

Causes for hypoglycemia in diabetes
▶ Drug overdose
  • Insulin
  • Sulfonyl ureas
▶ Insufficient carbohydrate supply after taking blood sugar lowering drugs
▶ Increase in exercise, physical activity
▶ Infections
▶ Surgery
▶ Trauma
▶ Vomiting
▶ Weight loss
▶ Incorrect absorption of insulin at the injection site
▶ Use of incorrect insulin
▶ Change of insulin medication
▶ Drug interactions
  • Alcohol
  • Betablockers
  • Glucagon deficit
  • NSAIDs
▶ Antibodies against insulin (sudden release of bound insulin)
▶ Reduced adrenaline secretion in polyneuropathy

Hypogonadism

Inadequate gonadal function, manifested by deficiencies in gametogenesis and/or the secretion of gonadal hormones. Manifested differently in males and in females, before and after the onset of puberty. If onset is in prepubertal males and testosterone replacement is not instituted, the individual has features of eunuchoidism, including sparse body hair, poor development of skeletal muscles, and delay in epiphyseal closure with long arms and legs. When hypogonadism occurs in postpubertal males, lack of energy and decreased sexual function are the usual concerns. In females with hypogonadism before puberty, failure to progress through puberty or primary amenorrhea is the most common presenting feature. When hypogonadism occurs in postpubertal females, secondary amenorrhea is the usual concern.

Hypogonadotropic hypogonadism (secondary hypogonadism)
Decreased secretion of the gonadotropic hormones LH and FSH by the anterior pituitary gland
▶ CNS disorders
  • Tumors
    ○ Craniopharyngioma
    ○ Germinoma
    ○ Other germ cell tumors
    ○ Hypothalamic glioma
    ○ Optic glioma
    ○ Astrocytoma
    ○ Pituitary tumor
  • Miscellaneous
    ○ Langerhans histiocytosis
    ○ Postinfectious lesions of the CNS
    ○ Vascular abnormalities of the CNS
    ○ Radiation therapy
    ○ Congenital malformations
      – Craniofacial anomalies
    ○ Head trauma
  • Genetic causes
    ○ Kallmann syndrome
    ○ Congenital adrenal hypoplasia
    ○ Congenital hypogonadotropic hypogonadism
    ○ Isolated LH deficiency
    ○ Isolated FSH deficiency
  ▶ Systemic, malnutrition
  • Exercise-induced amenorrhea
  • Miscellaneous
    ○ Prader-Willi syndrome
    ○ Laurence-Moon syndrome
    ○ Bardet-Biedl syndrome
    ○ Functional gonadotropin deficiency
    ○ Hyperprolactinemia
    ○ Marijuana use
    ○ Gaucher disease

Hypergonadotropic hypogonadism in males (primary hypogonadism, primary testicular failure)
▶ Klinefelter syndrome
▶ Inactivating mutations
  • LH beta subunit
  • FSH beta subunit
  • LH receptor
  • FSH receptor
▶ Other causes
  • Chemotherapy
  • Radiation therapy
  • Testicular biosynthetic defects
  • Sertoli-cell-only syndrome
  • LH resistance
  • Anorchism
  • Cryptorchidism

Hypergonadotropic hypogonadism in females (primary ovarian failure)
▶ Turner syndrome
▶ Inactivating mutations
  • LH beta subunit
  • FSH beta subunit
  • LH receptor
  • FSH receptor
▶ XX and XY gonadal dysgenesis
  • Familial and sporadic XX gonadal dysgenesis and its variants
  • Familial and sporadic XY gonadal dysgenesis and its variants
▶ Other causes of
  • Premature menopause
  • Radiation therapy
  • Chemotherapy
  • Autoimmune oophoritis

- Resistant ovary
- Galactosemia
- Glycoprotein syndrome type 1
- FSH-receptor gene mutations
- LH/human chorionic gonadotropin (hCG) resistance
- Polycystic ovarian disease
- Noonan syndrome

Hypokalemia

Abnormally low concentration of potassium ions in the circulating blood. Clinical symptoms seen particularly with a rapid drop in potassium. Indications for determination of the potassium level are cardiac dysrhythmias, acute or chronic renal failure, diarrhea, vomiting, known electrolyte disturbance, administration of diuretics and laxatives, and acid-base imbalance. ECG: repolarization disorders, ST depression, promin. U, may merge into TU waves. See ECG, Hypokalemia and Hyperkalemia → 117

Hypokalemia

Serum potassium < 3.5 mmol/l

Pseudohypokalemia

▶ Leukocytes > 100,000/µl: If the blood stands longer than 1 h, hypokalemia results, because the leukocytes absorb potassium from the plasma.

Decreased intake

▶ Anorexia nervosa
▶ Starvation
▶ Clay ingestion

Nonrenal losses

▶ Gastrointestinal
- Alcoholism with reduced intestinal absorption of potassium
- Chronic laxative abuse
- Diarrhea (→ 101)
  ○ Malabsorption syndrome
  ○ Chronic inflammatory bowel disease
  ○ Gastroenteritis
  ○ Villous adenoma of the rectum
  ○ Ureterosigmoidostomy
- Ileus (→ 206)
- Bulimia
- Vomiting
- Pyloric stenosis
- Acute pancreatitis
▶ Integumentary loss
- Sweat

Renal losses

▶ Drugs
- Antibiotics
  ○ Amphotericin
  ○ Carbenicillin
  ○ Gentamicin
  ○ Penicillin (high-dose therapy)
- Diuretics
  ○ Furosemide
  ○ Thiazides
  ○ Mannitol
▶ Mineralocorticoid excess
- Primary aldosteronism
  ○ Adenoma
  ○ Bilateral adrenal hyperplasia
- Secondary aldosteronism
  ○ Malignant hypertension
  ○ Renin-secreting tumor
  ○ Renal artery stenosis
  ○ Hypovolemia
- Apparent mineralocorticoid excess
  ○ Carbenoxolon
  ○ Chewing tobacco
  ○ Licorice excess
- Cushing's syndrome
  ○ Primary adrenal disease
  ○ Secondary to non-endocrine tumor
- Steroid therapy
- Adrenogenital syndrome
- Bartter's syndrome
▶ Renal tubular damage
- Renal tubular acidosis
- Leukemia
- Hereditary pseudohyperaldosteronism
▶ Chronic glomerulonephritis
▶ Polyuric phase after acute renal failure
▶ Heart failure

- Diabetes with glucosuria
- Diabetes insipidus
- Hypomagnesemia
- Liddle's syndrome

Redistribution into cells
- Metabolic alkalosis
- Drugs
  - Alpha-adrenergic antagonists
  - $Beta_2$-adrenergic agonists
  - Insulin
  - Vitamin B_{12} or folic acid (megaloblastic anemia)
- Total parenteral nutrition
- Hypokalemic periodic paralysis (Hereditary diseases with periodic potassium shift into the cells: hypokalemia and paralysis)
- Hypothermia
- Acute hyperventilation
- Stress (stimulation of beta adrenergic receptors results in potassium shift into the cells, e.g. with myocardial infarction)

Hypomagnesemia, See Magnesium → 232

Hypomelanosis
Depigmentation, hypopigmentation, leukoderma
Causes, associated disorders
- Vitiligo
- Diabetes mellitus
- Thyroid disease
  - Hyperthyroidism
  - Hypothyroidism
  - Hashimoto's thyroiditis
- Anemia
  - Pernicious anemia
- Drugs, toxins
  - Antibiotics + UV
  - Hydrochinone
  - Local corticosteroids
  - Mercury
  - Phenols
- Congenital

- Piebaldism
- Nevus depigmentosus
- Moles
- Postinflammatory hypomelanosis
- Tinea versicolor
- Albinism, oculocutaneous albinism
- Scleroderma
- Tuberous sclerosis
- Sarcoidosis
- Vogt-Kayanagi-Harada syndrome
- Psoriasis
- Infection
  - Secondary syphilis
  - Leprosy
- Collagen vascular disease
  - Rheumatoid arthritis
  - Systemic lupus erythematosus
- Neoplasm
  - Cutaneous T-cell lymphoma
  - Gastric carcinoma
  - Malignant melanoma
  - Lymphoproliferative diseases
- Metabolic
  - Homocystinuria
  - Phenylketonuria
  - Pituitary insufficiency
  - Addison's disease
  - Hypoparathyroidism
- Thrombopenia
- Dysgammaglobulinemia
- Myasthenia gravis
- Syringomyelia
- Candidiasis
- Varicosis

Hyponatremia
< 130 mmol/L
With a reduction in the extracellular fluid volume and low total body sodium
- Diuretics
  - Azosemid
  - Chlorthalidon
  - Ethacrynic acid
  - Furosemide

- Mefruside
- Thiazides
► Renal sodium losses
- Renal tubular acidosis
- Tubulointerstitial kidney disease
- Natriuresis caused by central disorder
  ∘ After pituitary surgery
  ∘ Subarachnoid bleeding
- Addison's disease
- NSAIDs
- Diuretics
► Mineralocorticoid deficiency
► Addison's disease
► Glucocorticoid deficiency
► Diabetic coma
► Osmotic diuresis
- Diabetics with glucosuria
- Patients with urea diuresis
► Metabolic acidosis
► Peritonitis
► Gastrointestinal loss
- Ileus (→ 206)
- Fistula
- Vomiting
- Gastric drainage
- Diarrhea
► Iatrogenic
- Ascites puncture
- Pleuracentesis
► Loss into the third space
- Burns
- Pancreatitis
- Large surgery
- Ketonuria

With a (slightly) increased extracellular fluid volume
► SIADH (syndrome of inappropriate antidiuretic hormone → 332)
- Paraneoplastic bronchial carcinoma (ectopic ADH secretion)
► Hypothyroidism
► After surgery
► Psychosis
► Drugs
- Amitryptilin

- Antidepressants
- Carbamazepine
- Carbamazepine
- Chemotherapeutics
- Clofibrates
- Cyclophosphamide
- Desipramine
- Fluoxetine
- Fluphenazine
- Haloperidol
- Isoproterenol
- Monaminoxidase inhibitors
- Morphine
- Neuroleptics
- Nicotine
- NSAIDs
- Somatostatins
- Thiothixene
- Tolbutamide
- Trifluorperazine
- Trimethoprim/sulfamethoxazole
- Vinblastine
- Vincristine

With increased extracellular fluid volume and high total body sodium
► Heart failure
► Hypotonic infusions
► Cirrhosis
► Nephrotic syndrome
► Renal failure
► Excessive hydration

Hypophosphatemia, See Phosphate → 283

Hypoproteinemia
See Protein in the Serum → 296

Hyposthenuria
See Urine Osmolality → 369

Hypotension
Reduced arterial blood pressure, lower than 90/60 mm Hg.

Primary hypotension (most common)
▶ Idiopathic hypotension
Secondary hypotension
▶ Shock
- Internal bleeding
- Overwhelming infection
- Heart failure
- Trauma
- All other forms of shock
▶ Endocrine
- Addison's disease
- Pituitary insufficiency
- Adrenocortical insufficiency
- Hypothyroidism
- Adrenogenital syndrome
- Bartter's syndrome
- Diabetes insipidus
▶ Cardiovascular
- Aortic stenosis
- Aortic arch syndrome
- Aortic isthmus stenosis
- Heart failure
- Dysrhythmias
- Pulmonary embolism
- Valsalva maneuver
- Myocardial ischemia
- Myocardial infarction
- Cardiac valve defect
- Perimyocarditis
- Pericardial effusion
- Constrictive pericarditis
- Carotid sinus syndrome
- Vagal syncope
- Fatigue
- Heat, hyperthermia
▶ Drugs, intoxications
- Alcohol
- (General) anesthetics
- Antianxiety drugs
- Antiarrhythmics
- Antidepressants
- Antihypertensives
- Betablockers
- Calcium channel blockers
- Diuretics

- Histamine
- Monoamine oxidase inhibitors
- Narcotic analgesics
- Nitrates
- Phenothiazines
- Recreational drugs
  ○ Alcohol
  ○ Cannabis
  ○ Opiates
- Sedatives
- Tranquilizers
- Tricyclic antidepressants
- Vasodilators
▶ Hypovolemia, dehydration (→ 93)
- Hemorrhage, bleeding
  ○ Gastrointestinal bleeding
- Anemia
- Fluid loss
- Hyponatremia
- Excessive fluid loss through dialysis
- Insufficient fluid intake
▶ Vasovagal
Response of blood vessels to stimulation of the vagus nerve
- Syncope, fainting (→ 344)
▶ Orthostatic
- Chronic
- Transient
  ○ After immobilization
  ○ Convalescence
  ○ During and after infections
  ○ Pregnancy
▶ Allergic reaction
- Anaphylaxis
▶ Neurogenic
- Guillain–Barré syndrome/ Polyradiculitis
- Parkinson's disease
- Tabes dorsalis
- Syringomyelia
- Polyneuropathy
- Shy-Drager syndrome
- Paraplegia
- Multiple CVA

H

Hypothyroidism

Inadequate supply of body cells with thyroid hormones. Symptoms in adults: general weakness, weight gain, constipation, hypothermia with cool skin and cold intolerance, hypotension, bradycardia, paresthesias, muscular spasms, deceleration of reflexes, apathy and other psychic impairment. In newborns: respiratory failure, cyanosis, jaundice, muscular hypotonia. In children: impairment of growth and physical development.

Causes
▶ Thyroiditis
- Hashimoto's thyroiditis (chronic)
- Subacute thyroiditis (De Quervain)
- Silent thyroiditis (pregnancy related)
- Suppurative thyroiditis (acute)
- Riedel's thyroiditis (invasive fibrous)
▶ Iatrogenic
- Thyreostatic therapy (treated Graves' disease)
  ○ Radioactive iodine therapy
  ○ Subtotal thyroidectomy
  ○ Antithyroid drugs
    - *Propylthiouracil*
    - *Methimazole*
- Head and neck surgery
- Radiation therapy to head, neck or chest area
- Drug therapy
  ○ Amiodarone
  ○ Butazolidin
  ○ Iodine
  ○ Interferon and IL-2
  ○ Lithium
▶ Iodine deficiency
▶ Infiltrative disorders
- Amyloidosis
- Cystinosis
- Dermatosclerosis
- Hemachromatosis
- Riedel's thyroiditis
- Sarcoidosis, granulomatous disease
- Scleroderma
- Neoplastic
▶ Congenital hy1pothyroidism
- Thyroid agenesis, dysgenesis, ectopy
- Hormone synthesis disorder
- Peripheral thyroid gland hormone resistance (end organ resistance)
- TSH deficiency
▶ Secondary hypothyroidism
(See Pituitary Insufficiency → 285)

Hypotonic dehydration
See Dehydration → 93

Hypovolemic shock, See Shock → 329

Hypoxemia, See Blood Gas Analysis → 57
See Arterial Hypoxemia → 40

Icterus,, See Bilirubin → 51,
See Cholestasis → 75

Ileus

Intestinal obstruction, bowel obstruction
Mechanical, dynamic or adynamic obstruction of the bowel, accompanied by colicky pain, abdominal distention, vomiting, absence of passage of stool, often fever and dehydration.

Mechanical obstruction
▶ Most common causes
- Adhesions
- Hernia
- Neoplasms
  ○ Ovarian cancer
  ○ Colon cancer
▶ Extraluminal compression
- Congenital abnormalities
  ○ Malrotation
  ○ Annular pancreas

- Neoplasm
  - Carcinomatosis
  - Sarcoma
- (Incarcerated) adhesions
  - Postoperative
  - Inflammatory
  - Intraabdominal abscess
  - Neoplastic
  - Traumatic
  - Congenital
- Ascites
- Others
  - (Incarcerated) hernia
  - Invagination, intussusception
  - Pregnancy
  - Volvulus
  - Intraabdominal hematoma
▶ Intrinsic bowel lesions
- Congenital abnormalities
  - Adhesive bands
  - Atresia
  - Bowel duplication
  - Cysts
  - Hirschsprung's disease
  - Imperforate anus
  - Meckel's diverticulum
  - Stenosis
- Neoplasms
  - Adenomatous polyps
  - Multiple polyposis syndromes
  - Colon carcinoma
- Inflammation
  - Crohn's disease
  - Ulcerative colitis
  - Diverticulitis
  - Diverticular stricture
  - Tuberculosis
  - Endometriosis
  - Ischemia
- Miscellaneous
  - Hematoma of the bowel wall
  - Surgical anastomosis
  - Pneumatosis intestinalis
  - Trauma
  - Radiation induced stenosis

- Iatrogen
  - NSAID
▶ Obstruction, occlusion
- Foreign body
- Biliary calculus/Gallstone ileus
- Diverticulitis
- Ascariades
- Scleroderma
- Endometriosis
- Megacolon
- Congenital megacolon
- Stool thickening/Coprolithiasis
  - Therapy with dietary fiber (wheat bran)

Nonmechanical obstruction (paralytic ileus)
Due to paralysis of the bowel wall. Usually result of peritonitis or shock.
▶ Peritoneal irritation
- Peritonitis
- Ulcer perforation
- Acute pancreatitis
- Mesenteric infarction
- Peritoneal carcinomatosis
- Trauma
  - Penetrating wounds
▶ Retro-/Extraperitoneal irritation
- Postoperative
- Cholecystolithiasis
- Pyelonephritis
- Renal colic
- Perinephric abscess
- Retroperitoneal hematoma
- Psoas abscess
- Ovarian torsion
- Testicular torsion
- Pancreatitis
- Lymphoma
- Cancer
▶ Infectious/Toxic/Metabolic causes
- Sepsis
  - Urosepsis
- Systemic infection
- Pneumonia
- Empyema

- Uremia
- Diabetic coma
- Porphyria
- Lead poisoning
- Severe electrolyte disturbance
  - Hyperparathyroidism
  - Hypokalemia
- Morphine
- Anticholinergics
- Antihistamines
- Catecholamines
- Narcotics
► Neurogenic causes
- Spinal cord disease
  - Injury
  - Tumor
  - Inflammation
- Cerebral diseases
  - Apoplexy
  - Brain tumor
► Miscellaneous
- Osteomyelitis of the spine
- Connective tissue disease
- Mechanical ventilation
- Vitamin deficiency
- Acid-base imbalance

Idiopathic intestinal obstruction (Pseudo-obstruction)
► Functional bowel disease
► Aerophagia

Immune neutropenia
See Leukopenia → 223

Immunoglobulins, monoclonal. See Paraproteinemia, Paraproteinuria → 275

Impaired consciousness, See Coma → 79

Impaired sensibility, See Paresthesias → 276, See Neuropathy, Peripheral → 258

Impotence

Impotentia coeundi is the inability to perform sexual intercourse, e.g. due to erectile dysfunction, ejaculatory impairment and/or premature ejaculation. Impotentia generandi is infertility in men who retain potentia coeundi. Erectile dysfunction represents the most common problem.

Impotentia coeundi
► Aging
► Psychic causes (very common)
- Relationship conflict
- Insecurity
- Repressed homoeroticism
- Stress
- Exhaustion
- Male menopause
- After sexual abuse
- Psychogenic
  - Depression
  - Schizophrenia
► Endocrine
- Hypogonadism
- Hyperprolactinemia
- Hyperthyroidism
- Acromegaly
- Addison's disease
- See Pituitary Insufficiency → 285
  - Pituitary adenoma
- Testosterone deficiency
- Diabetes mellitus
- Hyperadrenocorticalism
- Adiposogenital dystrophy
► Drugs, toxins
- Alcohol
- Nicotine
- Amphetamines
- Antihistamines
- Barbiturates
- Beta blockers
- Carbamazepine
- Cimetidine

- Clonidine
- Guanethidine
- Ketoconazole
- Cocaine
- Marijuana
- Methadone
- Methyldopa
- Metoclopramid
- MAO inhibitors
- Narcotics
- Phenothiazine
- Sedatives
- Spironolactone
- Thiazides
- Tricyclic antidepressants
► Vascular causes
- Arteriosclerosis
- Angiitis obliterans
- Leriche's syndrome
- Circulatory disorders
- Diabetes mellitus
  ○ Inadequate renal blood flow due to polyneuropathy
► Neurologic
- Iatrogenic
  ○ Surgery on the lesser pelvis, retroperitoneum or vertebral column
- Prolapsed disk
- Multiple sclerosis
- Apoplexy
- Trauma
  ○ Pelvic ring fracture
- Diabetes mellitus
  ○ Polyneuropathy
- Tabes dorsalis
- Paraplegia
- Pyelitis
- Conus medullaris syndrome
► Genital causes
- Prostatitis
- Priapism
- Balanitis
- Tumor of the genital organs
- Epispadia
- Hypospadia

- Phimosis
- Hydrocele
- Renal anomaly
► Testicular changes
- Tumor
- Bilateral anorchia/cryptorchidism
  ○ Gonadal agenesis
  ○ Cryptorchidism
  ○ Testicular trauma
  ○ Torsion
  ○ Tumor
  ○ Infection
    - *Mumps*
    - *Tuberculosis*
  ○ Surgery
  ○ Castration
- Varicocele
- Hydrocele
- Orchitis
- Epididymitis
- Klinefelter's syndrome
- Sertoli-cell-only syndrome
- Noonan's syndrome
- Lymphoma
- Chemotherapy
- Radiation therapy
- Idiopathic
- Reifenstein's syndrome
- Male pseudohermaphroditism (FSH, LH and testosterone elevated)
- Tubular sclerosis
► Miscellaneous
- Hypertension
- Chronic renal failure
- Lipid metabolism disorders
- Chronic hepatopathy
- Cirrhosis
- Severe systemic diseases
- Cachexia
- Heart failure

Impotentia generandi
► Sperm disorders
- Oligospermia
- Azoospermia
- Necrospermia

- ▶ Disorders of spermatogenesis
  - Testicular hypoplasia
  - Incomplete descent of one or both testes
  - After testicle injury or infection
  - After radiation therapy
  - Varicocele
  - Hydrocele
  - Cryptorchidism
- ▶ Obstruction of the seminal ducts
  - Infection
    ○ Orchitis
    ○ Epididymitis
    ○ Prostatitis
    ○ Urethritis
  - After surgery (urethral strictures, deferentectomy)
- ▶ Hormonal disorders
  - Hypogonadism
  - Hypothyroidism
  - Hypopituitarism
  - Hormone-secreting adrenocortical tumors
- ▶ Neurogenic
  - Paraplegia
  - After apoplexy
  - Multiple sclerosis
- ▶ Autoimmune
  - Autoantibodies against sperm
- ▶ Drugs, toxins
  - ACE inhibitors
  - Alcohol
  - Androgens
  - Corticosteroids
  - Nicotine
  - Sedatives
- ▶ Psychogenic
  - Stress
  - Relationship conflict
- ▶ Miscellaneous
  - Exogenous testosterone substitution
  - Advanced age
  - Spermatocystitis

Inappetence

See Nausea, Vomiting → 252
See Weight Loss → 382

Neurologic, psychogenic
- ▶ Anorexia. See Weight Loss → 382
- ▶ Depression
- ▶ Nausea
- ▶ Stress
- ▶ Alzheimer's disease
- ▶ Aerophagia

Systemic
- ▶ Neoplastic
- ▶ Infections
  - Influenza
  - Tuberculosis
  - Chronic bronchitis
  - Endocarditis
  - Sepsis
  - HIV
- ▶ Fever

Gastrointestinal
- ▶ Parenchymal liver diseases
  - Hepatitis
  - Cirrhosis
  - Neoplastic
  - Congested liver
- ▶ Stomach
  - Irritable stomach
  - Gastritis
  - Gastroduodenal ulcer disease
  - Carcinomas
- ▶ Bile duct disease
  - Stones
  - Neoplastic
- ▶ Pancreatopathy
- ▶ Intestinal
  - Inflammations
  - Inflammatory bowel disease
  - Neoplastic
  - Ileus (→ 206)

Metabolic
▶ Uremia
▶ Renal failure
▶ Hypercalcemia
▶ Malignant tumors

Endocrine
▶ Hypothyroidism
▶ Primary hyperparathyroidism
▶ Addison's disease

Drugs, toxins
▶ Adrenaline
▶ Alcohol abuse
▶ Aminophillin
▶ Antibiotics
▶ Antimycotics
▶ Chemotherapeutics
▶ Digitalis
▶ Diuretics
▶ Estrogens
▶ Lead poisoning
▶ Lithium
▶ Nicotine
▶ Opiates

Miscellaneous
▶ Anemia
▶ Pain

Incontinence, See Urinary Incontinence → 365, See Encopresis → 125

Infertility

Inability to conceive, in spite of regular unprotected intercourse. 50 % of infertility is found in women, 35 % of infertility is found in men, 15 % is attributable to both or undetermined.

Infertility in women
▶ Ovarial
  • Ovarian amenorrhea
    ○ Hypoplastic ovarium
    ○ Polycystic ovary syndrome
    ○ Ovarian tumor
    ○ After radiation
  • Anovulation
  • Corpus luteum deficiency
▶ Tubal
  • Tubal occlusion
    ○ After salpingitis
    ○ Tube adhesions
  • Endometriosis
  • Motility disorder
▶ Uterine
  • Uterus malformation
  • Malposition
  • Hysteromyoma
  • Endometrium damage (Asherman's syndrome)
▶ Cervical
  • Lack of secretion
  • Cervicitis
  • Anatomic changes
    ○ After conization
  • Autoimmune (sperm antibodies in the cervical mucus)
▶ Vaginal
  • Vaginal malformation
  • Vaginitis
  • Vaginismus
  • Imperforate hymen
▶ Extragenital causes (5%)
  • Metabolic and nutritional disorders
    ○ Thyroid disorders
    ○ Diabetes mellitus
    ○ Severe nutritional disturbances
      – *Anorexia nervosa*
    ○ Obesity
    ○ Hypophyseal impairment
  • Prolactinoma
  • Drug abuse
  • Stimulants (nicotine, alcohol)
  • Psychosexual problems
    ○ Frigidity
    ○ Neuroses
    ○ Dyspareunia
▶ Idiopathic or unexplained (<10%)

Infertility in men
See Impotence → 208

Inorganic phosphorus
See Phosphate → 283

Insomnia
Perception or complaint of inadequate or poor-quality sleep in the absence of external impediments, during the period when sleep should normally occur.

Transient, short-term insomnia
▶ Environmental
  • Noise
  • Light
  • Extremes of temperature
  • Poor bed
▶ Stress
  • New job
  • New school
  • Exams
  • Deaths

Chronic insomnia
▶ Medical
  • Chronic pain syndromes
    ○ Arthritis pain
    ○ Cancer pain
  • Chronic obstructive pulmonary disease (COPD)
  • Asthma
  • Chronic renal disease
  • Congestive heart failure
  • Reflux esophagitis
  • Hyperthyroidism
  • Chronic fatigue syndrome
  • Fibromyalgia
▶ Neurologic
  • Parkinson disease
  • Other movement disorders
  • Headache syndromes
    ○ Cluster headaches
▶ Psychiatric disorders
  • Depression
  • Schizophrenia
  • Bipolar disorder (manic phase)
  • Anxiety disorders
    ○ Nocturnal panic disorder
    ○ Posttraumatic stress disorder
▶ Drugs
  • Alcohol
  • Amphetamines
  • Barbiturates
  • Benzodiazepines
  • Caffeine
  • Cocaine
  • Sedatives

Primary sleep disorders
▶ Restless leg syndrome (RLS), periodic limb movement disorder
▶ Obstructive sleep apnea
▶ Circadian rhythm disorders
  • Sleep phase advance syndrome
  • Sleep phase delay syndrome
  • Shift workers

Primary insomnia
▶ Psychophysiologic insomnia
▶ Idiopathic insomnia
▶ Sleep state misperception

Insufficiency, respiratory
See Respiratory Failure → 319

Intention tremor, See Tremor → 358

Interstitial nephritis See Tubulointerstitial Diseases of the Kidney → 362

Intestinal circulation disorder
See Mesenteric Ischemia → 240

Intracerebral hemorrhage
See Bleeding, Intracranial → 56

Intracranial bleeding
See Bleeding, Intracranial → 56

Intracranial Pressure, Increased

Elevated ICP
Elevated pressure within the cranial cavity.

Vascular
- Venous drainage obstruction
  - Cerebral venous sinus thrombosis
    - Hypercoagulable state (aseptic)
    - Otitis media
    - Mastoiditis
  - Jugular vein cut (neck dissection)
  - Superior vena cava syndrome
    (→ 344)
  - Cor pulmonale (→ 85)
- Intracranial bleeding
  - Subdural hematoma
  - Epidural hemorrhage
  - Intraventricular hemorrhage
- Hypoxic-ischemic injury
- Arteriovenous malformation

Hydrocephalus (→ 186)

Metabolic, endocrine
- Diabetic ketoacidosis
- Cushing's disease
- Addison's disease
- Hypothyroidism
- Hypoparathyroidism
- Obesity
- Acromegaly
- Polycystic ovary syndrome

Encephalopathy
- Hepatic encephalopathy
- Reye's syndrome

Water, electrolytes
- Hypoosmolality
- Hyperosmolality

Trauma
- Severe head injury
- Battered child syndrome
- Focal traumatic lesion

Infection
- Meningitis
- Meningoencephalitis
- Encephalitis
- HIV infection
- Abscess

Neoplasm

Drugs, toxins
- Amiodarone
- Antibiotics
- Chlordecone
- Corticosteroids (withdrawal)
- Cyclosporine
- Growth hormone
- Lead poisoning
- Leuprolide
- Levothyroxine (children)
- Lithium
- Nalidixic acid
- Mineralcorticoids
- Oral contraceptives
- Progestins
- Retinoic acid (Vit.A)
- Sulfonamides
- Tetracyclines
- Vitamin A (hypervitaminosis A)

Idiopathic

Miscellaneous
- Pregnancy
- Iron deficiency anemia
- Orthostatic edema
- Water intoxication (psychogenic polydipsia)
- Systemic lupus erythematosus
- Antiphospholipid antibody syndrome
- Sleep apnea
- Turner's syndrome
- Decerebrate posture
- Decorticate posture

Intraocular Pressure

Increased
See Glaucoma → 155

Decreased
► Acute iridocyclitis
► Diabetic coma

Intrauterine Growth Retardation

Small for gestational age

Asymmetric IUGR
► Maternal hypertension
► Maternal preeclampsia
► Gestational diabetes mellitus
► Maternal collagen vascular disease
► Maternal infection
► Maternal cigarette smoking

Symmetric IUGR
► Maternal malnutrition
► Multiple gestation
► Maternal anemia
► Phenylketonuria
► Chromosomal abnormality
  • Trisomy 13
  • Trisomy 18
  • Trisomy 21
► Congenital malformation
► Early infection
  • TORCH virus infection
  • Syphilis
  • Listeria
  • Tuberculosis
► Drugs, toxins
  • Alcohol
  • Cigarette smoking
  • Illicit drug abuse
    ○ Heroin
    ○ Methadone
  • Phenytoin

Iridocyclitis, See Red Eye → 311

Iron

The iron content of the body is 38 mg/kg in women and 50 mg/kg in men. The iron depots in the body are: erythrocytes: approx. 3000 mg; myoglobin: approx. 120 mg; cytochromes: approx. 3-8 mg; liver/spleen: approx. 300-800 mg. Daily turnover through synthesis and conversion of hemoglobin is 25 mg. Uptake occurs mainly through resorption in the small intestine. Only bivalent iron is resorbed intestinally; bound iron is trivalent. Considerable iron loss is possible through menstruation and pregnancy.
See Ferritin → 142
See Transferrin Saturation → 358

Reference range	
Women	7-25 μmol/l
Men	9-27 μmol/l

Decreased serum iron
► Insufficient dietary iron
  • Malnutrition
    ○ Alcoholism
    ○ Vegetarian
    ○ Unbalanced nutrition
► Increased requirements
  • Pregnancy
  • Lactation
  • Infants or small children
► Inadequate iron absorption
  • Gastric and/or intestinal resection
  • Celiac sprue
  • Malabsorption/Maldigestion of siderous foods
► Hypo- and atransferrinemia
  • Nephrotic syndrome
  • Cirrhosis
  • Exudative enteropathy
  • Congenital deficiency
► Increased iron loss
  • Chronic gastrointestinal blood loss
  • Blood donor
  • Hemodialysis

- Menstrual bleeding
  - Occult bleeding
  - Heavy menstrual bleeding
- Massive hemoglobinuria
► Iron metabolism disorder
- Chronic inflammations
- Acute inflammations
- Infections
- Neoplasms
- Myocardial infarction
- Stress
- Uremia

Increased serum iron
► Idiopathic hemochromatosis1
► Secondary hemochromatosis
► Ineffective erythropoiesis with increased destruction of red blood cells in the bone marrow
► Vitamin B$_{12}$ deficiency
► Hemolysis
► Hemolytic anemia
► Hemosiderosis
► Sideroblastic anemia
► Homozygous thalassemia
► Megaloblastic anemia
► Porphyria cutanea tarda
► Frequent blood transfusions
► Nutritive iron overloading
► Hepatic hypersiderinemia in severe hepatopathy
- Release of stored iron through hepatocyte decay
► Cisplatin therapy

Ischemia, cerebral
See Cerebrovascular Accident → 71

Ischuria
See Urinary Tract Obstruction → 367

Isotonic dehydration
See Dehydration → 93

Jaundice (icterus), See Bilirubin → 51, See Cholestasis → 75

Joint Hypermobility

Causes
► Marfan syndrome
► Ehlers-Danlos syndrome
► Down syndrome
► Osteogenesis imperfecta
► Arthropathy in syphilis
► Homocystinuria
► Hyperlysinemia
► Rheumatoid arthritis
► Poliomyelitis
► Infantile cerebral palsy
► After joint effusion
► Genu recurvatum
► Idiopathic

Joint impairment, See Arthritis → 41

Jugular Venous Distention

Cardiac
► (Right) ventricular failure
► Cardiac tamponade
► Constrictive pericarditis
► Pericardial effusion
► Cardiomyopathy (restrictive)
► Right atrial myxoma

Pulmonary
► Tension pneumothorax
► Pulmonary hypertension
► COPD

Masses, tumor
► Goiter
► Mediastinal neoplasm
► Thymoma
► Aortic aneurysm
► Hodgkin's lymphoma

Miscellaneous
▶ Mediastinal emphysema
▶ Superior vena cava syndrome (→ 344)
▶ Valsalva maneuver

Karnofsky Performance Scale

Commonly used for assessing terminally ill patients.

Description	Percent (%)
Normal, no complaints, no evidence of disease	100
Able to carry on normal activity; minor signs and symptoms of disease	90
Normal activity with effort; some signs and symptoms of disease	80
Cares for self; unable to carry on normal activity or do work	70
Requires occasional assistance, but is able to care for most personal needs	60
Requires considerable assistance and frequent medical care	50
Disabled; requires special care and assistance	40
Severely disabled; hospitalization indicated although death not imminent	30
Very sick; hospitalization necessary; requires active support treatment	20
Moribund; fatal processes progressing rapidly	10
Dead	0

Kidney diseases, cystic
See Renal Cysts → 314

Knee Pain

Common causes
▶ Traumatic arthritis
  • Bone, ligament or cartilage damage
  • ACL injury
  • MCL injury
  • LCL injury
▶ Osteoarthritis
▶ Rheumatoid arthritis
Less common causes
▶ Acute gouty arthritis
▶ Adult Still's disease
▶ Baker cyst
▶ Bursitis
▶ Chondromalacia patellae
▶ Chronic gouty arthritis
▶ Gonococcemia
▶ Osgood-Schlatter disease
▶ Pseudogout
▶ Psoriatic arthritis
▶ Reiter's syndrome
▶ Scleroderma
▶ Systemic lupus erythematosus

Kyphoscoliosis

Abnormal curvature of the spine. Kyphosis (extensive flexion) combined with scoliosis, where spine curves to the side. Common causes are posture-related abnormalities, degenerative changes of the spine, and osteoporosis.
Causes: See Scoliosis → 326

Lactate in the Liquor

Increased
▶ Bacterial meningitis
▶ Viral meningitis
▶ Fungal meningitis
▶ Hemorrhagic insult
▶ Ischemic insults
▶ Seizures
▶ Syncope

Lactate, Lactic Acidosis

Main product of anaerobic reduction of pyruvate produced by glycolysis. Synthesized in the musculature, erythrocytes and brain. Severe lactate acidosis usually shows an acute life-threatening clinical picture.

See Acidosis, Metabolic → 11
See Acidosis, Respiratory → 12
See Anion gap → 34

Reference range	
Capillary blood	5–15 mg/dl
Deoxygenated blood	–16 mg/dl
CSF	11–19 mg/dl

Increased
▶ With hypoxia
• Circulatory insufficiency
  ○ Shock
    - *Hypovolemia*
    - *Sepsis*
    - *Myocardial infarction*
  ○ Heart failure
• Respiratory failure
  ○ Hypoventilation with hypercapnia
• Heavy exercise
• Seizures
• Hypothermia
• Severe anemia
▶ Without hypoxia
• Uncontrolled diabetes mellitus
• Drugs, toxins
  ○ Acetaminophen
  ○ Alcohol
  ○ Biguanides
  ○ Glucagon
  ○ High doses of insulin
  ○ Isoniazide
  ○ Norepinephrine
  ○ Paracetaldehyde
  ○ Salicylates
  ○ Sodium nitroprusside
• Infusions
  ○ Sodium bicarbonate
  ○ Glucose
  ○ Sorbitol
  ○ Fructose
  ○ Xylitol
• Miscellaneous
  ○ Postoperative
  ○ Postoperative recognition of acute intra-abdominal vascular occlusions

  ○ Fetal emergency situations during childbirth
  ○ Lever failure
  ○ Severe thiamine deficiency
  ○ End-stage renal failure
  ○ Leukemia
  ○ Tumors
  ○ Congenital enzyme deficiency
    - *Glycogen storage disease*

LAP See Leukocyte Alkaline Phosphatase (LAP) → 222

LDH

Lactate dehydrogenase.
Present in all tissues. The enzyme catalyzes the oxidation of lactic acid to pyruvic acid. Five isoenzymes (LDH1–LDH5) are known. LDH1–2: myocardial infarction, myocarditis, germ cell tumors, hemolytic anemia, renal infarct and muscular dystrophy. LDH3: pulmonary embolism and mononucleosis. LDH4–5: liver diseases, skeletal myopathies, metastatic neoplasms.

Increased
▶ Cardiac
• Myocardial infarction (increase begins after 6–12 h, reaches maximum after 24–60 h and is measurable up to 8 days after infarction)
• Myocarditis
• Acute heart failure
• Cardiac dysrhythmia
• After cardiac catheterization
• After cardiac valve substitution
▶ Pulmonary
• Embolism
• Infarction
• Pneumonia
• Congestive heart failure
▶ Hepatic
• Hepatitis
• Cirrhosis

- Toxic liver damage
- Portal hypertension
- Liver abscess
- Liver tumor (metastases)
▶ Red blood cell disease
  - Hemolytic anemia
  - Erythrocyte destruction from prosthetic heart valve
  - Megaloblastic anemia
▶ Malignant tumors (cytorrhexis)
  - Malignant lymphoma
  - Multiple myeloma
  - Leukemia
  - Liver tumor (metastases)
  - Neuroblastoma
  - Testicular tumors
▶ Musculoskeletal diseases
  - Myopathy
  - Progressive muscular dystrophy
  - Dermatomyositis
  - Neurogenic muscular atrophy
  - Muscular trauma
▶ Renal parenchymal disease
  - Infarction
  - Glomerulonephritis
  - Acute tubular necrosis
  - Kidney transplant rejection
▶ Intestinal ischemia, infarction
▶ Pancreatitis
▶ Postoperative
▶ Infectious mononucleosis

LDL Cholesterol

See Cholesterol → 77
See Hypercholesterolemia → 188
See Cholesterol hyperlipidemia → 188
See Coronary Risk Factor → 66
See HDL Cholesterol → 162
Calculation (accurate if triglycerides < 400 mg/dl): LDL = total cholesterol - HDL - (triglyceride / 5) or LDL = total cholesterol - HDL - VLDL. Normal range dependent on cardiac risk factors (→ 66).

Increased
▶ Primary hyperlipoproteinemia
▶ High fat diet
▶ Acute myocardial infarction
▶ Obstructive liver disease (primary biliary cirrhosis)
▶ Hypothyroidism
▶ Nephrotic syndrome
▶ Diabetes mellitus
▶ Drugs
  - Anabolic steroids
  - Progestins
  - Thiazide diuretics
Decreased
▶ Abetalipoproteinemia
▶ Advanced liver disease
▶ Malnutrition

Left axis deviation
See ECG, Cardiac Axis → 116

Leg Cramps

Water, electrolyte disorders
▶ Hypokalemia
▶ Hyponatremia
▶ Hypocalcemia
▶ Hypomagnesemia
▶ Hypophosphatemia
▶ Hyperkalemia
▶ Muscle overstrain (soreness)
▶ Metabolic acidosis
▶ Respiratory alkalosis
▶ Isotone dehydration
▶ Excessive sweating
▶ CO intoxication
Metabolic, endocrine
▶ Diabetes mellitus
  - Diabetic neuropathy
▶ Hypoglycemia
▶ Uremia
▶ Hemodialysis
▶ Hyperthyroidism
▶ Hypothyroidism

Vascular
- Peripheral arterial disease
- Deep venous thrombosis

Infection
- Influenza
- Salmonellosis
- Brucellosis
- Measles
- Malaria
- Toxoplasmosis
- Coxsackie B
- Leptospirosis
- Tetanus

Orthopedic
- Talipes planus-splay foot-talipes valgus
- Gonarthrosis
- Contractures

Drugs, toxins
- Alcohol
- Antihypertensives
- Betablockers
- Bronchodilators
- Contraceptives
- Corticosteroids
- Diuretics
- Fluor
- Isoniazid
- Methysergide
- Neuroleptics
- Nicotine
- Opiates
- Quinidine
- Scopolamine
- Succinylcholine

Neurologic
- Peripheral nerve injury
- Polyneuropathy
  - Diabetic polyneuropathy
- Radicular syndrome
- Spinal muscular atrophy
- Amyotrophic lateral sclerosis

Miscellaneous
- Myopathies
- Heat cramps

- Vitamin B_{12} deficiency

Leg edemas, See Leg Swelling → 220

Leg Length Discrepancy
Idiopathic
- Unilateral hyperplasia
- Unilateral hypoplasia

Growth plate injury
- Infection
- Trauma

Asymmetric paralysis
- Cerebral palsy
- Poliomyelitis

Mass induced growth
- Tumor
- Hypervascularity after fracture
- Juvenile rheumatoid arthritis

Leg Pain
Neurologic
- Lumbar canal stenosis (pseudoclaudication)
- Radiculopathy
- Plexopathy
- Peripheral neuropathy
- Restless leg syndrome

Musculoskeletal
- Baker cyst
- Muscle or tendon strain
- Ligament damage
- Arthritis
- Connective tissue disease
- Night cramps

Vascular
- Arterial disorders
  - Peripheral vascular disease (intermittent claudication)
  - Arterial thromboembolism
  - Cholesterol embolism
  - Obliterating endarteritis
  - Autoimmune vascular disorders

▶ Venous disorders
  • Deep vein thrombosis
  • Chronic venous insufficiency
  • Primary varicosis

Electrolyte disorders
▶ Hypocalcemia
▶ Hypokalemia
▶ Hyponatremia (diuretic therapy in hemodialysis)

Drugs, toxins
▶ Alcohol abuse
▶ Fluor intoxication
▶ Nicotine abuse

Infection
▶ Leptospirosis
▶ Coxsackie B

Leg Swelling

Leg swelling can occur with general edema, and may only involve one or both lower extremities.

Unilateral leg swelling
▶ Vascular causes
  • Venous insufficiency
  • Phlebothrombosis (DVT)
  • Post-thrombotic syndrome
  • Thrombophlebitis
  • Tumor compression
  • Varicosis
  • Arteriovenous fistula
  • Ischemia
  • Postischemic
▶ Lymphatic causes
  • After radiation therapy
  • Postoperative
  • Posttraumatic
  • Neoplastic
  • Parasites
    ○ Elephantiasis due to filariae
  • Secondary lymphatic blockage
    ○ Due to compression of the lymph vessels or veins: neoplastic
  • Hereditary lymphedema
▶ Allergic causes

  • Angioneurotic edema
  • Insect bites
▶ Miscellaneous
  • Compartmental syndrome
  • Sudeck's syndrome
  • Local trauma
  • Baker's cyst
  • Cellulitis
  • Erysipelas
  • Myorrhexis

Bilateral leg swelling
▶ Cardiac causes
  • Right ventricular failure
    ○ Mitral stenosis
    ○ Constrictive pericarditis
    ○ Cor pulmonale
  • Left ventricular failure
  • Cardiomyopathy
▶ Hypoproteinemia
  • Nephrotic syndrome
  • Glomerulonephritis
  • Liver disease with synthesis disorder or portal vein stasis
  • Malabsorption
  • Malnutrition
  • Exudative enteropathy/Protein-losing enteropathy
  • Uncompensated hypertension
▶ Constitutional causes
  • Premenstrual
  • Orthostatic
  • Heat
▶ Drugs
  • ACTH
  • Anticoagulants
  • Corticosteroids
  • Estrogen
  • Hydralazine
  • Laxative abuse
  • Licorice
  • Methyldopa
  • Minoxidil
  • Nifedipine-type calcium antagonists
  • Phenylbutazone
▶ Endocrine

- Hyperaldosteronism (Conn's syndrome)
- Hypothyroidism
- Hyperthyroidism
- Myxedema (Hypothyroidism)
- Premenstrual
► Water and electrolyte imbalances
- Hyperhydration
- Renal failure
- EPH gestosis
► Vascular causes
- Varicosis
- Thrombophlebitis
- Chronic venous insufficiency
- Systemic vasculitis
- Ischemic leg edemas
► Abdominal causes
- Thrombosis in the vena cava
- Tumor in the area of the hypogastrium
- Ascites
- Filariasis
► Miscellaneous
- Erysipelas
- Pernicious anemia
- Hereditary lymphedema
- Elephantiasis
- Idiopathic edema
- Allergic reaction

Leg Ulcer

Crural Ulcer
Ulcer of the lower leg. Most common cause is chronic venous insufficiency.

Vascular
► Arterial or ischemic causes
- Arteriosclerosis
- Peripheral vascular disease
- Thromboangiitis obliterans (Bürger's disease)
- AV malformation
- Raynaud's syndrome
- Embolism
► Venous
- Venous insufficiency

- Deep venous thrombosis
► Lymphatic disorders
- Lymphangitis
- Lymphedema

Collagen vascular disease
► Rheumatoid arthritis
► Systemic lupus erythematosus
► Scleroderma
► Polyarteritis

Hematologic
► Sickle cell anemia
► Thalasemia
► Polycythemia vera
► Leukemia
► Cold agglutinin disease
► Protein C deficiency
► Protein S deficiency
► Macroglobulinemia

Infection
► Cellulitis
► Osteomyelitis
► Furuncle
► Ecthyma
► Septic emboli
► Fungal
- Blastomycosis
- Coccidiomycosis
- Histoplasmosis
- Sporotrichosis
► Bacterial
- Syphilis
  ○ Tabes dorsalis (Charcot joint)
- Tuberculosis
- Lepra
► Protozoal

Dermatitis
► Contact dermatitis
► Other allergic condition
► Bullous disease

Drugs
► Ergotism
► Halogens
► Hydroxyureas
► Injection ulcer

K
L

▸ Methotrexate
▸ Oral coagulants (warfarin)

Positioning, trauma
▸ Decubitus ulcer (factitial pressure)
▸ Trauma
▸ Burns
▸ Cold injury
▸ Radiation dermatitis
▸ Insect bites

Systemic
▸ Diabetes mellitus
  • Diabetic neuropathy
▸ Congestive heart failure
▸ Gout
▸ Malnutrition
▸ Anemia
▸ Gaucher's disease

Neuropathy
▸ Diabetic neuropathy
▸ Tabes dorsalis
▸ Syringomyelia

Tumor
▸ Basal cell carcinoma
▸ Squamous cell carcinoma
▸ Melanoma
▸ Kaposi's sarcoma
▸ Mycosis fungoides
▸ Metastases

Leukocyte Alkaline Phosphatase (LAP)

Phosphomonoesterase occurring in mature cells of the neutrophilic granulocytopoiesis.

Increased
▸ Polycythemia vera
▸ Idiopathic thrombocytemia
▸ Osteomyelofibrosis
▸ Multiple myeloma
▸ Acute leukemia
▸ Malignant lymphomas
▸ Aplastic anemia

▸ Tissue necrosis
▸ Megaloblastic anemia
▸ Solid tumors

Decreased
▸ Chronic myelocytic leukemia (in all other myeloproliferative syndromes LAP activity increases)
▸ Anemia
▸ Hemolysis
▸ Iron deficiency anemia
▸ Sideroachrestic (= sidero-blastic) anemia

Leukocyte casts, See Cylindruria → 92

Leukocytosis

Granulocytosis, neutrophilia

An increase in leukocytes is mainly based on an increase of the neutrophilic polymorphic granulocytes or the lymphocytes. Very often caused by an infection. Viral diseases and particular bacterial infections can also lead to a leukopenia.

Reference range

4.3–10.0 x $10^3/\mu$l

Infections
▸ Bacterial infections
▸ Viral infections (leukopenia also possible)
  • Infectious mononucleosis
  • Infectious lymphocytosis
  • Mumps
  • Measels
  • Chickenpox
  • Viral hepatitis
▸ Parasitic infections
▸ Fungal infections

Physical stimuli
▸ Exercise
▸ Trauma
▸ Seizures

Neoplastic
▶ Polycythemia vera
▶ Malignant tumors
▶ Chronic myelocytic leukemia
▶ Acute leukemia
▶ Prolymphocytic leukemia
▶ Acute and chronic NHL with marrow involvment
▶ Hairy cell leukemia
▶ Myelofibrosis

Hematologic
▶ Hemorrhage
▶ Postsplenectomy
▶ Recovery from agranulocytosis
▶ Hemolytic anemia

Tissue necrosis
▶ Burns
▶ Gangrene
▶ Burns

Chronic inflammatory diseases
▶ Chronic polyarthritis
▶ Colitis
▶ Dermatitis
▶ Pyelonephritis
▶ Endocarditis
▶ Bronchitis

Drugs, toxins
▶ Aspirin
▶ Benzene
▶ CO
▶ Corticosteroids (!)
▶ Griseofulvin
▶ Growths factors
  • G-CSF
  • GM-CSF
▶ Isoniazide
▶ Lead
▶ Streptomycin
▶ Thallium
▶ Trimethoprim/sulfamethoxazole

Metabolic
▶ Gout
▶ Diabetic coma
▶ Uremic coma

▶ Hyperthyroidism
▶ Cushing´s syndrome

Congenital
▶ Down syndrome

Leukocyturia

White blood cells (leukocytes) in urine.
Leukocyturia + bacterial growth
▶ Urinary tract infection (UTI, → 114)
Leukocyturia without bacterial growth (= aseptic leukocyturia)
▶ Prostatitis
▶ UTI requiring special growth conditions
  • Urogenital tuberculosis
  • Chlamydia
  • Gonococci
  • Herpes viruses
  • Mycoplasma
▶ UTI under antibiotic therapy
▶ Sample contamination
▶ Vaginal discharge
▶ Acute fever
▶ Urinary stone
▶ Urinary tract tumor
▶ Chronic interstitial nephritis

Leukocyte count, See Leukopenia → 223,
See Leukocytosis → 222

Leukonychia, See Nail changes → 250

Leukopenia
Granulocytopenia, agranulocytosis, neutropenia.
Leukopenia: any situation in which the total number of leukocytes in the circulating blood is less than normal. Neutropenia is a reduction (< 1,500/µl) of the neutrophilic granulocytes. Values <500/µl increases the danger of infection greatly (especially opportunistic pathogens). Agranulocytosis is

K
L

characterized by a decrease in the white blood cell count < 2000/μl and a drop in granulocytes < 500/μl, or the total absence of granulocytes. The other hematopoietic cell lines can also be affected. Oral candidiasis is a common clinical sign of agranulocytosis.

Reduced granulocytopoiesis (aplastic disease)

▶ Bone marrow damage
- Drugs, toxins
  - Aminobenzene
  - Analgesics
  - Antibiotics
  - Anticonvulsants
  - Antidepressants
  - Antidiabetics
  - AZT
  - Benzene
  - Cardiovascular drugs
  - Chemotherapeutics
  - Chloramphenicol
  - Gold compounds
  - Griseofulvin
  - H_2 blockers
  - Hydantoin
  - Hypnotics
  - Immunsuppressives
  - Metamizol
  - Nitrophenol
  - Phenylbutazone
  - Pyramidon
  - Sulfonamides
  - Thyroid depressants
  - Vitamin A intoxication
  - Ionizing radiation
▶ Bone marrow infiltration, dysfunction
- (Acute) leukemia
- Malignant lymphomas
- Tumor infiltration
- Osteomyelosclerosis
- Agranulocytosis
- Aplastic anemia
- Myelofibrosis
  - Myeloproliferative disorders

- Infection
▶ Nutrition
- Vitamin B_{12} or folic acid deficiency
  - Pernicious anemia
- Iron deficiency anemia
- Alcoholism
- Cachexia
▶ Congenital
- Kostmann syndrome
- Cyclic neutropenia

Granulocytopenias caused by increased cell turnover

▶ Autoimmune
- Acute after certain infections (e.g. mononucleosis)
- Chronically in HIV infection
- Malignant lymphomas
- Systemic lupus erythematosus
- Sjögren's syndrome
- Drug-induced granulocytopenias
- Idiopathic (e.g. autoimmune granulocytopenia in children)
▶ Infection
- Bacterial infections
  - Tuberculosis
  - Brucellosis
  - Typhoid fever
  - Paratyphus
  - Diphtheria
  - Yellow fever
  - Ornithosis
  - Tularemia
- Viral infections
  - Varicella
  - Influenza
  - Infectious mononucleosis
  - Infectious hepatitis
  - Chickenpox
  - Poliomyelitis
  - Exanthema subitum
  - HIV
  - Parvovirus B19
  - EBV
- Protozoal
  - Malaria

  - Toxoplasmosis
  - Kala azar
  - Rickettsial
- Distribution disorder
  - Hypersplenism

Miscellaneous
- Benign neutropenia in black people
- Benign familial neutropenia
- Endocrine
  - Thyrotoxicosis
  - Hypopituitarism
  - Hypothyroidism
- Vasculopathy
  - Primary and secondary varicosis
  - Varicosis
  - Degenerative and inflammatory vasculopathies
  - Vein compression syndrome
- Hyperviscosity syndrome
  - Hyperglobulia
  - Paraproteinemia
  - Diuretics
- Lipid storage diseases

LH, See Gonadotropins → 158

Lipase

Splits triglyceride esters of long-chain fatty acids. It is not absolutely organ-specific to the pancreas.
Main indications are diagnosis and followup of pancreatitis.

Reference range
< 190 U/l

Increased
- Acute pancreatitis
- Chronic relapsing pancreatitis
- Pancreatic cancer
- Pancreatic pseudocyst
- Acute cholecystitis
- Cholangitis
- Extrahepatic duct obstruction
- After ERCP

- Peptic ulcer disease
- Bowel obstruction or infarction
- Salivary gland inflammation or tumor
- Parotitis epidemica
- Renal failure
- Diabetic ketoacidosis
- Sarcoidosis

Lipid metabolism disorders,
See Triglycerides → 360
See Hypercholesterolemia → 188
See Cholesterol hyperlipidemia → 188 See Coronary Risk Factor → 66
See LDL Cholesterol → 218
See HDL Cholesterol → 162

Lipoprotein (a) (Lp (a))

A type of lipoprotein that is elevated in certain types of hyperlipoproteinemia and associated with increased risk of coronary disease.

Reference range
< 300 mg/l

Causes of increased Lp (a)
- Uremia
- Nephrotic syndrome
- Uncontrolled diabetes mellitus
- Hypothyroidism
- Acute phase of myocardial infarction

Causes of reduced Lp (a)
- Hyperthyroidism
- Drugs
  - Estrogen
  - Neomycin

Liver diseases

Hepatopathies

Infection
▶ Viral **hepatitis**
- Hepatitis A-G
- Epstein-Barr virus
- Cytomegalovirus
- Varicella-zoster
- Coxsackie
- Herpes simplex
  ○ HSV1
  ○ HSV2
- Measles
- Rubella

▶ Comcomitant hepatitis in infectious diseases
- HHV6
- Parainfluenza
- Yellow fever
- German measles
- Coxsackie
- Mumps
- Tuberculosis
- Leptospirosis
- Brucellosis
- Rickettsiosis
- Yellow fever
- Amebiasis
- Malaria
- Toxoplasmosis
- Schistosomiasis
- Trypanosomiasis
- Parasitic infection of the bile ducts
  ○ Ascariasis lumbricoides
  ○ Liver flukes
  ○ Trichinella spiralis

▶ Helminth infections of the liver
- Ascariasis lumbricoides
- Echinoccocus granulosus
- Echinoccocus multilocularis
- Schistosoma japonicum
- Schistosoma mansoni
- Liver flukes
- Canine roundworm

▶ Protozoiasis of the liver
- Toxoplasma gondii
- Trypanosoma cruzi
- Entamoeba histolytica
- Plasmodium falciparum
- Plasmodium vivax
- Plasmodium ovale

▶ Abscess
- Klebsiella
- Proteus
- Staph. aureus
- E. coli
- Leptospirosis
- Salmonella
- Rickettsia
- Tuberculosis
- Brucellosis

Metabolic
▶ **Alcohol abuse**
▶ Wilson's disease
▶ Hemochromatosis
▶ α_1-antitrypsin deficiency
▶ Cystic fibrosis
▶ Protoporphyria
▶ Galactosemia
▶ Hypertyrosinemia
▶ Glycogenosis
▶ Fructose intolerance
▶ Gaucher's disease
▶ Histiocytosis X
▶ Niemann-Pick disease
▶ Hyperthyroidism

(Cardio-)vascular
▶ Budd-Chiari syndrome
▶ Congestive heart failure
▶ Constrictive pericarditis
▶ Thrombosis
▶ Shock
▶ Hypoxia

K
L

- ► Tumor
- ► Inferior vena cava web

Drugs, toxins (selection only!)
- ► Acetaminophen
- ► Alcohol (!)
- ► Allopurinol
- ► Anabolic steroids
- ► Aspirin
- ► Chloroethylene
- ► Dantrolene
- ► Estrogens
- ► Halothan
- ► Isoniazide
- ► Methyldopa
- ► Nitrofurantoin
- ► Oxacillin
- ► Phenylbutazone
- ► Tetracyclines
- ► Thyroid depressants

Autoimmune, systemic
- ► Autoimmune hepatitis
- ► Primary sclerosing cholangitis
- ► Primary biliary cirrhosis
- ► Inflammatory bowel disease
- ► Sarcoidosis
- ► Amyloidosis
- ► Chronic myelocytic leukemia
- ► Polycythemia
- ► Osteomyelofibrosis
- ► (Non-)Hodgkin's lymphoma
- ► Hyperthermia
- ► Burns

Cholestatic (→ 75)
- ► Intrahepatic cholestasis (impairment of the bile flow in the liver)
- ► Extrahepatic cholestasis

Miscellaneous
- ► Alcoholic hepatitis
- ► Fatty liver (→ 142)

Localized liver changes
- ► Abscess (see infection)
- ► Benign tumors
  - • Focal nodular hyperplasia
  - • Hemangiomas
  - • Adenomas
  - • Hemangioendothelioma
    - ○ Hepatomas
- ► Malignant tumors
  - • Hepatocellular carcinoma
  - • Cholangiocarcinoma
  - • Angiosarcoma
  - • Metastases
    - ○ Colon cancer
    - ○ Pancreatic cancer
    - ○ Gastric carcinoma
    - ○ (Non-)Hodgkin's lymphoma
- ► Cysts (See Hepatic Cysts → 178)
- ► Hematoma
  - • Postoperative
  - • Trauma
  - • Bleeding

Diffuse liver changes
- ► Fatty liver (→ 142)
- ► Chronic hepatitis
  - • Chronic viral hepatitis
  - • Granulomatous hepatitis
  - • Autoimmune hepatitis
  - • Alcoholic hepatitis
  - • Drug-induced hepatitis
  - • Biliary hepatitis (→ 75)
  - • Wilson's disease
  - • Hepatitis in systemic diseases
- ► Cirrhosis (→ 78)

Loss of appetite, See Anorexia → 36

Loss of hearing. See Hearing Loss, Hearing Impairment → 165

Low voltage ECG
See ECG, QRS Complex → 118

Lumbago, See Back Pain → 49,
See Sciatica → 324

K
L

Lung Disease

Impaired lung function.

Physiologic categories
▶ Obstructive lung disease (→ 262)
▶ Restrictive lung disease (→ 320)
▶ Oxygenation disorders (→ 40)

Major lung diseases
▶ Asthma
▶ Bronchiolitis obliterans organizing pneumonia (BOOP)
▶ Chronic bronchitis
▶ COPD (chronic obstructive pulmonary disease)
▶ Emphysema
▶ Interstitial lung disease
▶ Pulmonary fibrosis
▶ Sarcoidosis

Luteinizing Hormone
See Gonadotropins → 158

Lymph Node Enlargement, Localalized

Lymph node enlargement, generalized
See Lymphadenopathy → 229

Axillary
▶ Breast cancer
▶ Mastitis
▶ Hodgkin's lymphoma
▶ Lymphatic leukemia
▶ Systemic lupus erythematosus
▶ Waldenström's syndrome
▶ Cat scratch fever
▶ Toxoplasmosis
▶ Erysipelas
▶ Lymphangitis
▶ Vaccination
▶ Anthrax
▶ Brucellosis
▶ Tularemia
▶ Idiopathic

Subauricular
▶ Infections
  • Angina
    ○ A. catarrhalis
    ○ Streptococcal tonsillitis
    ○ Vincent's angina
  • Infectious mononucleosis
  • Measles
  • Mumps
  • German measles
  • Varicella
  • Three-day fever
  • Aphthous stomatitis
  • Influenza
  • Tuberculosis
  • Toxoplasmosis
  • Listeriosis
▶ Neoplasms
  • Hodgkin's lymphoma
  • Leukemia

Supraclavicular
▶ Infections
  • Toxoplasmosis
  • Histoblastosis
▶ Neoplasms
  • Hodgkin's lymphoma
  • Pancoast tumor
  • Reticulosis
  • Hemoblastosis
  • Metastatic tumor
    ○ Esophageal/stomach/laryngeal/thyroid/bronchial/breast cancer

Lymph Node Metastases
See Lymphadenopathy → 229

Cervical lymph nodes
▶ Carcinoma in the oral cavity area
▶ Carcinoma in the throat area
▶ Carcinoma in the nasal area
▶ Carcinoma in the laryngeal area
▶ Esophageal cancer
▶ Lung cancer
▶ Salivary carcinoma
▶ Thyroid cancer

- ► Bronchial cancer
- ► Malignant lymphoma
- ► Neuroendocrine carcinoma
- ► Malignant melanoma

Supraclavicular lymph nodes
- ► Lung cancer
- ► Laryngeal cancer
- ► Esophageal cancer
- ► Gastric carcinoma
- ► Thyroid cancer
- ► Bronchial cancer
- ► Malignant lymphoma
- ► Neuroendocrine carcinoma
- ► Breast cancer
- ► Malignant melanoma

Axillary lymph nodes
- ► Breast cancer
- ► Lung cancer
- ► Carcinoma of the GI tract
- ► Malignant melanoma
- ► Malignant lymphoma
- ► Cervical cancer
- ► Uterine cancer
- ► Ovarian cancer
- ► Prostate cancer
- ► Testiclular (embryonal) carcinoma
- ► Gastric carcinoma
- ► Carcinoma in the GI tract
- ► Pancreatic cancer
- ► Kidney cancer
- ► Bladder cancer

Inguinal lymph nodes
- ► Cervical cancer
- ► Bladder cancer
- ► Rectal cancer
- ► Vaginal cancer
- ► Uterine cancer
- ► Ovarian cancer
- ► Prostate cancer
- ► Testicular (embryonal) carcinoma
- ► Malignant melanoma

Lymphadenopathy

Generalized lymph node enlargement.

Malignant diseases
- ► Hematologic
  - Lymphoma
    - ○ Hodgkin's lymphoma
    - ○ Non-Hodgkin's lymphoma
  - Waldenström's syndrome
  - Angioimmunoblastic lymphadenopathy
  - Leukemia
    - ○ Acute lymphocytic leukemia
    - ○ Chronic lymphocytic leukemia
    - ○ Acute leukemias
    - ○ Sézary syndrome
    - ○ Hairy cell leukemia
  - Malignant histiocytosis
  - Amyloidosis
- ► Metastatic
  - Breast cancer
  - Laryngeal cancer

Infections
- ► Bacterial
  - Actinomycosis
  - Atypical mycobacterial infection
  - Bang's disease (brucellosis)
  - Cat scratch disease
  - Chancroid
  - Chlamydia (lymphogranuloma venerum, trachoma)
  - Diphtheria
  - Glanders
  - Leprosy
  - Listeriosis
  - Lymphogranuloma venerum (Chlamydia)
  - Melioidosis
  - Plague
  - Salmonella
  - Scarlet fever
  - Staphylococci
  - Streptococci
  - Syphilis

K
L

- Tonsillitis
- Trachoma (Chlamydia)
- Tuberculosis
- Tularemia
- Vincent's angina
▶ Fungal
- Coccidioidomycosis
- Histoplasmosis
- Paracoccidioidomycosis
▶ Viral
- Adenovirus
- Epidemic keratoconjunctivitis
- German measles
- Hepatitis
- Herpes viruses
  ○ HSV
  ○ ZMV
  ○ VZV
  ○ Mononucleosis (EBV, CMV)
  ○ HV-6
  ○ HV-8
- HIV
- Measles
- Rubella
- Vaccinia
▶ Parasitic
- Filariasis
- Leishmaniasis
- Toxoplasmosis
- Trypanosomiasis
▶ Rickettsial
- rickettsialpox
- scrub typhus

Autoimmune
▶ Angioimmunoblastic lymphadenopathy
▶ Dermatomyositis
▶ Drug hypersensitivity
- Allopurinol
- Carbamazepine
- Diphenylhydantoin
- Gold
- Hydralazine
- Phenytoin
- Primidone
▶ Felty's syndrome

▶ Juvenile rheumatoid arthritis
▶ Rheumatoid arthritis
▶ Sharp syndrome
▶ Foreign tissue
- Arthroplasty
- Breast prosthesis
- Silicone
▶ Graft-vs.-host disease
▶ Mixed connective tissue disease
▶ Polymyositis
▶ Primary biliary cirrhosis
▶ Serum sickness
▶ Systemic lupus erythematosus
▶ Sjögren's syndrome
▶ Stimulation of the immune system

Miscellaneous
▶ Castleman's disease (giant lymph node hyperplasia)
▶ Cervical cyst
▶ Dermatopathic lymphadenitis
▶ Eosinophilic granuloma
▶ Familial mediterranean fever
▶ Histiocytosis X
▶ Hyperthyroidism
▶ Inflammatory pseudotumor of lymph node
▶ Kawasaki's disease (mucocutaneous lymph node syndrome)
▶ Kikuchi's disease (histiocytic necrotizing lymphadenitis)
▶ Lipid storage disease
- Fabry's disease
- Gaucher's disease
- Niemann-Pick disease
- Tangier disease
▶ Lymphomatoid granulomatosis
▶ Rosai-Dorfman disease (sinus histiocytosis)
▶ Sarcoidosis
▶ Severe hypertriglyceridemia
▶ Vascular transformation of sinuses

Idiopathic lymph node enlargement

Lymphedema

Accumulation of excessive lymph fluid and swelling of subcutaneous tissues due to obstruction, destruction, or hypoplasia of lymph vessels. See Edema → 122, See Leg Swelling → 220

Primary lymphedema
► Congenital lymphedema (at birth)
► Lymphedema praecox (during puberty)
► Lymphedema tarda (later in life)

Secondary lymphedema
► Tumor obstruction (regional lymph nodes)
  • Prostate cancer
  • Lymphoma
► Iatrogenic
  • Postoperative
    ○ Axillary node dissection
  • After radiation therapy
► Posttraumatic
► Infection of regional lymph nodes
  ○ Filariasis (Wuchereria bancrofti)
  ○ Tuberculosis
► Edema (→ 122)
► See Leg Swelling → 220
► Venous
  • Chronic venous insufficiency
  • Postphlebitic syndrome
► Myxedema (hypothyroidism)
► Lipedema
  • Seen in women with onset after puberty
  • Increased subcutaneous fat between pelvis and ankle
► Malignant lymphedema
  • Rapid, painful cancer-related edema begins centrally

Lymphocytopenia

Absolute reduction of the lymphocytes < 1000/μl.

Infections
► HIV
► Tuberculosis
  • Miliary tuberculosis
► After influenza
► Measles
► Scarlet fever

Drugs, toxins
► Antilymphocyte globulin
► Chemotherapeutics
► Corticosteroids
► Radiation

Depressed immune system
► Congenital immune deficiency
► Antibody deficiency syndrome
► HIV

Miscellaneous
► Acute stress
  • Trauma
  • Postoperative
  • Burns
  • Heavy exercise
  • Pregnancy
  • Severe pain
► Aplastic anemia
► Sarcoidosis
► Hodgkin's lymphoma
► Single non-Hodgkin's lymphomas
► Polycythemia
► Uremia
► Systemic lupus erythematosus
► Felty's syndrome
► Cushing's disease
► Dermatomyositis
► Inflammatory bowel disease
► After snakebite
► Paroxysmal nocturnal hemoglobinuria
► After burns
► Anesthesia
► Surgery

K
L

- Banti's syndrome (idiopathic portal hypertension)
- Secondary hypersplenia
- Zinc deficiency
- Whipple's disease
- Exudative enteropathy
- Lymphocyte phthisis

Lymphocytosis

Lymphocytosis (> 5000/µl and/or > 40% in the differential blood count)

Lymphocytosis > 15,000/µl
- Pertussis
- Infectious mononucleosis
- Chronic and acute lymphocytic leukemia

Infections
- Viral
  - Cytomegalovirus
  - Varicella
  - Infectious mononucleosis
  - Viral pneumonia
  - Herpes virus
  - HIV
  - Mumps
  - Measles
  - Chickenpox
  - Adenovirus
  - Hepatitis viruses
- Bacterial
  - Pertussis
  - Brucellosis
  - Tuberculosis
- Protozoan
  - Toxoplasmosis
- Spirochetal
  - Syphillis

Leukocytosis with shift to the left (increase in the percentage of immature cells)
- Polycythemia
- Acute leukemia
- Chronic granulocytic leukemia
- Osteomyelofibrosis

- Chronic erythroleukemia

Acute transient
- Trauma
- Stress
- Postoperative
- Pain
- Exertion

Drug hyersensitivity
- p-aminosalicylic acid
- Phenytoin

Miscellaneous
- Immunocytoma
- Hairy cell leukemia
- Waldenström's syndrome
- Hyperthyroidism
- Addison's disease
- Inflammatory bowel disease
- Sarcoidosis

Macroglossia See Tongue Swelling → 356

Magnesium

Distribution within the body similar to potassium, with approx. 1% (mainly in ionized form) in the serum, approx. 40% in the skeletal muscles and approx. 60% in the osseous tissue. Best known function is the activation of Na+ K+ ATPase (significant for cardiac dysrhythmias), adenylate cyclase, pyruvate dehydrogenase, calcium ATPase and others. **Hypomagnesemia** leads to an increased cell membrane permeability, which leads to a reduced potassium/sodium gradient between intra- and extracellular space, as well as intracellular calcium increase. The clinical symptoms of hypomagnesemia and of hypocalcemia are similar. Discomfort starts only at very low plasma levels of < 0.4 mmol/l. Indications for determination of the magnesium level are neuromuscular hyperexcitability (vertigo, ataxia, convulsions, tetany,

tremor, muscular twitching, increased tendon reflexes) as well as gastrointestinal and cardiac discomfort.
Normal daily requirement 10–15 mmol/d

Reference range
women: 1.9–2.5 mg/dl
men: 1.8–2.6 mg/dl

Hypomagnesemia
▶ Malnutrition or GI loss
  • Malabsorption syndromes (→ 233)
  • Maldigestion syndromes (→ 233)
  • Parenteral nutrition
  • Alcoholism
  • Chronic inflammatory bowel diseases
  • Short bowel syndrome
  • Sprue
▶ Renal losses
  • Chronic renal disease
  • Diabetic acidosis
  • Diuretics
  • Nephrotoxic drugs
    ○ Aminoglycosides
    ○ Cyclosporin
    ○ Foscarnet
    ○ Methotrexate
▶ Endocrine disorders
  • Hyperthyroidism
  • Diabetic ketoacidosis
  • Hyperaldosteronism
  • Hyperparathyroidism
▶ Increased sequestration of magnesium from the extracellular space
  • Increased uptake into the intracellular space
  • Increased uptake into the bones
  • Respiratory alkalosis
  • Precipitation in the tissue
▶ Familial hypomagnesemia

Hypermagnesemia
Clinical symptoms > 6 mg/dl; respiratory paralysis possible > 12 mg/dl)
▶ Renal insufficiency
▶ Uncontrolled diabetes mellitus

▶ Addison's disease
▶ Hypothyroidism
▶ Drugs
  • Antacids
  • Magnesium-containing enema, salts

Malabsorption syndrome
See Malassimilation → 233

Malassimilation
Maldigestion, malabsorption
Syndrome based on maldigestion and/or malabsorption with the cardinal symptoms chronic diarrhea (steatorrhea) and weight loss. Maldigestion is imperfect predigestion in the stomach, breakdown of the nutritional components by pancreatic enzymes or emulsification of fats by bile. Malabsorption is understood to be an impairment of food transport from the intestinal lumen into the blood and lymph. Symptoms include weight loss, massive feces, muscle weakness, skin and mucosa changes as well as anemia.
See Weight Loss → 382.

Maldigestion
▶ Lack or inactivity of pancreatic lipase
  • Exocrine pancreatic insufficiency (→ 269)
    ○ Chronic pancreatitis
    ○ Pancreatic cancer
    ○ Pancreatectomy
    ○ Cystic fibrosis
    ○ Zollinger-Ellison syndrome
▶ Steatorrhea after gastrectomy
▶ Decreased intestinal bile acid (with faulty formation of lipid micelles)
  • Deficiency in conjugated bile acids/ liver diseases
    ○ Parenchymal liver diseases
    ○ Cholestasis
    ○ Obstructive jaundice
    ○ Ileal resection
    ○ Bacterial overgrowth in the small

intestine in blind loop syndrome
- Interrupted enterohepatic circulation of the bile acids
  - Ileal resection
  - Crohn's disease
- Irregular bacterial growth in the small intestine
  - Diverticulosis in the small intestine
  - Fistula
  - Stricture
  - Afferent loop syndrome
  - Hypomotility states
    - *Diabetes mellitus*
- Drugs
  - Calcium carbonate
  - Cholestyramine
  - Neomycin

Malabsorption
▶ Small intestine
- Inflammatory bowel disease
- Gluten-sensitive enteropathy
- Tropical sprue
- Whipple's disease
- Chronic intestinal infections and parasitosis
- Amyloidosis
- Radiation enteritis
- Malignant intestinal lymphomas and lymph node metastases

▶ Short bowel syndrome
- Massive resection
- Gastroileostomy
- Enteroenteric fistulas

▶ Vascular
- Angina intestinalis
- Severe right ventricular failure or constrictive pericarditis

▶ Inflammation, infiltration
- Crohn's disease
- Becet's disease
- Infectious enteritis
- Eosinophilic enteritis
- Radiation enteritis
- Amyloidosis
- Collagen-vascular diseases

  - Scleroderma
  - Systemic lupus erythemaosus
  - Rheumatoid arthritis
  - Vasculitis
- Lymphomas
- Retroperitoneal malignancy

▶ Biochemical or genetic changes
- Lactase deficiency
- Congenital glucose-galactose malabsorption
- Congenital fructose malabsorption
- Celiac sprue
- Cystinuria
- Hypogammaglobulinemia
- Abetalipoproteinemia
- Hartnup syndrome (monoaminomonocaroxyl-acid transport defect)

▶ Inadequate absorptive area
- Gastroileostomy
- Jejunal bypass
- After multiple or extensive intestine resections
  - Crohn's disease
  - Diseases of the mesenteric vessels

▶ Lymphatic blockade
- Intestinal lymphangiectasis
- Lymphoma
- Whipple's disease

Endocrine and metabolic impairment
▶ Diabetes mellitus
▶ Zollinger-Ellison syndrome
▶ Verner-Morrison syndrome
▶ Hyperthyroidism
▶ Hypoparathyroidism
▶ Adrenal failure
▶ Carcinoid syndrome

Cardiovascular diseases
▶ Congestive heart failure
▶ Constrictive pericarditis
▶ Chronic mesenteric vascular insufficiency
▶ Collagen diseases with vasculitis

Drugs
▶ Broad-spectrum antibiotics

- Colchicin
- Cytotoxic drugs
- Iron salts
- Laxatives
- NSAIDs

Miscellaneous
- Food allergy
- Mastocytosis
- Iron deficiency
- Protein-losing gastropathy
- Psoriasis
- Dermatitis herpetiformis
- Immunodeficiency

Mechanical ileus, See Ileus → 206

Mediastinal Mass

Most common mediastinal tumors
- Goiter
- Thymom
- Lymphoms
- Neurogenic mediastinal tumors
- Dermoid
- Teratoma
- Mesothelial cysts
- Diaphragmatic hernia
- Esophageal diverticulum
- Aortic aneurysm
- Pericardial diverticulum

Anterior mediastinum
- Substantial thyroid
- Parathyroid tumor
- Thymoma
- Mesenchymal neoplams
  - Lipoma
  - Fibroma
  - Sarcoma
  - Lymphoma
  - Hemangioma
- Germinal cell neoplasm
  - Dermoid
  - Seminoma
  - Teratoma
- Aortic aneurysm

- Cardiac aneurysm
- Pericardial fat necrosis
- Pleuropericardial cyst
- Enlarged left atrium
- Bronchogenic cys
- Hiatal hernia
- Lipoma
- Mediastinal phlegmon

Central mediastinum (bifurcation)
- Enlarged lymph nodes
  - Infectious
    - Bacterial
      - *Tuberculosis*
    - Histoplasmosis
  - Neoplastic
    - Bronchial carcinomas
    - Metastases
    - Malignant lymphoma
      - *Hodgkin's lymphoma*
    - Leukemia
  - Granulomatous disease
    - Sarcoidosis
    - Histiocytosis X
    - Pneumoconiosis
    - Silicosis
- Vascular dilataion
  - Pulmonary artery
  - Mediastinal veins
  - Superior vena cava
- Primary tracheal neoplasms
- Bronchiogenic cyst
- Esophageal cysts
- Esophageal diverticulum

Posterior mediastinum
- Esophageal lesions
  - Neoplasm
  - Diverticulum
  - Megaesophagus (Achalasia)
  - Hiatal hernia
- Diseases of the thoracic spine
  - Neoplasm
  - Infectious spondylitis
  - Fracture with hematoma
- Cystic lesions
  - Bronchiogenic cysts

M
N

- Thoracic duct cysts
- Neurenteric cysts
- Gastroenteric cysts
▶ Tumors
  - Neurinom
  - Neurofibrom
  - Neurosarcom
  - Schwannom
  - Gangliocytom
  - Meningiom
  - Chondrom
  - Sympathicoblastoma
▶ Meningocele
▶ Paraganglion
▶ Diaphragmatic hernia
▶ Descending aortic aneurysm
▶ Mediastinal abscess
▶ Hematom
▶ Pancreatic pseudocyst

Melanism

Melanosis, hyperpigmentation, diffuse hypermelanosis

Chemical, physical causes
▶ Sun exposure
▶ UV
▶ Burns
▶ Caustic burns
▶ Heat radiation
▶ X-radiation

Dermatologic
▶ Scars
▶ Scleroderma
▶ Psoriasis
▶ Neurodermitis
▶ Systemic lupus erythematosus
▶ Lichen ruber planus
▶ Pityriasis versicolor
▶ Xeroderma pigmentosus
▶ Contact dermatitis
▶ Herpes zoster
▶ Dermatitis herpetiformis

Endocrine, metabolic
▶ Cushing's disease

▶ Grave's disease
▶ Hyperthyroidism
▶ Addison's disease
▶ Pheochromocytoma
▶ Acromegaly
▶ Porphyria
▶ Diabetes mellitus
▶ ACTH-/MSH-producing pituitary tumor
▶ Whipple's disease
▶ Uremia

Liver
▶ Cirrhosis
▶ Hemochromatosis

Spleen
▶ Felty's syndrome

Genitalia
▶ Heller-Nelson syndrome

Hematologic, neoplasm
▶ Pernicious anemia
▶ Folic acid deficiency
▶ Neoplasm

Nutrition
▶ Malnutrition
▶ Starvation
▶ Pellagra (niacin deficiency)
▶ Scurvy
▶ Vitamin A deficiency
▶ Vitamin B_{12} deficiency

Drugs, toxins
▶ ACTH
▶ Amiodarone
▶ Amitriptyline
▶ Arsenic
▶ Arsenic
▶ Betaxolol
▶ Busulfan
▶ Chlorpromazine
▶ Clozapine
▶ Dibromomannitol
▶ Estrogen
▶ Gold
▶ Haloperidol
▶ Hydantoin
▶ Lead

► Mercury
► Minocycline
► Oral contraceptives
► Perfumes
► Perphenazine
► Phenacetin
► Phenothiazine
► Progesterone
► Quinidine
► Selenium sulfide lotion
► Silver
► Thioridazine

Melena, See Gastrointestinal Bleeding → 152, See Occult Blood → 262

Meningismus

Stiff neck with resistance to neck flexion, with Kernig's sign (patient in supine position, hip and knee flexed, pain induced by attempt to extend leg) and Brudzinski's sign (passive flexion of neck results in spontaneous flexion of hip and knees).

Meningitis (→ 237)

Noninfectious causes
► Tumor
  • Meningiosis carcinomatosa
  • Brain tumors
  • Lymphomas
► Intracranial hemorrhage
  • Subarachnoid hemorrhage
  • Cerebral hemorrhage
► Miscellaneous
  • Emboli
  • Thrombi
  • Ischemia
  • Associated meningitis
    ○ Intracerebral abscesses
    ○ Sinusitis
    ○ Otitis
  • Porphyrias
  • Intoxications
    ○ Lead
  • Cerebellar tumors

• Tetanus
• Muscular tenseness of the cervical spine

Meningitis

Inflammation of the leptomeninges and underlying subarachnoid cerebrospinal fluid (CSF) due to infection by bacteria, viruses, fungi, other organisms, or non-infectious causes, such as trauma. Symptopms include fever, headache, stiff neck (See Meningismus → 237) also vomiting, seizures and impaired consciousness. It can be useful to divide symptom onset into acute, subacute, and chronic categories. Diagnosis: lumbar puncture and cerebrospinal fluid.

Cerebrospinal Fluid (CSF)

	Normal levels	Acute bact.M.	Acute viral M.	TB M.	Neuro-borrell.
Cells/µl *	< 5	in the 1000s	in the 100s	in the 100s	some 100
Cells	lymph./monos 7:3	gran.> lymph.	lymph.> gran.	various leukos	lymph.-mono-cytic
Total protein mg/dl	45 - 60	typically 100-500	typically normal	typically 100-200	typically up to 350
Glucose ratio (CSF/plasma)	typically > 0.5	< 0.3	> 0.6	< 0.5	normal
Lactate mmol/l	< 2.1	> 2.1	< 2.1	> 2.1	-
Others	ICP: 6-22 cm H₂O		PCR of HSV-DNA	PCR of TBC-DNA	IgG/IgM CSF/serum ratio

*with treated bacterial meningitis, immunodepression or aseptic meningitis, fewer cells possible

Common causes
► Neonates
  • Group B streptococci
  • Escherichia coli
  • Listeria monocytogenes
  • Non-group B streptococci
► Infants and children
  • Haemophilus influenzae

- Neisseria meningitidis
- Streptococcus pneumoniae
▶ Adults
  - Streptococcus pneumoniae
  - Haemophilus influenzae
  - Neisseria meningitidis
  - Staphylococci
  - Gram-negative bacilli
  - Streptococci
  - Listeria species
▶ Elderly adults
  - Streptococcus pneumoniae
  - Escherichia coli
  - Klebsiella pneumoniae
  - Streptococcus agalactiae (Group B Streptococcus)
  - Listeria monocytogenes

Infectious
▶ Bacterial meningitis
  - Neisseria meningitidis
  - Haemophilus influenzae
  - Streptococcus pneumoniae
  - Streptococcus agalactiae (Group B streptococcus)
  - Staphylococcus aureus
  - Staphylococcus epidermidis
  - Escherichia coli
  - Klebsiella pneumoniae
  - Proteus
  - Pseudomonas
  - Listeria monocytogenes
  - Streptococci
  - Mycobacteriae
  - Leptospira
  - Syphilis
  - Borrelia
  - Tuberculosis
  - Whipple's disease (Tropheryma whippeli)
▶ Viral (aseptic) meningitis
  - Enterovirus
    ○ Coxsackie viruses
    ○ Echo viruses
  - Herpes viruses
    ○ HSV
    ○ EBV
    ○ VZV
    ○ CMV
  - HIV
  - Mumps
  - Measles
  - Polio
  - Rabies
  - Rubella
  - Adenovirus
  - Influenza
  - Arboviruses (CEE)
▶ Nonviral agents
  - Rickettsia
  - Chlamydia psittaci
  - Mycoplasma pneumoniae
▶ Fungal meningitis
  - Oral candidiasis
  - Aspergillosis
  - Histoplasmosis
  - Cryptococcosis
  - Coccidioidomycosis
▶ Parasites
  - Toxoplasmosis
  - Triquinine
  - Malaria
  - Cysticercosis
  - Schistosomiasis

Noninfectious
▶ Drugs, toxins
  - Azathioprine
  - Carbamazepine
  - Lead
  - NSAIDs
  - Trimethoprim-sulfamethoxazole
▶ Meningeal disease
  - Behçet's syndrome
  - Meningeal carcinomatosis
  - Meningeal leukemia
  - Sarcoidosis
▶ Parameningeal disease
  - Abscess
  - Brain tumor
  - Cerebrovascular accident
  - Multiple sclerosis

- Chronic otitis
- Chronic sinusitis
▶ Iatrogenic
- Reaction to intrathecal injection
- Vaccine reaction
  ○ Pertussis
  ○ Rabies
  ○ Smallpox
  ○ Others

Menstrual pain, See Dysmenorrhea → 109

Mental Disorders

Anxiety disorders
▶ Panic disorder
▶ Agoraphobia
▶ Social phobia
▶ Specific phobia
▶ Obsessive-compulsive disorder
▶ Posttraumatic stress disorder
▶ Acute stress disorder
▶ Generalized anxiety disorder

Childhood disorders
▶ Asperger's disorder
▶ Attention-deficit disorder
▶ Autistic disorder
▶ Conduct disorder
▶ Oppositional defiant disorder
▶ Separation anxiety disorder
▶ Tourette's disorder

Cognitive disorders
▶ Delirium (→ 95, confusion (→ 81)
▶ Dementia (→ 96)
  - Multi-Infarct dementia
  - Dementia in alcoholism
  - Dementia of Alzheimer type
  - Other dementia

Eating disorders
▶ Anorexia nervosa
▶ Bulimia nervosa

Mood disorders
▶ Major depressive disorder
▶ Bipolar disorder

▶ Cyclothymic disorder
▶ Dysthymic disorder

Personality disorders
▶ Paranoid personality
▶ Schizoid personality
▶ Schizotypal personality
▶ Antisocial personality
▶ Borderline personality
▶ Histrionic personality
▶ Narcissistic personality
▶ Avoidant personality
▶ Dependent personality
▶ Obsessive-compulsive personality

Schizophrenia and other
▶ Psychotic disorders
▶ Schizophrenia
▶ Delusional disorder
▶ Brief psychotic disorder
▶ Schizoaffective disorder
▶ Schizophreniform disorder
▶ Shared psychotic disorder

Substance-related disorders
▶ Alcoholism
▶ Amphetamines
▶ Cannabis
▶ Cocaine
▶ Hallucinogens
▶ Inhalants
▶ Nicotine
▶ Opioids
▶ Phencyclidines
▶ Sedatives

Mental Retardation

Below-average general intellectual
function with deficits in adaptive behavior
before age 18.
See Dementia → 96
See Confusion → 81
See Coma → 79

Idiopathic

Trauma
▶ Intracranial hemorrhage
▶ Lack of oxygen

- Before birth
- During birth
- After birth
▶ Head injury

Infections
▶ Congenital
  - Rubella
  - CMV
  - Toxoplasmosis
▶ Congenital and postnatal
  - Meningitis
  - Encephalitis
  - Listeriosis
  - HIV infection

Chromosomal abnormalities
▶ Down's syndrome
▶ Fragile X syndrome
▶ Angelman syndrome
▶ Prader-Willi syndrome
▶ Cri du chat syndrome

Genetic and inherited metabolic disorders
▶ Galactosemia
▶ Tay-Sachs disease
▶ Phenylketonuria
▶ Hunter syndrome
▶ Hurler syndrome
▶ Sanfilippo syndrome
▶ Metachromatic leukodystrophy
▶ Adrenoleukodystrophy
▶ Lesch-Nyhan's syndrome
▶ Rett syndrome
▶ Tuberous sclerosis

Metabolic
▶ Reye's syndrome
▶ Congenital hypothyroidism
▶ High bilirubin levels in babies
▶ Hypoglycemia

Toxins
▶ Intrauterine exposure
  - Alcohol
  - Cocaine
  - Amphetamines
  - Other drugs

▶ Methylmercury poisoning
▶ Lead poisoning

Malnutrition

Environmental
▶ Low socioeconomic status
▶ Deprivation syndrome

Mesenteric Ischemia

Intestinal ischemia
Interruption in blood flow to all or part of the small intestine or the right colon with abdominal pain or unexplained GI symptoms.

Causes
▶ Superior mesenteric artery embolism
  - Cardiac thrombus
  - Cardiac arrhythmia
    ○ Atrial fibrillation
  - Congestive heart failure (CHF)
  - Myocardial infarction
  - Valvular disease
  - Endocarditis
  - Aortic aneurysm
▶ Superior mesenteric artery thrombosis
  - Vasculitis
  - Atherosclerosis
  - Polycythemia vera
  - Neoplasm (compressing tumor)
  - Coagulation disorder
▶ Nonocclusive mesenteric ischemia
  - Congestive heart failure
  - Hypotension
  - Hypovolemia
  - Shock
  - Hemorrhagic blood loss
  - Sepsis
  - Atherosclerosis
  - Drugs
    ○ Digitalis
    ○ Pressors
▶ Mesenteric venous thrombosis
  - Cirrhosis
  - Hypercoagulable state
  - Peritonitis

- Trauma
- Vasculitis
- Polycythemia vera
▶ Collagen vascular disease
- Reiter's syndrome
- Behçet's syndrome
- Progressive systemic sclerosis
- Polyarteritis nodosa
- Systemic lupus erythematosus
- Rheumatoid arthritis
- Dermatomyositis
- Sjögren's syndrome (drying up of salivary, lacrimal and sebaceous glands)
- Wegener's granulomatosis
- Henoch-Schönlein purpura

Metabolic acidosis
See Acidosis, Metabolic → 11

Metabolic alkalosis
See Alkalosis, Metabolic → 18

Metanephrine
See Urine Catecholamines → 368

Methemoglobinemia, See Cyanosis → 91

Microcytes, See Anemia → 28

Miosis

Contraction of the pupil, pupil constriction, near reaction, consensual light reaction.
See Anisocoria → 35, mydriasis (→ 245).
Causes
▶ Normal response
- Parasympathetic stimulation
- Bright light reaction
- Near reaction
▶ Cerebral
- Pontine bleed

- Pontine lesion
- Encephalitis
- Neurosyphilis
- Oculomotor nerve (CN 3) disease
▶ Congenital
▶ Horner's syndrome
▶ Cavernous sinus thrombosis
▶ Inflammation
- Cornea
- Conjunctiva
- Iris
▶ Drugs, toxins
- Benzodiazepines
- Cholinergics
- Clonidine
- Hypnotics
- Morphine
- Opiates
- Organophosphates
- Phenothiazines
- Pilocarpine
- Sedatives

Mitral Regurgitation

Stages
▶ Acute
▶ Chronic compensated
▶ Chronic decompensated
Pathophysiology
▶ Chordae tendineae rupture
▶ Papillary muscle dysfunction
▶ Mitral valve prolapse
▶ Myxomatous degeneration
▶ Mitral annular calcification
▶ Left ventricular dilation
Causes
▶ Rheumatic heart disease
▶ Mitral valve prolapse (ie, myxomatous degeneration)
▶ Myxomatous degeneration
▶ Coronary heart disease
▶ Myocardial infarction
▶ Left ventricular dilation
▶ Hypertrophic cardiomyopathy

M
N

- ▶ Mitral annular calcification
- ▶ Heart failure
- ▶ Infective endocarditis
- ▶ Congenital mitral regurgitation
- ▶ Trauma
- ▶ Miscellaneous
  - Prosthetic valve
  - Ehlers-Danlos syndrome
  - Marfan syndrome
  - Osteogenesis imperfecta
  - Systemic lupus erythematosus

Mitral Stenosis

Causes
- ▶ Rheumatic fever
- ▶ Congenital mitral stenosis
- ▶ Bacterial endocarditis
- ▶ Heart tumor (myxoma)
- ▶ Carcinoid syndrome
- ▶ Lupus erythematosus
- ▶ Amyloidosis
- ▶ Rheumatoid arthritis

Mitral Valve Diseases

See Mitral Stenosis → 242
See Mitral Regurgitation → 241
See Mitral Valve Prolapse → 242

Mitral Valve Prolapse

Causes
- ▶ Congenital
- ▶ Marfan's syndrome
- ▶ Acquired
- ▶ Papillary muscle dysfunction
  - Infarction
  - Trauma
- ▶ Myxomatous degeneration of the mitral valve

Monocytosis

Increased monocytes in the differential blood count: > 8% of leukocytes. Consider chronic myelomonocytic leukemia (CMML) and acute monoblastic leukemia.

Reference range

Monocytes 0-0.8 × 10^3/μl
See Lymphocytosis → 232

Infections
- ▶ Mononucleosis
- ▶ Cytomegalovirus
- ▶ Infectious hepatitis
- ▶ Whooping cough
- ▶ Tuberculosis
- ▶ Bacterial endocarditis
- ▶ Infectious endocarditis
- ▶ Brucellosis
- ▶ HZV
- ▶ Syphilis
- ▶ Malaria
- ▶ Relapsing fever
- ▶ Trypanosomiasis
- ▶ Kala azar

Hematologic
- ▶ Melodyspastic syndromes
- ▶ Acute nonlymphocytic leukemia
  - Acute monocytic leukemia
  - Acute monoblastic leukemia
- ▶ Myeloproliferative disease
- ▶ Lymphoproliferative disease
  - Hodgkin's disease
  - Non-Hodgkin's disease
  - Myeloma
- ▶ Recovery from neutropenia
  - After chemotherapy
  - G-CSF
  - GM-CSF
  - Convalescence after infections and agranulocytosis
- ▶ Benign familial neutropenia
- ▶ Other malignant lymphomas
- ▶ Carcinoma

Gastrointestinal
▶ Cirrhosis
▶ Ulcerative colitis

Miscellaneous
▶ Sarcoidosis
▶ Systemic lupus erythematosus
▶ Inflammatory bowel disease
▶ Drugs
▶ Convalescence after infections and agranulocytosis
▶ Lipid storage disorders
▶ Gaucher's disease

Mouth, dry, See Xerostomia → 384

Mucosa Hemorrhage

See Hemorrhagic Diathesis → 176
See Purpura → 309

Infections
▶ Stomatitis aphthosa
▶ Herpes zoster
▶ Yellow fever
▶ Recurring fever
▶ Diphtheria
▶ Abdominal typhoid fever
▶ Brucellosis
▶ Trichinosis
▶ Kala-azar

Hematologic
▶ Hemorrhagic diathesis (→ 176)
  • Vascular
    ○ Osler's disease
    ○ Henoch-Schönlein purpura
    ○ Moschcowitz' disease
    ○ Avitaminosis C
  • Thrombocytes
    ○ Thrombopenia
    ○ Idiopathic-thrombocytopenic purpura (Werlhof's disease)
    ○ Willebrand-Juergen's thrombopathy
    ○ Glanzmann's thrombasthenia
    ○ Essential hemorrhagic thrombocythemia
  • Plasma

    ○ Hemophilia
    ○ Afibrinogenemia
▶ Leukocytopoiesis
  • Acute leukemia
  • Chronic granulocytic leukemia
▶ Lymphoreticular system
  • Chronic lymphatic leukemia
  • Disorder of the reticuloendothelial cells
  • Letterer-Siwe disease
  • Hand-Schüller-Christian disease
  • Waldenström's macroglobulinemia

Skin diseases
▶ Erythema multiforme
▶ Pemphigus
▶ Epidermolysis bullosa
▶ Fuchs' syndrome

Gastrointestinal
▶ Ulcerative colitis
▶ Cirrhosis
▶ Amyloidosis
▶ Other diseases
▶ Autoantibody thrombocytopenia
▶ Spinalioma
▶ Drug allergy
  • Bismuth
  • Pyrazolone
  • Quinine
  • Sulfonamides

Toxins
▶ Benzol
▶ Boron
▶ Chloroform
▶ Mercury
▶ Phosphorus
▶ Radiation injury

Muscle Weakness

Acute or chronic muscular strength reduction. Muscle weakness is usually caused by systemic, neurologic or vascular diseases, rarely by an independent myopathy.

MN

Acute, subacute
▶ Metabolic
  • Hypokalemia
  • Hyperkalemia
  • Hypophosphatemia
  • Hypercalcemia
  • Hypermagnesemia
  • Hypoglycemia
▶ Rhabdomyolysis (→ 322)
▶ Connective tissue diseases
  • Polymyositis
  • Dermatomyositis
▶ Infection
  • Viral
    ○ Coxsackie
    ○ Herpes zoster
    ○ Influenza
    ○ HIV
    ○ Poliomyelitis
    ○ Rabies
  • Other
    ○ Botulism
    ○ Brucellosis
    ○ Tuberculosis
    ○ Toxoplasmosis
    ○ Diphtheria
    ○ Leprosy
    ○ Trichinosis
▶ Miscellaneous
  • Acute peripheral neuropathy
  • Thyrotoxicosis
  • Uremia
  • Liver failure
  • Corticosteroids
  • Organophosphates

Chronic muscle weakness
▶ Physical deconditioning
▶ Low cardiac output
  • Mitral stenosis
  • Mitral regurgitation
▶ Muscular dystrophies
  • Steroid myopathy
  • Alcoholic myopathy
  • Oculopharyngeal
  • Facioscapulohumeral

  • Myotonic
  • Duchenne's disease
  • Myasthenia gravis
  • Eaton-Lambert syndrome
▶ Endocrine, metabolic
  • Adrenocortical insufficiency
  • Hyperthyroidism
  • Hypothyroidism
  • Hyperparathyroidism
  • Vitamin D deficiency
  • Cushing's syndrome
  • Acromegaly
  • Hypoglycemia
  • Diabetic neuropathy
▶ Inflammatory myopathy
▶ Connective tissue disease
  • Lupus erythematosus
  • Rheumatoid arthritis
  • Polymyositis
  • Dermatomyositis
  • Sarcoidosis
  • Sjögren's syndrome
  • Mixed connective tissue disease
▶ Drugs, toxins
  • Alcohol (alcoholic myopathy)
  • Aminoglycosides
  • Arsenic
  • Chloroquine
  • Clofibrates
  • Corticosteroids
  • Lead
  • Organophosphates
▶ Electrolyte abnormalities
  • Hypokalemia
  • Hyperkalemia
  • Hypophosphatemia
  • Hypercalcemia
▶ Hematologic
  • Pernicious anemia
  • Other anemia
  • Beriberi
▶ Psychiatric
  • Depression
  • Somatization syndrome
  • Chronic fatigue syndrome

- ▶ Progressive neural-muscular atrophy
  - Amyotrophic lateral sclerosis
  - Multiple sclerosis
  - Peroneal muscular atrophy (Charcot-Marie-Tooth)
  - Chronic peripheral neuropathy (see drugs)
- ▶ Miscellaneous
  - Chronic infections
  - Malignant tumor/cachexia
  - Malnutrition
  - Uremia
  - Liver failure
  - Mitochondrial myopathy
  - Rhabdomyolysis (→ 322)
  - Glycogen storage disease
  - Lipid storage disease

Muscular Atrophy, Hand

Frequent causes
- ▶ Carpal tunnel syndrome
- ▶ Ulnar nerve paralysis
- ▶ Radial nerve paralysis
- ▶ Brachial paralysis
- ▶ Pancoast tumor
- ▶ Neurogenic muscular atrophy
- ▶ Syringomyelia
- ▶ Amyotrophic lateral sclerosis (ALS)

Muscular spasms, See Tetany → 348

Myalgia
Muscular pain
Connective tissue disease
- ▶ Fibrositis
- ▶ Rheumatoid arthritis
- ▶ Polymyalgia rheumatica
- ▶ Dermatomyositis
- ▶ Lupus erythematosus
- ▶ Scleroderma
Systemic infection
- ▶ Influenza
- ▶ Coxsackievirus

- ▶ Arbovirus
- ▶ Dengue fever
- ▶ Rabies
- ▶ Polymyelitis
- ▶ Rheumatic fever
- ▶ Typhoid fever
- ▶ Campylobacter
- ▶ Salmonellosis
- ▶ Brucellosis
- ▶ Leprospirosis
- ▶ Trichinosis

Endocrine
- ▶ Hypothyroidism
- ▶ Hyperparathyroidism
- ▶ Hypoglycemic myopathy

Drugs
- ▶ Abphotericin B
- ▶ Chloroquine
- ▶ Cimetidine
- ▶ Clofibrate
- ▶ Glucocorticoids
- ▶ Oral contraceptives

Miscellaneous
- ▶ Ischemic atheroscerotic disease
  - Intermittent claudication
- ▶ Trauma
- ▶ Tumor
- ▶ Rhabdomyolysis
- ▶ Polyneuropathy
- ▶ Congenital enzyme deficiency
  - McArdle's disease

Mydriasis
Pupil dilation, pupil dilitation
See Anisocoria → 35, miosis (→ 241)
Causes
- ▶ Normal response
  - Sympathetic stimulation
  - Dark lighting
- ▶ Drugs, toxins
  - Anticholinergics
  - Atropine
  - Amphetamines
  - Antihistamines

M
N

- Cocaine
- CO
- Epinephrine
- Mydriatic drug (atropine)
- Sympathomimetics
- Tricyclic antidepressants
► Coma
► Trauma
  - Ocular trauma
  - Head trauma
► Acute glaucoma
► Optic atrophy
► Oculomotor nerve (CN III) paralysis
► Aneurysm of the posterior communicating artery
► Brain tumor (→ 58)

Myocarditis

Inflammation of the muscular walls of the heart. Symptoms include palpitations, tachycardia, cardiac pain (pericardial affection), arrhythmia or heart block, dilated cardiomyopathy, dyspnea, even shock symptoms (pericardial tamponade; AV block). It may present with symptoms similar to those seen in myocardial infarction. Frequently, however, the disease is nonapparent. In the ECG sinus tachycardia and ST segment changes are common. In the majority of the cases, there is a viral cause, mostly Coxsackie viruses or ECHO viruses.

Infectious causes
► Viruses
  - Coxsackie virus B1-B5
  - Coxsackie virus A
  - ECHO virus
  - Adenoviruses
  - Epstein-Barr virus
  - Flavivirus
  - HIV
  - Influenza virus
  - Measles virus
  - Mumps virus
  - Polio virus
  - Rabies virus
  - Variella zoster virus
  - CMV
  - Hepatitis viruses
  - Psittacosis
  - Arboviruses
► Bacteria
  - Salmonella
  - Menigococci
  - Gonococci
  - Staphylococci
  - Enterococci
  - Beta-hemolyzing streptococci
  - Clostridium
  - Psittacoses
  - Legionella
  - Borrelia burgdorferi
  - Syphilis
  - Diphtheria
  - Typhoid fever
  - Tuberculosis
  - Rheumatic fever
  - Brucella
  - Tetanus
  - Pertussis
  - Tularemia
  - Spirochetes
    ○ Syphilis
    ○ Leptospirosis
    ○ Lyme disease
  - Rickettsia
    ○ Rocky Mountain spotted fever
    ○ Q fever
    ○ Typhoid fever
► Fungi
  - Oral candidiasis
  - Aspergillosis
  - Actinomycosis
  - Blastomycosis
  - Histoplasmosis
  - Coccidioidomycosis
  - Cryptococcosis
► Protozoa
  - Malaria

- Echinoccocosis
- Toxoplasmosis
- Trypanosomiasis (Chagas' disease)
- Amebiasis
- Leishmaniasis
- Sacrosporidiosis
► Helminths
- Echinoccocosis
- Schistosomiasis1
- Ascariasis
- Filariasis
- Cysticercosis
- Trichinosis

Secondary cardiomyopathy
► Drugs, toxins, physical causes
- Adriamycin
- After radiation
- Alcohol
- Bleomycin
- Catecholamines
- Chemotherapeutics
- Chloroquine
- Cobalt
- Cocaine
- Cyclophosphamide
- Daunorubicin
- Doxorubicin
- Emetine
- Lead
- Lithium
- Phenothiazines
- Tetanus
► Metabolic, nutritional
  ○ Vitamin B$_1$ deficiency
  ○ Niacin deficiency
  ○ Selenium deficiency
  ○ Uremia
  ○ Gout
  ○ Obesity
► Endocrine
  ○ Pheochromocytoma
  ○ Hypothyroidism
  ○ Hyperthyroidism
  ○ Cushing's disease
  ○ Diabetes mellitus

  ○ Acromegaly
► Systemic
  ○ Scleroderma
  ○ Dermatomyositis
  ○ Polyarteritis nodosa
  ○ Kawasaki's syndrome
  ○ Systemic lupus erythematosus
► Granulomatous, infiltrative
  ○ Sarcoidosis
  ○ Wegner's granulomatosis
  ○ Malignant heart diseases
  ○ Metastases
  ○ Hemochromatosis
  ○ Amyloidosis
  ○ Endomyocardial fibrosis
► Neuromuscular
  ○ Myotonia dystrophica
  ○ Muscular dystrophy
► Hypersensitivity
  • Drugs
    ○ Acetazolamide
    ○ Amytriptilin
    ○ Chlorthalidon
    ○ Hydrochlorothiazide
    ○ Indomethacin
    ○ Indomethacin
    ○ Methyldopa
    ○ Penicillin
    ○ Phenylbutazone
    ○ Phenytoin
    ○ Spironolactone
    ○ Sulfonamides
    ○ Sulfonyl ureas
    ○ Tetracyclines
  • Graft-vs.-host disease
  • Giant cell arteritis
► Hereditary disorders
  • Glycogen storage diseases
  • Niemann-Pick disease
  • Hand-Schüller-Christian disease
  • Fabry's disease
  • Gangliosiderosis
  • Gaucher's disease
  • Mucopolysaccharidosis
  • Hunter's syndrome

MN

- Hurler's disease
▶ Miscellaneous
  - Hypokalemia
  - Carnitine deficiency

Myoglobin

Myoglobin is an oxygen carrying protein present in skeletal and cardiac muscle. It is a marker of ischemic injury. Due to its low molecular weight it is released into the peripheral circulation earlier than other markers. Myoglobin levels begin to rise within 2 hours (CK-MB after 4–6 hours) after cardiac injury. To differentiate between myoglobin from cardiac muscle and skeletal muscle, test CK-MB or troponin I and/or C. Indication in the early diagnosis of acute myocardial infarction (AMI), skeletal myopathies, risk assessment of pending renal failure, in rhabdomyolysis or polytrauma; in sports medicine for the assessment of muscular fitness level.
See Creatine Kinase (CK) → 88
See Troponin I and Cardiac Troponin T → 361.

Reference range
Women	7–64 µg/l
Men	16–76 µg/l

Increased
▶ Myocardial infarction
▶ Skeletal myopathy
  - Myopathies
  - Rhabdomyolysis
  - Crush syndrome
  - Muscular ischemia
  - Muscular fatigue
▶ Physical
  - Malignant hyperthermia
  - Burns
  - Heatstroke
  - Frostbite
▶ Endocrine causes
  - Conn's syndrome
  - Hypothyroidism
  - Hyperthyroidism
  - Diabetic coma
▶ Electrolyte imbalance
  - Hypokalemia
  - Hypophosphatemia
  - Hypernatremia
▶ Drugs, toxins
  - Acute alcoholism
  - Amphetamines
  - Amphotericin B
  - CO
  - Fibrate
  - Halothane
  - Heroin
  - HMG-CoA reductase inhibitors
  - Insecticides
  - Neuroleptics
  - Sedatives (overdose with coma)
▶ Febrile infections
  - Influenza
  - Adenoviruses
  - Coxsackie viruses
  - HSV
  - Infectious mononucleosis
  - Typhoid fever
  - Tetanus
  - Legionnaires' disease
  - Toxic shock syndrome

Myopathy, Muscle Diseases

Inflammatory diseases of the musculature. Clinical signs of a myopathy are usually muscle pains and/or weakness.
See Myoglobin → 248
Primary/hereditary myopathies
▶ Progressive muscular dystrophy
▶ Congenital myopathy
▶ Opthalmoplegia externa
Localized myopathies
▶ Muscle trauma
▶ Pulled muscle
  - Sports
  - Poor posture
  - Overwork

- Compartmental syndrome
- Tumors
- Inflammation
  - Bacteria
    - Tetanus
    - Gas gangrene
    - Leprosy
    - Staphylococci
    - Borrelia stage III
  - Parasites
    - Toxoplasmosis
    - Trypanosomiasis
    - Echinococcal cysts
    - Sacrosporidiosis
    - Trichinella spiralis
    - Schistosomiasis
    - Cestoda
    - Nematodes
  - Viruses
    - Coxsackie
    - Influenza
    - German measles
- Fibromyalgia syndrome (syndrome with musculo-skeletal pains but without concrete evidence of muscle, bone or joint inflammation. Clinical picture: multifocal pain, fatigue and sleep disturbance. Affects mainly middle-aged women)

Generalized myopathies

- Collagen vascular disease
  - Dermatomyositis in adults
  - Dermatomyositis/polymyositis in malignant tumors
  - Sjögren's syndrome (→ 332)
  - LE
  - Rheumatic fever
  - Chronic polyarthritis
  - Scleroderma
  - Polyarteritis nodosa
  - Myositis associated with other diseases
- Granulomatous diseases
  - Sarcoidosis
  - Wegner's granulomatosis

- Myasthenia gravis
- Inflammatory myopathies
  - Eosinophilic myositis
  - Drug-induced myopathy
- Endocrine
  - Hyperaldosteronism
  - Hyperparathyroidism
  - Hyperthyroidism
  - Thyrotoxicosis
  - Hypothyroidism
  - Cushing's syndrome
  - Hyperadrenocorticalism
  - Addison's disease
- Drugs, toxins
  - Alcohol (alcoholic polymyopathy)
  - Botulism
  - Chloroquine
  - Cimetidine
  - Clofibrate
  - Colchicine
  - Corticosteroids
  - D-Penicillamine
  - Hydroxyurea
  - Ipecac
  - NSAIDs
  - Organophosphates
  - Pravastatin
- Neurologic
- Miscellaneous
  - Malignant tumors
  - Paraneoplasia
  - McArdle's disease
  - Xanthine oxidase deficiency
  - Phosphofructokinase deficiency
  - Carnitine deficiency
  - Progressive muscular dystrophy, Bekker type
  - Muscular phosphofructokinase deficiency
  - Phosphorylase B kinase deficiency
  - Progressive muscular dystrophy
  - Congenital myopathy
  - Malignant hyperthermia

Myositis
See Myopathy, Muscle Diseases → 248

Nail changes
Nail changes furnish supplementary information, especially in advanced age. Clinically most important: hippocratic nails and clubbed fingers (→ 78).

Hippocratic nails
Large, curved nails, usually in combination with clubbing (→ 78).
▶ Lung diseases
  - Infections
    ◦ Lung abscess
    ◦ Empyema
    ◦ Bronchiectases
    ◦ Tuberculosis
  - Neoplasms
    ◦ Bronchial carcinomas
    ◦ Pulmonary metastases
    ◦ Mesothelioma
  - Pulmonary fibrosis
  - Silicosis
  - Arteriovenous shunts
  - Pulmonary artery sclerosis
▶ Cardiac
  - Congenital cyanotic cardiac disease
  - Infectious endocarditis
  - Heart failure
▶ Intestinal
  - Ulcerative colitis
  - Crohn's disease
  - Sprue
▶ Liver diseases
  - Biliary cirrhosis
  - Liver tumors
▶ Miscellaneous
  - Cerebrovascular accident
  - Idiopathic hypertrophic osteoarthropathy
  - Pachydermoperiostosis

Koilonychia
Malformation of the nails in which the outer surface is concave. Often associated with hypochromic anemia.
▶ Iron deficiency
▶ Hypochromic anemia
▶ Pellagra
▶ Vitamin B_{12} deficiency
▶ Malnutrition
▶ Diabetes
▶ Raynaud's syndrome
▶ Multiple myeloma
▶ Graves' disease
▶ Addison's disease
▶ Cushing's disease
▶ Hereditary

Onychogryphosis
Claw-like, thickened nails, mostly in advanced age.
▶ Onychomycosis
  - Candida
  - Molds
  - Dermatophytes
▶ Chronic eczema
▶ Pachyonychia congenita
▶ Idiopathic

Onchorrhexis
Brittle, split nails
▶ Chronic chemical damage
  - Frequent washing
  - Nail polish
  - Nail polish remover
  - Potassium hydroxide
▶ Thyroid diseases
▶ Lichen ruber
▶ Anemia

Onychodystrophy
Deformed, brittle, rough, discolored nails
▶ Eczema
▶ Fungal infection
▶ Psoriasis

Onycholysis
Painless loss of the nail
▶ Psoriasis
▶ Eczema
▶ Onychomycosis

- Reiter's disease
- Thyroid diseases
- Circulation disorders
- Diabetes
- Tumor
- Hematoma under the nail
- Drugs

Beau's lines
Transverse furrows. Sign of a previous arrest of growth
- Severe infectious diseases
- Surgery
- Trauma
- Malnutrition
- Coronary occlusion
- Psychiatric
  - Shock
  - Depression
  - Delirium
- Traumatic damage to nail matrix
- Toxins
  - Arsenic
  - Chemotherapeutics
  - Fluoride
  - Lead
  - Thallium
- Reiter's disease
- Gout

Mees lines
Horizontal white bands of the nails
- Drugs, toxins
  - Arsenic
  - Chemotherapeutics
  - Thallium
- Fluorosis
- Occasionally in leprosy

Pitted nails
Pinpoint depressions in the nails
- Psoriasis
- Neurodermatitis
- Rheumatic fever
- Lichen ruber
- Lupus erythematosus
- Alopecia areata

Leukonychia
White coloration of the nails
- Leukonychia punctata (white dots)
  - Trauma (nail care!)
- Leukonychia striata longitudinalis (white longitudinal stripes)
  - Darier's disease
- Leukonychia totalis (total discoloration)
  - Anemia
  - Cirrhosis
  - Cardiac diseases
  - Fever
  - Hypoalbuminemia
  - Mycosis
  - Noxa
  - Potassium nitrate solution
  - Nitrite solution
  - Silver solution
  - Hereditary

Yellow nails
Yellow-greenish discoloration of some or all nails with subsequent oncholysis.
- Congenital hypoplasia/dysplasia of peripheral lymph vessels
- Diseases of the bronchial tubes
- Disease of the nasal sinuses
- Smoker's fingers

Half-and-half nails
Reversible white (proximal), brown (distal) coloration of the nails
- Uremia

Green-black discoloration
- Infection with Pseudomonas aeruginosa

Brown-black discoloration
- Moles
- Acral lentiginous melanoma
- Hematoma under the nail (grows out with the nail)
- Ochronosis
- Alcaptonuria

Blue discoloration
- Argyria (accumulation of silver sulfide)
- DADPS

Paronychia
Inflammations of nail bed/fold
► Bacterial
► Candida
► Syphilis

Narcolepsy

Sleep disorder consisting of recurring episodes of unexpected sleep during the day, and often disrupted nocturnal sleep.
Causes
► Hereditary (related to DR-2)
► Secondary
  • Head trauma
  • Encephalopathy
  • Brain tumor
  • Cerebrovascular insufficiency

Nausea, Vomiting

Nausea is the sensation leading to the urge to vomit. It is associated with altered physiologic activity, including gastric hypomotility and increased parasympathetic tone that precede and accompany vomiting. Vomiting should be distinguished from regurgitation, which is spitting up of gastric contents without associated nausea or forceful abdominal muscular contractions.
See Inappetence → 210
Main causes
► Gastroenteritis
► Spoiled foods
► Drugs, toxins
Gastrointestinal
► Inflammation
  • Gastroenteritis
  • Hepatitis
  • Pancreatitis
  • Peptic ulcer disease
  • Gastroesophageal reflux diesease
  • Appendicitis
  • Cholecystitis
  • Crohn's disease
  • Peritonitis
► Bowel obstruction
  • Ileus (→ 206)
    ○ Mechanical obstruction
    ○ Non-mechanical obstruction
  • Subileus
  • Stenosis
    ○ Scars
    ○ Inflammation
    ○ Malignant
  • Foreign bodies
  • Volvulus
  • Hernia
  • Pseudo-obstruction
  • Gastric outlet obstruction (→ 151)
  • Esophageal stenosis
  • Achalasia
  • Diabetic gastroparesis
► Visceral pain
  • Biliary colic
  • Ischemic enterocolitis
  • Pancreatitis
  • Appendicitis
  • Peritonitis
► Stomach operation
  • Post-gastrectomy syndrome (after Billroth II or Roux-Y anastomosis)
  • Vagotomy without pyloroplastic
► Gastroparesis
  • Diabetes mellitus
  • Scleroderma
  • Amyloidosis
  • Metabolic
  • Postoperative
  • Postviral
  • Idiopathic
► Miscellaneous abdominal causes
  • Gastric carcinoma
  • Esophageal diverticulum
  • Esophagitis
  • Mesenteric infarction
  • Gastrocolic fistula
  • Zollinger-Ellison syndrome
  • Cholecystolithiasis

- Cholecystitis
- Gall bladder hydrops
- Peritonitis
- See Acute abdomen → 7
- Pancreatitis
- Urolithiasis
- Renal colic
- Pyelonephritis
- Twisted ovarian cyst
- Testicular torsion
- Dysmenorrhea

Infections
▶ Acute infections (especially in children)
▶ Food poisoning
▶ Gastroenteritis
  - Viral
  - Bacterial
  - Eosonophilic
  - Parasitic
▶ Meningitis
▶ Meningoencephalitis
▶ Hepatitis
▶ Malaria
▶ Q fever
▶ Spotted fever
▶ Cholecystitis
▶ Appendicitis
▶ Pancreatitis
▶ Peritonitis
▶ AIDS

Drugs, toxins
▶ Alcohol abuse
▶ Antiarrhythmics
▶ Antibiotics
▶ Carbonic anhydrase inhibitors
▶ Chemotherapeutics
▶ Colchicine
▶ Digitalis
▶ Drug abuse
▶ Drug side-effects
▶ Ergot alkaloids
▶ Estrogens
▶ Food allergy
▶ Gastroenteritis
▶ Heavy metals

▶ Ipecac
▶ Mushroom poisoning
▶ Narcotics
▶ Opiates
▶ Plant-protection agents
▶ Solvents
▶ Theophylline

Metabolic, endocrine
▶ Hepatic coma
▶ Metabolic acidosis
▶ Addison's disease
▶ Renal failure
▶ Uremia
▶ Precoma diabeticum
▶ Thyrotoxicosis
▶ Hypothyreosis
▶ Diabetic ketoacidosis
▶ Hyperemesis gravidarum/Pregnancy
▶ Fructose intolerance hypoglycemia
▶ Adrenal failure
▶ Hepatic porphyria
▶ Hypercalcemia/Hyperparathyroidism
▶ Hyponatremia
▶ SIADH

Postoperative
▶ Dumping syndrome
▶ Vagotomy
▶ Anastomosis stenosis
▶ Afferent loop syndrome

Nervous system, vestibular disorders
▶ Motion sickness
▶ Menière's disease
▶ Acoustic neurinoma
▶ Inflammation in the area of the vestibular organ
▶ Vestibular neuronitis
▶ Labyrinthitis
▶ Vertebro-basilar syndrome
▶ Ear infection
▶ Heat stroke
▶ Increased intracranial pressure
  - Tumor
  - Head trauma
  - Hemorrhage
  - Edema

M
N

- Meningitis, encephalitis
- Hydrocephalus
- Migraine
- Tabes dorsalis
- After brain radiation

Eyes
- Refractive error
- Glaucoma

Cardiovascular
- Myocardial infarction
- Heart failure
- Orthostatic reaction
- Hypertension
- Pulmonary embolism
- Cardiac dysrhythmia

Psychiatric
- Anxiety
- Depression
- Self-induced
  - Anorexia nervosa
  - Bulimia
- Psychogenic vomiting
- Concealed vomiting
- Erotic vomiting
- Drug withdrawal

Miscellaneous
- Morning sickness
- Kinetosis
- Acute altitude sickness
- After radiation therapy

Neck pain, See Back Pain → 49

Neck stiffness, See Brudzinski's Sign → 60
See Meningismus → 237,
See Meningitis → 237

Neck Swelling

Infection, inflammation
- Pharyngitis
- Tonsillitis
- Parotitis
- Laryngitis
- Abscess
- Phlegmon
- Lymphadenitis
- Odontopathies
- Stomatitis
- Cheilitis
- Sialadenitis submandibularis
  - Chronic
  - Bacterial
- Perichondritis of the larynx
- Bacterial infection
  - Scarlet fever
  - Tuberculosis
    - Tuberculous lymphadenitis
  - Brucellosis
  - Listeriosis
  - Syphilis
  - Cat-scratch disease
  - Vincent's angina (necrotizing tonsillitis through fusobacteria and borrelia)
- Fungal infection
  - Cervicofacial actinomycosis
- Viral infections
  - Infectious mononucleosis
  - Herpes viruses
  - German measles
  - Mumps
  - Tularemia
  - HIV
- Tropical diseases
  - Lepra
  - Leishmaniasis
  - Trypanosomiasis
- Zoonoses
  - Toxoplasmosis

Thyroid disorder
- Goiter
- Nodular goiter
- Cysts
- Thyroiditis
  - Hashimoto's
  - Subacute
  - Acute-purulent
- Thyroid cancer

Lymphadenopathy ((→ 229))

Cysts, deformations
- Cyst of the floor of the mouth
- Ranula of the sublingual gland
- Lateral or medial cervical cysts
- Dermoid cyst
- Epidermoid cyst
- Hypopharyngeal diverticulum
- Laryngocele
- Cystic lymphangiomas
- Turner's syndrome
- Dystope thyroid tissue

Neoplasm
- Hodgkin's lymphoma
- Non Hodgkin's lymphoma
- Lipoma
- Fibroma
- Leukemia
- Lymph node metastasis
- Lymphosarcoma
- AML
- CML
- Osteomyelosclerosis
- Multiple myeloma
- Carcinoma in the area of the
  - Submandibular gland
  - Floor of the mouth
  - Tonsils
  - Larynx
  - Pharynx
  - Hypopharynx
  - Parotis
- Parathyroid adenoma
- Tumor of the mandible
- Tumor of the submandibular gland
- Neurinoma
  - Schwannoma
  - Neurofibroma

Miscellaneous
- Hemorrhage
- Hematoma
- Jugular venous distention
- Thrombophlebitis of the internal jugular vein
- Glomus tumor

- Carotid paraganglion
- Collagen vascular disease
  - Systemic lupus erythematosus
  - Rheumatoid arthritis
  - Still's disease (juvenile form of rheumatoid arthritis)
  - Felty's syndrome (splenomegaly with rheumatoid arthritis and leukopenia)
- Boeck's disease
- Sialolithiasis (submandibular gland)
- Reactive lymphadenopathy through drugs
- Cutaneous emphysema (after rib fracture)
- Degenerative changes of the cervical spine

Nephrolithiasis

Kidney stones
Formation of calculi in kidney, renal pelvis and ureter. 75-80% are calcium stones and radiopaque. Affects 3-4 times more men than women. See Uric Acid → 364, See Hyperglycemia → 189 See Urolithiasis → 371

M
N

Calcium (oxalate/phosphate) stones
- Idiopathic hypercalciuria 50%
- Hyperuricuria 15%
- Hypercalcemia ((→ 187))
  - Primary and secondary hyperparathyroidism
  - Vitamin D intoxication
  - Tumor hypercalcemias
  - Bone metastases
    ○ Multiple myeloma
  - Paget's disease
  - Sarcoidosis
  - Osteoporosis
  - Cushing's syndrome
  - Hyperthyroidism
  - Leukemia
  - Milk-alkali syndrome
- Distal renal tubular acidosis
- Hyperoxaluria

- Congenital
- Excessive vitamin C intake
- Increased intestinal absorption of oxalates
  - Crohn's disease
  - Ulcerative colitis
  - Pancreatitis
  - Cirrhosis
  - Small intestinal resection
  - Steatorrhea
  - Sprue
  - Diabetic enteropathy
▶ Hyperphosphaturia
- Hyperparathyroidism
- Fanconi's syndrome
- Phosphate diabetes
▶ Idiopathic calculosis

Magnesium ammonium phosphate stones (infectious stones) 20%
▶ Chronic infection (usually with urea-splitting organisms)
- Proteus
- Pseudomonas
- Klebsiella

Uric acid stones
▶ Idiopathic
▶ Gout
▶ Alcohol abuse
▶ Purine metabolism (enzyme deficiency)
- Lesch-Nyhan syndrome
- Glycogen storage disease
- Xanthinuria
▶ Tumor
- Leukemia/Lymphoma especially after chemotherapy
▶ Dehydration
▶ Drugs
- Amino acids (infusion)
- Aspirin
- Estrogens
- Probenecid
- Uricosurics

Cystine calculi (hereditary)
▶ Cystinuria

Nephrotic Syndrome

Proteinuria > 3.5 g/24, hypoproteinemia, hypalbuminemia (with or without edemas) and hyperlipoproteinemia with increase of cholesterol and triglycerides.

GN with nephrotic syndrome
▶ Membranous GN (most frequent form)
- Autoimmune diseases
  - Systemic lupus erythematosus
  - Thyroiditis
  - Mixed connective tissue disease
  - Diabetes mellitus
- Hepatitis B
- Carcinomas
- Captopril
- Penicillamine
▶ Minimal-change-GN
- Hodgkin's lymphoma
- Drug-toxic (NSAID !)
- After throat infections
▶ Focal and segmental GN
▶ Membranoproliferative GN (after throat infections)

Acute glomerulonephritis, with nephritis and usually smaller proteinuria (< 3.5 g/24 h)
▶ IgA glomerulonephritis (most frequent form, often after throat infections)
- Berger's disease (IgA)
- Henoch-Schönlein purpura
▶ Acute postinfectious glomerulonephritis
- Post streptococci-GN
▶ Rapid progressive glomerulonephritis
- Systemic lupus erythematosus
- Goodpasture's syndrome
- Wegener's granulomatosis
- Subacute endocarditis
- Shunt infections
  - Cryoglobulinemias

Secondary
▶ Systemic diseases
- Diabetes mellitus
- Systemic lupus erythematosus

- Sjögren's syndrome
- Rheumatoid arthritis
- Polyarteritis nodosa
- Sarcoidosis
- Amyloidosis
- Vasculitis
- Henoch-Schönlein purpura
- Goodpasture's' syndrome
- Dermatomyositis
- Mixed cryoglobulinemia
▶ Hereditary diseases
- Lipoatrophy
- Sickle cell anemia
- Congenital nephrotic syndrome
- Alport's syndrome (hereditary nephritis with chronic interstitial nephritis, nerve deafness and eye anomalies)
- Fabry's disease
- Orthostatic proteinuria
▶ Infections
- Streptococcus
- Hepatitis A, B, C
- HIV
- Toxoplasmosis
- Infectious mononucleosis
- Malaria
- Syphilis
- Shunt nephritis
- Endocarditis
▶ Neoplasm
- Multiple myeloma
- Lymphomas
- Solid tumors
▶ Drugs
- Antiepileptics
- Captopril
- Contrast media
- Gold
- Heroin
- Mercury
- NSAIDs
- Penicillamine
- Probenecide

▶ Miscellaneous
- Thyroiditis
- Hypothyroidism
- Renovascular hypertension
- Renal vein thrombosis
- Pre-eclampsia
- Severe obesity
- Graft-vs.-host disease
- Chronic interstitial nephritis
- After beesting

Consequences due to protein loss
See Protein in the Serum → 296
▶ Albumin
- Ascites
- Edemas
- Pleural effusions
▶ Antithrombin
- Renal vein thrombosis
- Arterial thrombosis
- Thrombosis of peripheral veins
▶ Immunoglobulins
- Immune deficiency
▶ Transferrin
- Iron deficiency anemia
▶ Ceruloplasmin
- Copper deficiency
▶ Thyroxin-binding globulin
- False thyroid test results
▶ Vitamin D-binding globulin
- Vitamin D_3 deficiency
▶ Miscellaneous changes
- Altered plasma protein binding of drugs
- Increase of LDL, IDL, VLDL, triglycerides, lipoprotein(a)
- Decreased HDL

Neuron-specific enolase
See NSE → 260

M
N

Neuropathy, Peripheral

Disease of peripheral neurons and their envelopes due to direct toxic or hypoxic damage (vasa nervorum). Symptoms include distal paresthesia and sensory disturbances. It usually begins in the lower extremities, followed by flaccid paralysis, areflexia, muscular atrophy, trophic impairment of the skin.

Most common causes
- Diabetic polyneuropathy
- Alcoholic polyneuropathy

Endocrine, metabolic
- Diabetes mellitus
- Hypothyroidism
- Acromegaly
- Uremic/chronic renal failure
- Porphyria
- Primary biliary cirrhosis
- Dysproteinemia
- Paraproteinemia
- Multiple myeloma

Malnutrition, malabsorption
- Pernicious anemia
- Thiamine deficiency
- Vitamin B_1 deficiency
- Vitamin B_6 deficiency
- Vitamin B_{12} deficiency
- Sprue

Infection
- Infectious mononucleosis
- German measles
- Herpes zoster
- Diphtheria
- Syphilis
- Dysentery
- Typhoid fever
- Paratyphus
- Lyme disease
- Tuberculosis
- Mycosis
- Malaria
- Viral hepatitis
- Botulism
- HIV
- Spotted fever
- Brucellosis

Drugs, toxins
- Alcohol
- Arsenic
- Carbon monoxide
- Chloramphenicol
- Cisplatin
- Colchicin
- Gold
- High-dose pyridoxine
- Hydralazine
- Industrial solvents
- Isoniazid
- Isoniazide
- Lead
- Lithium
- Meprobamate
- Mercury
- Metronidazole
- Nitrofurantoin
- Phenytoin
- Platinum
- Thallium
- Trichloroethylene
- Vinblastine

Mechanical
- Spinal process
- Trauma
- Compression
- Carpal tunnel syndrome
- Congenital causes

Hereditary disease
- Charcot-Marie-Tooth disease
- Refsum's disease
- Hereditary ataxia
- Metachromatic leukodystrophy
- Fabry's disease

Systemic disorders
- Sarcoidosis
- Rheumatoid arthritis
- Polyarteritis nodosa

- Amyloidosis
- Systemic lupus erythematosus
- Scleroderma
- Sjögren's syndrome
- Atherosclerosis
- Nonsystemic vasculitic neuropathy
- Lymphoma
- Leukemia

Miscellaneous
- Guillain-Barré syndrome/Polyradiculitis
- Paraneoplasia
  - Bronchial carcinomas
- After tetanus shot
- Idiopathic

Neutrocytosis, See Leukocytosis → 222

Neutropenia, See Leukopenia → 223

Night Blindness

Nyctalopia, nocturnal amblyopia
Limited ability to see in reduced illumination due to impaired rod function.
Causes
- Hereditary
- Vitamin A deficiency (→ 321)
  - Impaired bile flow
  - Fat resorption disorder
  - Protein deficiency
- Retinitis pigmentosa
- Uncorrected myopia (nearsightedness)
- Glaucoma
- Cataracts
- Gyrate atrophy
- Xerophthalmia
- Zinc deficiency
- Siderosis retinae
- Retinal detachment
- Peripheral chorioretinitis
- Optic atrophy
- Hypoxia
- Cirrhosis
- Albinism

- Oguchi's disease
- Laurence-Moon-Biedl syndrome

Night sweats, See Hyperhidrosis → 191

Nocturia

Excessive urinating at night.
Causes
- Congestive heart failure
- Renal/urinary tract disorders
  - Benign prostatic hyperplasia
  - Urethral stricture
  - Urinary tract infection (UTI)
    ○ Acute cystitis (uncomplicated UTI)
    ○ Chronic UTI
    ○ Recurrent UTI
  - Chronic renal failure
  - Nephrotic syndrome
- Excessive fluid intake before bedtime, particularly:
  - Alcohol
  - Caffeinated beverages
  - Coffee
  - Tea
- Drugs
  - Cardiac glycosides
  - Demeclocycline
  - Diuretics
  - Lithium
  - Methoxyflurane
  - Phenytoin
  - Propoxyphene
  - Vitamin D
- Miscellaneous
  - Diabetes mellitus
  - Cirrhosis with ascites
  - Hypercalcemia
  - Diabetes insipidus
  - Non-cardiac edemas

Normetanephrine
See Urine Catecholamines → 368

M
N

NSE

Neuron-specific enolase
Enzyme of glycolysis. Tumor marker, especially for small cell lung cancer.

Reference range

< 10 µg/l

Increased

▶ Benign diseases
- Pulmonary fibrosis
- Bronchopneumonia
- Liver diseases
- Hemolysis

▶ Malignant diseases
- Small cell lung cancer!
- Neuroblastoma
- Medullary thyroid cancer
- Pancreatic endocrine tumors
- Carcinoid
- Melanoma
- Seminoma
- Breast cancer
- Kidney cancer

Nystagmus

Rhythmical, persistent, involuntary horizontal, vertical or rotatory oscillation of the eyeballs, either pendular or jerky. The direction of the nystagmus is named for the quick component of the nystagmus.

Physiologic nystagmus
▶ Optokinetic (attempt to fix on moving objects)
▶ Labyrinthine stimulation (e.g. with cold water in auditory canal)
▶ Extreme lateral gaze

Congenital nystagmus
▶ Idiopathic infantile nystagmus
▶ Latent nystagmus
▶ Sensory deficit nystagmus
- Early visual deprivation
  ○ Congenital cataracts
  ○ Severe glaucoma
  ○ Peters anomaly
- Albinism (as a result of multifactorial visual impairment)
- Foveal hypoplasia
  ○ Aniridia
  ○ Albinism
- Retinal disease
  ○ Leber congenital amaurosis
  ○ Achromatopsia
  ○ Mmacular toxoplasmosis
- Retinal detachment
  ○ Severe retinopathy of prematurity
  ○ Posterior persistent hyperplastic primary vitreous
  ○ Familial exudative vitreoretinopathy
- Optic nerve abnormality
  ○ Hypoplasia
  ○ Coloboma
  ○ Atrophy
- Cortical visual impairment
  ○ Perinatal insult
  ○ Structural CNS abnormality

▶ Spasmus nutans (fine nystagmus associated with head-nodding)

Acquired nystagmus
▶ Seesaw nystagmus
- Rostral midbrain lesions
- Parasellar lesion
  ○ Pituitary tumors
- Visual loss due to retinitis pigmentosa

▶ Downbeat nystagmus
- Lesions of the vestibulocerebellum and underlying medulla
  ○ Arnold-Chiari malformation
  ○ Vertebrobasilar insufficiency
  ○ Multiple sclerosis
  ○ Wernicke encephalopathy
  ○ Encephalitis
  ○ Lithium intoxication
- Heat stroke
- Idiopathic

▶ Upbeat nystagmus
- Medullary lesions
  ○ Perihypoglossal nuclei

o Medial vestibular nucleus
o Nucleus intercalatus
- Lesions of the anterior vermis of the cerebellum
- Benign paroxysmal positional vertigo
▶ Periodic alternating nystagmus
- Arnold-Chiari malformation
- Demyelinating disease
- Spinocerebellar degeneration
- Lesions of the vestibular nuclei
- Head trauma
- Encephalitis
- Syphilis
- Posterior fossa tumors
- Binocular visual deprivation
▶ Pendular nystagmus
- Demyelinating disease
- Monocular visual deprivation
- Binocular visual deprivation
- Oculopalatal myoclonus
- Internuclear ophthalmoplegia
- Brainstem dysfunction
- Cerebellar dysfunction
▶ Spasmus nutans
- In healthy children
- Gliomas
  o Chiasmal glioma
  o Suprachiasmal glioma
  o Third ventricle glioma
▶ Torsional
- Lateral medullary syndrome (Wallenberg syndrome)
▶ Abducting nystagmus of internuclear ophthalmoplegia
- Demyelinating disease
- Brain stem stroke
▶ Gaze evoked
- Drugs, toxins
  o Alcohol
  o Anticonvulsants
  o Carbamazepine
  o Phenobarbital
  o Phenytoin

Obesity

State of excess adipose mass with abnormal increase of fat in the subcutaneous connective tissues. Obesity is gauged by the body mass index (BMI), which is equal to weight/height^2 in kg/m^2.

BMI (kg/m^2)	
Appropriate weight	19–25
Overweight	> 25
Obesity	> 30

A high body mass index is associated with increased risk of death at all ages among both men and women.
See Weight Gain → 382

Contributory factors
▶ Familial influences
▶ Physical inactivitiy
▶ Dietary factors
- Eating patterns
- Type of diet
▶ Socioeconomic
▶ Educational
- Maternal nutritional factors
- Infant feeding practices
▶ Cultural-ethnic
▶ Psychologic
- Anxiety-related obesity
- Depression-related obesity

Genetic factors
▶ Inherited predisposition
▶ Genetic disorders associated with obesity
- Alström's syndrome
- Dystrophia adiposogenitalis (Fröhlich's syndrome)
- Klinefelter's syndrome (gynecomastia, small testicles)
- Laurence-Moon-Bardet-Biedl syndrome (internal hyperostosis frontalis with obesity, debility, syndactyly, retinitis pigmentosa, hypogonadotropic hypogonadism)

- Prader-Willi syndrome (microsomia, obesity, imbecility, muscular hypotension, bilateral cryptorchidism, hypogonadotropic hypogonadism)
- Pseudohypoparathyroidism
- Stewart-Morel-Morgagni syndrome

Hypothalamic dysfunction
- Tumor
- Inflammation
- Trauma
- Surgery
- Increased intracranial pressure

Endocrine
- Hypothyroidism
- Cushing's syndrome (excess glucocorticoids)
- Hypopituitarism
- Hyperinsulinism
  - Insulinoma
  - Excess exogenous insulin
- Hypogonadism
  - Menopause
  - Stein-Leventhal syndrome (hirsutism, menstrual abnormalities, infertility, enlarged "polycystic ovaries")
- Pubertal obesity

Lipomatosis
Excessive local accumulation of fat
- Multiple lipomas
- Madelung's disease
- Launois-Bensaude syndrome
- Adiposis dolorosa (Anders' disease, Dercum's disease)

Drugs
- Antiemetics
- Antiepileptics
- Antihypertensives
- Appetite stimulants
- Corticosteroids
- Estrogens
- Insulin
- Isoniazide
- Lithium
- Phenothiazines
- Progesterones
- Tricyclic antidepressants

Miscellaneous
- Glycogen storage disorders
- Pregnancy

Obstructive Lung Disease

Decrease in the exhaled air flow due to narrowing or obstruction of the airways.

Types
- Asthma
- Chronic obstructive pulmonary disease (COPD)
  - Chronic bronchitis
  - Emphysema
- Bronchiectasis
- Cystic fibrosis
- Bronchiolitis

Occult Blood

Occult gastrointestinal bleeding, hidden gastrointestinal bleeding, occult fecal blood, occult stool blood

Blood in the feces in amounts too small to be seen, but detectable by tests.
See Gastrointestinal Bleeding → 152

Causes
- Esophageal varices
- Inflammation
  - Esophagitis
  - Gastritis
  - Duodenitis
  - Inflammatory bowel disease
- Peptic ulcer
- Gastrointestinal trauma
- Recent gastrointestinal surgery
- Tumors
  - Colorectal cancer
  - Intestinal polyp
  - Gastric carcinoma
  - Gastrointestinal tumor
  - Esophageal cancer
- Hemorrhoids

► Fissures
► Infections
  • Amebiasis
  • Nematodes
  • Scarlet fever
► Miscellaneous
  • Arteriovenous malformation
  • Löffler's syndrome
  • Hiatal hernia
  • Diverticula
  • Angiodysplasia of the colon
  • Portal hypertension
  • NSAID
  • GM-CSF therapy
► Idiopathic

Oligospermia, See Azoospermia,
Oligospermia → 48, See Impotence → 208

Onychogryphosis, Onychorrhexis,
Onychodystrophy, Onycholysis
See Nail changes → 250

Ophthalmoplegia
Paralysis of one or more of the ocular
muscles, pupillary paralysis.
Causes
► Infection, inflammation
  • Meningitis
  • Virus encephalitis
  • Diphtheria
  • Tetanus (toxoid)
  • Botulism
► Vasculitis
► Midbrain lesion
► Brainstem stroke
► Bilateral third nerve involvement
► Acute cranial polyneuropathy
► Myasthenia gravis
► Adie's pupils
► Iris injury
► Drugs, toxins
  • Alcoholism (thiamine deficiency,

    Wernicke's encephalopathy)
  • Benztropine
  • Lead poisoning
  • Topical mydriatic

Optic nerve inflammation
See Optic Neuropathy → 263

Optic neuritis
See Optic Neuropathy → 263

Optic Neuropathy
Demyelinating optic neuropathy, retrobulbar optic neuritis
Optic neuritis
► Multiple sclerosis (!)
► Encephalomyelitis
► Posterior uveitis
► Optic nerve vascular lesions
  • Central retinal artery occlusion
  • Central retinal vein occlusion
  • Anterior ischemic optic neuropathy
► Neoplasm
  • Optic nerve glioma
  • Neurofibromatosis
  • Meningioma
► Fungal infections
► Drugs , toxins
  • Alcohol
  • Aminosalicylic acid
  • Benzene
  • Cigarette smoking
  • Chloramphenicol
  • Ethambutol
  • Isoniazid
  • Lead
  • Penicillamine
  • Phenothiazines
  • Phenylbutazone
  • Quinine
  • Streptomycin
Anterior ischemic optic neuropathy
► Vasculitis

O
P

- Giant cell arteritis
- Systemic lupus erythematosus
- Polyarteritis nodosum
- Bürger disease
- Allergic vasculitis
- Postimmunization
- Postviral vasculitis
- Syphilis
- Radiation necrosis
▶ Systemic vasculopathies
- Hypertension
- Arteriosclerosis
- Diabetes mellitus
- Migraine
- Takayasu's disease
- Carotid occlusive disease
▶ Hematologic
- Polycythemia vera
- Sickle cell anemia
- Acute hypotension
- Glucose-6-phosphate dehydrogenase deficiency
▶ Ocular
- Postcataract
- Low tension glaucoma

Compressive optic neuropathy
▶ Primary malignancies
▶ Metastases
▶ Optic nerve tumors
- Optic nerve gliomas
- Optic nerve meningiomas
▶ Thyroid ophthalmopathy
▶ Cavernous hemangiomas
▶ Sarcoidosis
▶ Trauma
▶ Solid orbital tumors
- Meningiomas
- Hemangiomas
- Schwannoma
▶ Cystic tumors
- Dermoid cysts
- Cholesterol granuloma
- Mucoceles
- Conjunctival orbital cysts
▶ Inflammatory and infiltrative processes

- Sarcoidosis
- Lupus

DDx
▶ Branch retinal artery occlusion
▶ Central retinal artery occlusion
▶ Acute angle closure glaucoma
▶ Meningioma
▶ Multiple sclerosis
▶ Optic neuritis
▶ Anterior ischemic optic neuropathy
▶ Compressive optic neuropathy
▶ Sarcoidosis
▶ Sudden visual loss
▶ Syphilis
▶ Thyroid ophthalmopathy

Orbitopathy, See Proptosis → 294

Orthostatic hypotension, See Syncope → 344, See Hypotension → 204

Osmolality, plasma
See Hypertonic dehydration → 93

Osmolality, urinary
See Urine Osmolality → 369

Osteolysis
Softening, absorption, and destruction of bony tissue.
Causes
▶ Tumors
- Multiple myeloma
- Metastases
- Leukemia
- Osteolytic sarcoma
- Eosinophilic bone granulation tumor
- Lymphogranuloma
- Central chondroma
- Bone hemangioendothelioma
- Extraosseous soft tissue tumors
▶ Osteomyelitis (Brodie's abscess)
▶ Syphilitic gumma

- Chondromatosis
- Hand-Schüller-Christian disease (cholesterol lipidosis: exophthalmus, diabetes insipidus and irregular bone defects; mostly in children)

Osteomalacia

Defective uptake of minerals into the normal or overgrowing protein bone matrix (osteoid) as a secondary bone formation impairment. The increased elastic bone matrix mass results in increased softness and curvature tendency of the bones. X-ray findings: thinning of the basal lamina and end plates, loss of definition of trabecular details, separation of the compact bone layers, indistinct border to the medullary spongiosa.

Lack of circulating vitamin D metabolites

See Vitamin D → 379
- Malnutrition
  - Undernourishment
  - Vegetarian diet
  - Malnutrition in advanced age
- Vitamin D malabsorption
  - Gastrectomy
  - Faulty bile function
  - Exocrine pancreatic insufficiency
  - Small intestinal disease
- Insufficient sun exposure
- Disordered vitamin D metabolism (defective hydroxylation to active metabolites)
  - Chronic liver diseases
  - Chronic renal failure
  - Prostatic cancer
  - Mesenchymal tumors
  - Anticonvulsant therapy
  - Vitamin D-dependent rickets (25-hydroxyvitaminD_1-hydroxylase deficiency)
- Renal loss
  - Nephrotic syndrome

Peripheral resistance to vitamin D
- Vitamin D-dependent rickets
- Chronic renal failure
- Anticonvulsant therapy

Hypophosphatemia
- Malnutrition
- Malabsorption
  - Gastrointestinal impairment
  - Phosphate-binding antacids
- Renal loss
  - Hereditary (X-chromosomal/autosomal recessive)
  - Congenital renal phosphate loss with hypercalciuria, renal stones, osteomalacia and rickets
  - Fanconi syndrome (hereditary impairment of amino acid metabolism with cystine storage in various organs, rachitic microplasia and nephropathy)
  - Primary hyperparathyroidism
  - Tumor phosphaturia
  - Neurofibromatosis
  - Toxins
    - Cadmium
    - Aluminium
    - Lead
- Chronic dialysis

Miscellaneous
- Calcium deficiency
  - Biphosphonates
- Calcification inhibitors
  - Sodium fluoride
- Hypoparathyroidism
- Chronic acidosis
- Total parenteral nutrition
- Renal transplantation

Osteomyelitis

Acute osteitis, usually due to bacterial infection. In children the long tubular bones are more frequently affected, in adults the vertebral bodies.

Common agents
- Gram-positive cocci

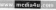

- Staphylococcus aureus
- S. epidermis
- S. pyogenes
- S. pneumoniae
▶ Gram-negative bacteria
- Pseudomonas
- Klebsiella
- Serratia
- E.coli
▶ Anaerobic bacteria
- Bacteroides
- Fusobacterium
- Actinomycetes
- Peptococcus
▶ Other germs

Causes
▶ Infectious foci (50%)
- Surgical interventions
- Decubitus
- Sinusitis
- Tonsillitis
- Otitis
▶ Peripheral vasculopathies (30%)
- Vasculitis
- Diabetic angiopathy
▶ Hematogenous spread (20%)
- Skin infection
- Urinary tract infections
- Gastrointestinal infections
- Pneumonia

Osteoporosis

Quantitative reduction of bone tissue with preserved bone structure due to increased bone catabolism and/or reduced bone formation.

Primary osteoporosis
▶ Postmenopausal osteoporosis (Type 1)
▶ Senile osteoporosis (Type 2)

Secondary osteoporosis
▶ Immobilization
▶ Endocrine
- Estrogen deficiency
- Testosterone deficiency

- Steroid excess
  ○ Cushing's syndrome
  ○ Steroid therapy (> 1 year 7.5 mg prednisolone equivalent/day)
- Thyrotoxicosis
- Primary hyperparathyroidism
- Diabetes mellitus
- Hypogonadism
- Acromegaly
- Hypopituitarism
▶ Nutritional
- Protein deficiency
- Vitamin C deficiency
- Calcium/Viramin D deficiency
- Malabsorption/Maldigestion
- Anorexia
- Postgastrectomy
- Total parenteral nutrition
- Pregnancy and lactation
▶ Malignancies
- Leukemia
- Lymphoma
- Multiple myeloma
- Waldenström´s macroglobulinemia
- Generalized mastocytosis
▶ Drugs, toxins
- Alcoholism
- Antiepileptics
- Cigarette smoking
- Dihydrotachysterol
- Heparin therapy (long-term)
- Laxatives
- Methotrexate
▶ Genetic
- Homocystinuria
- Osteogenesis imperfecta
- Ehlers-Danlos syndrome
- Marfan syndrome
- Down syndrome
▶ Miscellaneous
- Rheumatoid arthritis
- Ankylosing spondylitis
- Chronic obstructive pulmonary disease
- Chronic liver diseases
- Chronic hypophosphatemia

- Chronic renal failure (renal osteodystrophy)
- Chronic acidosis
- Paget's disease
- Cystic fibrosis
- Juvenile osteoporosis
- Pregnancy
- Idiopathic

Overeating
Hyperorexia, excessive eating
▶ Diabetes mellitus
▶ Hyperthyroidism
▶ Insulinoma
▶ Tapeworm
▶ Pregnancy
▶ Drugs
  - Corticosteroids
  - Estrogens
▶ Encephalopathy
  - Tumor in the hypothalamus
  - Other tumor
  - Trauma
▶ Dumping syndrome
▶ Bulimia nervosa
▶ Glycogenosis
▶ Hereditary fructose intolerance

Overweight, See Obesity → 261

Oxygen partial pressure
See Blood Gas Analysis → 57

Oxygen saturation
See Blood Gas Analysis → 57

Pain, abdominal
See Abdominal Pain, Acute → 7

Pain, anal, See Anorectal pain → 35

Pain, back, See Back Pain → 49

Pain, bone, See Bone Pain → 58

Pain, eye, See Eye pain → 138

Pain, Diffuse
Musculoskeletal pain, aches, chronic pain
Collagen vascular disease, rheumatic
▶ Rheumatoid arthritis
▶ Sjögren's syndrome
▶ Polymyalgia rheumatica
▶ Ankylosing spondylitis
▶ Reiter's syndrome
▶ Vasculitis
▶ Polymyositis
▶ Dermatomyositis
▶ Eosinophilia myalgia syndrome
▶ Silicone implants
▶ Psychogenic rheumatism
▶ Fibromyalgia
▶ Myofascial pain syndrome
▶ Bilateral soft tissue rheumatism
Miscellaneous
▶ Postviral arthralgia, myalgia
▶ Hyperthyroidism
▶ Hypothyroidism
▶ Hypophosphatemia
▶ Osteomalacia
▶ Metabolic bone disease
▶ Paraneoplastic snydrome
▶ Hypermobility
▶ Chronic fatigue syndrome
▶ Multiple sclerosis
▶ Overuse syndromes
▶ Entrapment neuropathy

Pain, facial, See Facial pain → 140

Pane, flank, See Flank Pain → 146

Pain, genital

OP

Pain, menstruation

Pain, Radiation

Into the arm
► Angina pectoris
► Myocardial infarction
► Thoracic vertebrae syndrome
► Scapulohumeral arthritis
► Pancoast tumor

Into the left shoulder
► Scapulohumeral arthritis
► Scapulocostal syndrome
► Cervical spondylosis
► Polymyalgia rheumatica
► Lung neurinoma
► Pancoast tumor
► Acute pancreatitis
► Splenic rupture
► Diaphragmatic hernia
► Tubal rupture

Into the right shoulde
► Scapulohumeral arthritis
► Scapulocostal syndrome
► Cervical spondylosis
► Polymyalgia rheumatica
► Lung neurinoma
► Pancoast tumor
► Cholelithiasis
► Liver rupture
► Liver abscess
► Subphrenic abscess

► Pancreas head carcinoma
► Tubal rupture

Into the groin
► Inguinal hernia
► Femoral hernia
► Kidney diseases
  • Nephrolithiasis
  • Acute pyelonephritis
  • Intrarenal abscess
  • Genitourinary tuberculosis
► Vasculopathy
  • Pelvic venous thrombosis
  • Terminal aorta occlusion
► Orthopedic causes
  • Disk prolapse
  • Coxarthrosis
  • Genitofemoral nerve neuralgia
► Cryptorchism
► Prostatitis
► Appendicitis
► Perityphlitic abscess

Into the thigh
► Femoral hernia
► Inguinal hernia
► Coxarthrosis
► Sciatica (→ 324)
► Meralgia paraesthetica
► Osteoporosis
► Peripheral iliac thrombosis
► Parametritis

Into the back
► Posterior myocardial infarction
► Aortic aneurysm
► Terminal aortic occlusion
► Lung neurinoma
► Bronchial carcinoma
► Hiatus hernia
► Acute pancreatitis
► Osteoporosis

Pain, urination, See Dysuria → 114

Paleness, Pallor

Loss of normal skin or mucous membrane color.
► Normal fair appearance
► Lack of exposure to the sun
► Anemia (→ 28)
  • Blood loss
  • Poor nutrition
► Hypotension
► Shock
► Edema
► Frostbite
► Infectious diseases
► Intoxication
► Cancer
► Kidney diseases (uremia)
► Chronic liver diseases
► Addison's disease

Palpitations

Irregular heartbeat, heartbeat sensations, heart pounding
Conscious, unpleasant awareness of one's own heartbeat.
Without arrhythmia
► Cardiac disorders
  • Aortic regurgitation
  • Aortic stenosis
  • Patent ductus arteriosus
  • Ventricular septal defect
  • Atrial septal defect
  • Cardiomegaly
  • Hyperkinetic heart syndrome
  • Tricuspid insufficiency
  • Perimyocarditis
  • Prosthetic heart valve
  • Pacemaker
► Noncardiac disorders
  • Exercise
  • Anxiety

• Anemia
• Dehydration
• Fever
• Hypoglycemia
• Pheochromocytoma
• Postural hypotension
• Menopausal syndrome
• Aortic aneurasm
• Migraine
• Arteriovenous fistula
• Respiratory acidosis
• Metabolic acidosis
• Hyperventilation
• Hypoxemia
• Hyperthyroidism
► Drugs
• Alcohol
• Aminophylline
• Antiarrhythmics
• Antiasthmatics
• Antidepressants
• Atropine
• Beta blockers
• Cocaine
• Caffeine
• Cardiac glycosides
• Neuroleptics
• Nicotine
• Nitrates
• Sympathomimetics
• Theophylline
• Thyroid drugs
With arrhythmia
• Extrasystoles
• Bradyarrhythmias
• Tachyarrhythmias

Pancreatic Insufficiency, Exocrine

Reduction of exocrine pancreatic function with maldigestion. Symptoms include fatty stools, weight loss, weakness and muscle atrophy.
See Pancreatitis, Acute → 270

O P

Causes
► Chronic alcoholism
► Cystic fibrosis
► Neoplasm
  • Pancreas
  • Duodenum
► Pancreatectomy
► Hyperparathyroidism
► Lipid metabolism disorders
► Congenital pancreatic dysfunction
► Idiopathic pancreatitis
► Trauma
► Shwachman syndrome (pancreatic insufficiency with bone marrow damage)
► Stomach surgery
  • Billroth I/II
  • Vagotomy with pyloroplasty
► Gastrinoma (Zollinger-Ellison syndrome)
► Hemochromatosis
► Dietary protein deficiency with hypoalbuminemia
► Enzymes
  • Protrypsin deficiency
  • Enterokinase deficiency
  • α_1-antitrypsin deficiency
  • Isolated amylase, lipase or protease deficiency

Pancreatic Polypeptide (PP)

Peptide secreted by islet cells of the pancreas in response to a meal. Physiologic function uncertain.

Increased
► VIPoma
► Ppoma
► Insulinoma
► Gastrinoma (Zollinger-Ellison syndrome)
► Advanced age

Pancreatitis, Acute

Acute inflammation of the pancreas, when factors involved in maintaining cellular homeostasis (to avoid digesting itself) are out of balance.

Alcoholism

Bile duct obstruction (→ 75)
► Cholelithiasis
► Stenosis
► Tumor
► Edema
► Spasms
► Cysts
► Ascarides

Trauma
► Blunt trauma
► Penetrating trauma
► Postoperative
► After ERCP (endoscopic retrograde cholangiopancreatography)

Metabolic, endocrine
► Hypertriglyceridemia
► Hypercalcemia
► Renal failure
► Porphyria
► Hemochromatosis
► Aminoaciduria
► Acute gestational fatty liver

Infections
► Bacterial
  • Legionella
  • Mycoplasma
  • Cambylobacter jejuni
  • Leptospirosis
  • Rickettsia
  • Salmonella
  • Tuberculosis
► Viral
  • Mumps
  • Hepatitis
  • Infectious mononucleosis
  • Coxsackievirus
  • ECHO virus

- HIV
- CMV
▶ Fungal
  - Aspergillosis
  - Candidiasis (C. albicans)
  - Cryptococcus
▶ Parasitic
  - Ascariasis
  - Toxoplasmosis

Collagen vascular disease
▶ Systemic lupus erythematosus
▶ Necrotizing vascular angiitis
▶ Thrombotic thrombocytopenic purpura
▶ Henoch-Schönlein purpura

Drugs
▶ ACE inhibitors
▶ Azathioprine
▶ Dideoxyinosine
▶ Estrogens
▶ Furosemide
▶ Oral contraceptives
▶ Pentamidine
▶ Sulfonamides
▶ Tetracyclines
▶ Thiazides
▶ Valproic acid

Obstruction of the ampulla Vateri
▶ Crohn's disease
▶ Duodenal diverticulum

Miscellaneous
▶ Penetrating gastrointestinal ulcer
▶ Pancreas divisum
▶ Partial pancreas resection
▶ Posttransplantation
▶ Cystic fibrosis
▶ Hereditary pancreatitis

Risk factors
▶ Advanced age
▶ Hypotension
▶ Tachycardia
▶ Fever
▶ Leukocytosis
▶ Lung disease

Pancytopenia
Aplastic anemia
Pronounced reduction in the number of erythrocytes, all types of white blood cells, and the blood platelets in the circulating blood. The major causes of morbidity and mortality from aplastic anemia include infection and bleeding.

Congenital, hereditary
▶ Fanconi's anemia (hereditary refractory anemia characterized by pancytopenia and hypoplasia of the bone marrow with impairment of the amino acid metabolism, cystine storage in miscellaneous organs, rachitic microplasia and nephropathy)
▶ Dyskeratosis congenita
▶ Cartilage hair hypoplasia
▶ Pearson syndrome
▶ Amegakaryocytic thrombocytopenia (TAR syndrome)
▶ Shwachman-Diamond syndrome
▶ Dubowitz syndrome
▶ Diamond-Blackfan syndrome
▶ Familial aplastic anemia

Aquired (80%)
▶ Toxic-allergic marrow damage
  - Drugs, toxins
    ○ Arsenics
    ○ Benzol
    ○ Chemotherapeutics
    ○ Chloramphenicol
    ○ Gold
    ○ Hydantoins
    ○ Organic arsenics
    ○ Phenylbutazone
    ○ Sulfonamides
  - Radiation
▶ Bone marrow infiltration, repression
  - Infection
    ○ Tuberculosis
    ○ Fungal
  - Metastases

- Myelofibrosis
- Reticulosis
- Bone marrow tumor
- Albers-Schönberg disease
- Gaucher's disease and other lipid storage disease
- Osteopetrosis
▶ Hematologic
- Leukemia
- Lymphoproliferative disorders
- Lymphoma with marrow involvement
- Multiple myeloma
- Myeloproliferative disorders
- Myelodysplastic syndromes
▶ Infections
- Severe infection
- Brucellosis
- Hepatitis A and B
- Tuberculosis
- Brucellosis
- Syphilis
- Epstein-Barr virus (EBV)
- HIV
- CMV
- Parvovirus
- Mycobacterial infections
▶ Splenic disorder
- Lymphoma
- Gaucher's disease
- Niemann-Pick disease
- Splenomegaly due to congestion
- Kala-Aza
▶ Miscellaneous
- Pernicious anemia
  ◦ Vitamin B_{12} deficiency
  ◦ Folate deficiency
- Banti's syndrome (idiopathic portal hypertension)
- Thymoma
- Systemic lupus erythematosus
- Felty's syndrome (splenomegaly with rheumatoid arthritis and leukopenia)
- Sarcoidosis
- Cirrhosis
- Paroxysmal nocturnal hemoglobinuria

- Graft-versus-host reaction
- Pregnancy

paO2, See Blood Gas Analysis → 57

Papilledema

Edema of the optic disk, often due to increased intracranial pressure (→ 213).

Causes

▶ Intracranial masses
- Brain tumor
- Brain cyst
- Hydrocephalus (→ 186)
- Foster Kennedy's syndrome
▶ Intracranial bleeding
- Subarachnoid hemorrhage
- Subdural hematoma
- Epidural bleeding
▶ Infection, inflammation
- Meningoencephalitis
- Cerebral abscess
- Extradural abscess
- Subdural empyema
- Syphilis
- Neuropapillitis
▶ Obstruction of retinal veins
- Cavernous sinus thrombosis
- Central retinal vein occlusion
▶ Hypertensive encephalopathy
▶ Drugs
- Cisplatin
- Corticosteroids
- Lithium
- Tetracyclines
▶ Head trauma
▶ Orbital lesions
▶ Metabolic endocrine
- Thyrotoxicosis
- Hypoparathyroidism
- Hypocalcemic tetany
- Cushing's syndrome
▶ Miscellaneous
- Hypercapnia
- Sarcoidosis

- Infectious endocarditis
- Eclampsia
- Paget's disease
- Dysostosis craniofacialis (Crouzon's disease)
- Arnold-Chiari malformation
- Systemic lupus erythematosus
- Osteoma
- Chondroma

Paradoxical Pulse

Pulsus paradoxus

Exaggerated inspiratory decrease in systolic blood pressure (> 10 mm Hg).

Cardiovascular
▶ Cardiac tamponade
▶ Pericardial effusion
▶ Constrictive pericarditis
▶ Adhesive pericarditis
▶ Endocardial fibrosis
▶ Myocardial amyloidosis
▶ Mitral stenosis with right heart failure
▶ Tricuspid stenosis

Pulmonary
▶ Pulmonary emphysema
▶ Pulmonary embolism
▶ Severe asthma

Miscellaneous
▶ Paramediastinal effusion
▶ Scleroderma
▶ Hypovolemia

Paralytic ileus, See Ileus → 206

Paraneoplastic Syndromes

Symptom complexes directly resulting from a malignant neoplasm, but not resulting from the presence of tumor cells.

Pathophysiology (endocrine impairment, ectopic hormone production)
▶ Hormone production by benign cells (e.g. adenomas)

▶ Hormone production by tumor disease of an endocrine organ (e.g. pheochromocytoma)
▶ Changes in hormone production due to infiltration of an endocrine gland
▶ Changes in hormone production by drugs or infections

Types
▶ Cushing's syndrome (ACTH, CRH, MSH)
▶ Hypercalcemia (PTH)
▶ SIADH (Schwartz-Bartter's syndrome, ADH; frequently occurring after metastatic spread)
  • Lung cancer
  • Breast cancer
  • Melanoma
▶ Gynecomastia (gonadotropins)
▶ Acromegaly (GH, GHRH)
▶ Hyperthyroidism (TSH)
▶ Galactorrhea (prolactin)
▶ Hyperglobulia (erythropoetin)
▶ Diarrhea/ metabolic impairment (VIP)
▶ Hypokalemia
▶ Hypoglycemia
▶ Carcinoid syndrome
▶ Osteoarthropathy (vasoactive substances, GHRH)
▶ Precocious puberty (chorion gonadotropins)
▶ Hypercalcemia (cholecalciferol , IL-1 , PG E2 , PTH , TNF-α, TNF-β, in tumors with development of bone metastases)
  • Breast cancer
  • Lung cancer
  • Carcinoma of kidney
  • Ovarial carcinoma
  • Pancreas carcinoma

Paraneoplastic endocrinopathies
▶ Hypertension (pheochromocytoma)
▶ Hyponatremia (Schwartz-Bartter's syndrome)
▶ Gynecomastia (testicular tumors [β-HCG])
▶ Ulcer disease (Zollinger-Ellison syndrome; tumor usually limited to the

O
P

pancreas or duodenum, frequently malignant, gastrin-producing, associated with MEN)
► Hyperglycemia (glucagenoma)
► Hypoglycemia (insulinoma, liver cell carcinoma)
► Hypercalcemia (bronchial carcinomas, multiple myeloma, breast cancer, hypernephroma, parathyroid carcinoma)
► Cushing's syndrome (small-cell bronchial carcinomas, adrenal cortex carcinomas)
► Amenorrhea (ovarial carcinoma, prolactinoma)

Hematologic changes
► Effects on the erythropoiesis
  • Polycythemia (renal tumors)
  • Autoimmune hemolytic anemia
  • Microangiopathic hemolytic anemia (fragmentocytes, in gastric carcinoma)
  • Aplastic anemia (pure red cell anemia; in thymomas, gastric carcinoma, breast cancer, T-lymphoproliferative diseases)
► Effects on the leukocytopoiesis
  • Eosinophilia
  • Leukocytosis (in Hodgkin's and non-Hodgkin's lymphoma, bronchial carcinomas, gastric carcinoma, pancreas carcinoma, soft tissue sarcomas)
  • Sweet's syndrome
  • Leukopenia (thymoma)
► Effects on the megakaryopoiesis
  • Thrombocytosis (in non-small-cell bronchial carcinomas, tumors of the gastrointestinal tract, pleural mesothelioma, Hodgkin's and non-Hodgkin's lymphoma)
  • Thrombocytopenia (in Hodgkin's lymphoma, immunoplastic lymphoma, bronchial carcinomas, breast cancer, tumors of the rectum and the gallbladder)
► Effects on the coagulation
  • DIC

• Thrombosis (pancreas carcinoma, bronchial carcinomas)

Vascular impairment
► Thrombophlebitis
► Thrombocytopenic purpura
► Endocarditis

Neuromuscular impairment
► Peripheral polyneuropathy (in bronchial carcinomas, ovarial carcinoma, gastric carcinoma, breast cancer, prostate carcinoma, cervical carcinoma, colon carcinoma, uterus carcinoma, rectal carcinoma)
► Eaton-Lambert syndrome (myasthenia gravis like syndrome in carcinomas, especially in bronchial carcinomas)
► Polymyositis
► Myasthenia gravis (in thymoma, pancreas carcinoma, breast cancer, prostate carcinoma, ovarial carcinoma, cervical carcinoma and lymphomas)
► Polymyositis (bronchial carcinoma, prostate carcinoma, rectal carcinoma, tumors of the female genital organs, the nose and the thyroid gland as well as in lymphomas)
► Subacute cerebellar degeneration
► Cortex degeneration
► Subacute necrotic myelopathy
► Encephalomyelitis
► Cerebral symptoms
► Amyotrophic lateral sclerosis (in lung cancer, breast cancer, gastric carcinoma and colon carcinoma)
► Limbic encephalitisis (Hodgkin's lymphoma, small-cell bronchial carcinomas)
► Progressive multifocal leukoencephalopathy (in neoplasias of the lymphoreticular system)
► Neuropapillitis
► Spinocerebellar degeneration (in bronchial carcinomas)

Skeletal manifestations
► Digital glubbing (small-cell bronchial

carcinomas)
► Hypertrophic pulmonary osteoarthropathy

Skin manifestations
► Hyperpigmentation
► Acanthosis nigricans (in intra-abdominal tumors: adenocarcinoma of the stomach)
► Paraneoplastic acrokeratosis (Bazex's syndrome, in carcinomas of the oropharyngeal/gastrointestinal tract)
► Hypertrichosis
► Glucagenoma syndrome in α-cell-carcinoma of the pancreas with necrolytic erythema that spreads peripherally
► Dermatomyositis (in lung cancer, breast cancer, gastric carcinoma)
► Pruritus (Hodgkin's lymphoma, polycythemia)
► Gardner's syndrome (colon carcinoma)

Paraproteinemia, Paraproteinuria

Presence of paraproteins in the blood or urine. Paraproteins are monoclonal immunoglobulins or immunoglobulin light chains resulting from a clonal proliferation of plasma cells or B-lymphocytes.

Causes
► Malignant lymphoproliferative diseases
  • Waldenström's syndrome
  • Malignant lymphomas
► Multiple myeloma
  • Bence-Jones plasmocytoma
  • IgA-plasmocytoma
  • IgG-plasmocytoma
  • IgD-plasmocytoma
  • IgM -plasmocytoma
  • IgE-plasmocytoma
► Chronic idiopathic cold agglutinin disease
► Primary amyloidosis
► Benign gammopathy

► Heavy chain disease (Franklin's disease)
► Cirrhosis
► Amyloidosis (primary form)
► Cryoglobulins
► Associated with malignant tumor
  • Bronchial carcinoma
  • Prostate carcinoma
  • Malignant melanoma
► Monoclonal gammopathy of unclear origin

Parathyroid Hormone

Parathormone, parathyrin, PTH
Peptide hormone formed in the parathyroid glands, raising the serum calcium by causing bone resorption.

Reference range	
PTH	1–7 pmol/l

Increased
► Primary hyperparathyroidism
  • Parathyroid adenoma
  • Gland hyperplasia
  • Parathyroid malignancy
  • Familial hyperparathyroidism
    ∘ MEN I
    ∘ MEN II
  • Lithium therapy
  • Familial hypocalciuric hypercalcemia
► Secondary hyperparathyroidism
► Pseudohypoparathyroidism (congenital PTH receptor defect)
► Vitamin D deficiency
► Rickets
► Osteomalacia
► Age

Decreased
► PTH < 2–20 pg/ml and Ca^+< 2.1 mmol/l: hypoparathyroidism
► PTH < 2–20 pg/ml and Ca^{++}> 2.6 mmol/l: hypercalcemia due to tumor
► Cancer
► Granulomatous disease

Paresthesias

Abnormal sensation like burning, pricking, tickling, or tingling, often in the absence of external stimuli.

Neuropathies
▶ Local injury to the nerves
▶ Pressure on the nerves
  • Herniated disk
  • Tumors
  • Abscesses
  • Arthritic bones
▶ Lack of blood supply to the area
▶ Inflammation
  • Acute idiopathic polyneuritis
  • Chronic relapsing polyneuropathy
▶ Entrapments
  • Carpal tunnel syndrome (→ 69)
  • Ulnar entrapment (cubital tunnel)
  • Thoracic outlet syndrome
  • Lateral femoral cutaneous syndrome
  • Peroneal palsy
  • Tarsal tunnel

Central nervous system
▶ Cerebrovascular insult
▶ Transient ischemic attack (TIA)
▶ Migraine
▶ Seizures
▶ Brain tumor
▶ Head trauma
▶ Brain abscess
▶ Encephalitis
▶ Multiple sclerosis

Metabolic
▶ Diabetes mellitus
▶ Nutritional deficiencies
  • Vitamin B_{12} deficiency
  • Thiamin deficiency
  • Folic acid deficiency
▶ Hypothyroidism
▶ Alcoholism
▶ Uremia
▶ Porphyria
▶ Amyloidosis

Inflammation
▶ Local trauma
▶ Acute idiopathic polyneuritis
▶ Chronic relapsing polyneuropathy

Infections
▶ HIV
▶ Lyme disease
▶ Herpes zoster
▶ Diphtheria
▶ Leprosy

Collagen vascular diseases
▶ Polyarteritis nodosa
▶ Sjögren syndrome
▶ Systemic sclerosis
▶ Systemic lupus erythematosis
▶ Autoimmune vasculitis
▶ Rheumatoid arthritis

Hereditary
▶ Charcot-Marie-Tooth syndrome
▶ Denny-Brown's syndrome
▶ Familial amyloiditic polyneuropathy

Neoplasm
▶ Tumor compression
▶ Paraneoplastic syndrome
▶ Lymphoma
▶ Cancer
  • Stomach cancer
  • Lung cancer
  • Breast cancer
  • Ovary cancer
▶ Plasma cell dyscrasias
  • Multiple myeloma
  • Osteoclastic myeloma
  • Monoclonal gammopathy
  • Waldenström's macroglobulinemia

Drugs, toxins
▶ Alcohol
▶ Acetazolamide
▶ Amiodarone
▶ Amitriptyline
▶ Arsenic
▶ Chemotherapeutics
▶ Chloramphenicol
▶ Chloroquine

- Cigarette smoking
- Cisplatin
- Cyanide
- Dapsone
- Disulfiram
- D-penicillamine
- Gold
- HIV drugs
  - Didanosine
  - Zalcitabine
  - Stavudine
- Hydralazine
- Isoniazid
- Lead
- Lithium
- Mercury
- Metronidazole
- Nitrofurantoin
- Organophosphates
- Phenytoin
- Pyridoxine
- Sulfonamides
- Thallium

Miscellaneous
- Long-term radiation
- Sarcoidosis
- Malnutrition

Parkinsonism

Abnormal condition of the nervous system due to degeneration of dopaminergic neurons in the substantia nigra (basal ganglia), resulting in rigor, akinesia and tremor.

Primary Parkinsonism
- Parkinson's disease (80-90%, primary degeneration of substantia nigra)

Secondary Parkinsonism
- Infection
  - Encephalitis
  - Meningitis
  - Postencephalitic
- Drugs, toxins
  - Carbon monoxide

- Flunarizine (reversible)
- Manganese
- Methyl alcohol
- Methyldopa
- Neuroleptics
- Nifedipine (reversible)
- Reserpine
- Hypoxic and traumatic brain damage
  - Cerebral insults
    - Infarctions
    - Hemorrhages
  - Brain tumor
  - Apallic syndrome
  - Psychic traumas
  - Boxer trauma
- Miscellaneous
  - Kernicterus
  - Wilson's disease
  - Syphilis
  - Hypoparathyroidism
  - Hydrocephalus

Paronychia, See Nail changes → 250

Parosmia

Subjective perception of nonexistent odors.

Causes
- Chronic rhinitis (ozena)
- Empyema of the nasal sinuses
- Aura of an epileptic seizure
- Hallucination
  - Schizophrenia
  - Hysteria

Parotid Gland Enlargement

Uni- or bilateral, painless or painful, localized as well as diffuse enlargement of the parotid gland.

Painless
- Mainly unilateral
  - Dysgenetic cysts
  - Acquired cysts

O
P

- Cystadenolymphomas
- Benign salivary gland tumors
  (→ 324)
- Malignant salivary gland tumors
  (→ 324)
▶ Mainly bilateral
- Sarcoidosis
- Sialadenosis
- Myoepithelial parotitis (Sjögren's syndrome)

Painful

▶ Mainly unilateral
- Acute bacterial parotitis
- Chronic relapsing parotitis
- Sialolithiasis of the parotid gland
▶ Mainly bilateral
- Acute viral parotitis
  ∘ Mumps
  ∘ Cytomegalovirus
  ∘ Coxsackie
  ∘ Influenza

Paroxysmal Cold Hemoglobinuria

Paroxysmal cold hemoglobinuria is a rare disease associated with intravascular hemolysis and hemoglobinuria following exposure to cold. It is due to a specific antibody - the Donath-Landsteiner antibody. The antibody sticks to the red blood cells in the cold and causes a complement-mediated lysis on rewarming.

Causes

▶ Congenital syphilis
▶ After viral infection
- Measles
- Mumps
- Glandular fever
- Chicken pox
▶ Idiopathic
See Anemia → 28

Partial Thromboplastin Time
PTT

Screening test in case of f suspected congenital or acquired hemorrhagic diathesis (→ 176). Screening test to prove hyper-coagulability (reduced PTT), monitoring of a heparin therapy. Concerns the factors of the endogenous coagulation system. If platelet count, bleeding time, thromboplastin time and thrombin time are normal, a prolonged partial thromboplastin time suggests hemophilia. Although the PTT also responds to the activation of factor X, it nevertheless reacts primarily to the anti-thrombin effects of heparins.
See Thromboplastin time → 352

Reference range
Around 35-55 sec.
Under heparin therapy according to indication: 1.5-2.5x longer .
PTT is not prolonged under therapy with low-molecular heparins

▶ Prolonged
- Heparin
- Warfarin/Prothrombin complex deficiency (warfarin therapy)
  ∘ PTT is prolonged with gradual reduction in prothrombin complex (factor IX deficiency). The correlation is not, however, as precise as with thromboplastin time (→ 352).
- Thrombolytics
- Von Willebrand's disease
- Clotting factor deficiency
  ∘ Factor I deficiency
  ∘ Factor II deficiency
  ∘ Factor V deficiency
  ∘ Factor VIII deficiency (Hemophilia A)
  ∘ Factor IX deficiency (Hemophilia B)
  ∘ Factor X deficiency
  ∘ Factor XI deficiency
  ∘ Factor XII deficiency
- Therapy with unfractionated heparin

- Subcutaneous heparin injection
- Inhibition of factors V, VIII, IX, XI and XII
- Liver disease
- Vitamin K deficiency
- Circulating anticoagulants or specific factor inhibitor
  ○ Penicillin reaction
  ○ Rheumatoid factor
- Disseminated intravascular coagulation (DIC)
- Fibrinolytic states
- Fibrinogen deficiency
- Impaired fibrin polymerization
- Fibrin polymerization inhibitors
  ○ Multiple myeloma
  ○ Collagen vascular disease
  ○ Cirrhosis
- Hypoalbuminemia
- Drugs, toxins
  ○ Penicillin overdose
  ○ Protamine chloride
- Newborns

pCO2, See Blood Gas Analysis → 57

PCV, See Hematocrit → 172

Pelvic Inflammatory Disease

PID

Ascending infection of the female upper genital tract. Serious complication of sexually transmitted diseases (STD).

Etiology

▶ Chlamydia trachomatis
▶ Neisseria gonorrhea
▶ Mycoplasma
▶ Streptococci
▶ Staphylococci
▶ Enterococci
▶ Bacteroides

DDx

▶ Hemorrhagic or ruptured ovarian cyst
▶ Ectopic pregnancy
▶ Appendicitis
▶ Urinary tract infection
▶ Ovarian torsion
▶ Septic abortion
▶ Ovarian tumor
▶ Myoma

Penis ulcer, See Genital Ulcer → 154, See Sexually Transmitted Diseases → 329

Peptic Ulcer Disease

Ulceration in the stomach or duodenum due to imbalance between mucosal protective factors and various mucosal-damaging mechanisms.
Duodenal ulcer: gastric ulcer = 4:1.

Drugs

▶ Alcohol
▶ Cigarette smoking
▶ Glucocorticoids
▶ NSAIDS

Infection

▶ Helicobacter pylori

Acid

▶ Idiopathic
▶ Zollinger-Ellison syndrome

Stress

▶ Severe systemic disease
▶ Surgery
▶ Trauma
▶ Cerebral trauma
▶ Burns
▶ Chronic debilitated conditions

Miscellaneous

▶ Incompetent pylorus or lower gastroesophageal sphincter
▶ Chronic obstructive pulmonary disease
▶ Cystic fibrosis
▶ Alpha-1-antitrypsin deficiency (→ 20)
▶ Systemic mastocytosis
▶ Hyperparathyroidism

O
P

▶ Basophilic leukemia
▶ Chronic renal failure
▶ Cirrhosis

Perceptive deafness. See Hearing Loss, Hearing Impairment → 165

Percussion of the Lungs

Dullness
▶ Infiltration
  • (Lobar) pneumonia
  • Tuberculous infiltrate
  • Lung abscess
  • Pulmonary infarction
  • Pulmonary edema
  • Lung tumor
▶ Atelectasis
  • Congenital
  • Foreign body
  • Bronchiolitis obliterans
  • Tumor
  • Pleural effusion
  • Pericardial effusion
  • Pneumothorax
▶ Pleural effusion
▶ Pleural tumor

Flatness
▶ Large pleural effusion

Resonance
▶ Chronic bronchitis

Hyperresonance
▶ Emphysema
▶ Status asthmaticus
▶ Pneumothorax

Tympany
▶ Large pneumothorax
▶ Lung caverns
▶ Lung cyst
▶ Intestinal loop

Pericardial Effusion

Increased amounts of fluid within the pericardial sac. Greater amounts can lead to a life-threatening tamponade.

Serous
▶ Infection
  • Viral pericarditis
  • Bacterial pericarditis
  • Tuberculous pericarditis
▶ Congestive heart failure
▶ Hypoalbuminemia
▶ Cirrhosis
▶ Acute pancratitis
▶ Nephrotic syndrome
▶ Malnutrition
▶ Chronic disease
▶ Irradiation
▶ Chemotherapeutics
▶ Hypothyroidism
▶ Dressler's syndrom

Blood
▶ Iatrogenic
  • Heart surgery
  • Cardiac catheter
  • Anticoagulants
  • Chemotherapeutics
▶ Trauma
▶ Neoplasm
▶ Acute myocardial infarction
▶ Cardiac rupture
▶ Aortic or pulmonary artery rupture
▶ Perforation
  • Spontaneous
    ○ Dissecting aortic aneurysm
    ○ Ventricle perforation
  • Iatrogenic
    ○ Cardiac catheter
    ○ Pacemaker probes
    ○ Postpericardiotomy syndrome
▶ Uremia
▶ Coagulopathy

Lymph or chylus
▶ Congenital

- Idiopathic
- Neoplasm
- Benign obstruction of thoracic duct
- After cardiothoracic surgery

Metastatic tumor
- Lung
- Breast
- Leukemia
- Lymphoma
- Pericarditis

Miscellaneous
- Systemic lupus erythematosus
- Cardiomyopathy

Pericarditis

Inflammation of the visceral and parietal layers of the pericardium. Macroscopic fibrinous, serous, hemorrhagic and purulent pericarditis are distinguished. The progress can be acute (< 6 weeks), subacute (6 weeks to 6 months) or chronic (> 6 months). A cardiac tamponade can occur as a life-threatening complication. Symptoms include retrosternal pain with radiation into the front chest wall and the shoulder region, fever, pericardial rub, ECG changes (ST-T, low voltage).

Pericarditis, acute
- Infections
  - Viral
    - Coxsackie A
    - Coxsackie B
    - Mumps virus
    - ECHO virus
    - Adeno virus
    - Cytomegalovirus
    - Epstein-Barr virus
    - Varicella virus
    - HIV
    - Influenza virus
  - Bacterial
    - Streptococci
    - Staphylococci
    - Tuberculosis
    - Pneumococci
    - Legionella
    - Meningococci
    - Neisseria gonorrhoe
    - Treponema pallidum
    - Borrelia
    - Francisella
    - Rickettsia
  - Fungal
    - Histoplasmosis
    - Coccidioidomycosis
    - Candida infection
    - Blastomycosis
  - Other infections
    - Echinococcosis
    - Amebiasis
    - Actinomycosis
    - Mycoplasma infection
    - Toxoplasmosis
- Tumors
  - Primary tumors (benign or malignant)
  - Tumors metastatic to pericardium
    - Lung
    - Breast
    - Lymphoma
    - Leukemia
- Metabolic
  - Renal failure
  - Uremia
  - Hypothyroidism
  - Diabetic coma
  - Hypothyroidism
  - Addison´s crisis
  - Cholesterol pericarditis
- Myocardial infarction
  - Early pericarditis
  - Late pericarditis (Dressler's syndrome)
- Collagen vascular diseases, inflammation
  - Postmyocardial infarction (Dressler's syndrome)
  - Postpericardiotomy
  - Acute rheumatic fever
  - Mixed connective tissue disease
  - Scleroderma

O P

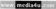

- Wegener's granulomatosis
- Sarcoidosis
- Amyloidosis
- Rheumatoid arthritis
- Systemic lupus erythematosus
- Dermatosclerosis
- Dermatomyositis
- Polyarteritis nodosa
- Polymyositis
- Reiter's syndrome
- Ankylosing spondylitis
- Inflammatory bowel disease
- Whipple's disease
- Behçet's disease
- Infectious mononucleosis
- Familial Mediterranean fever
▶ Allergic
- Serum sickness
- Drugs
  ○ Dantrolen
  ○ Doxorubicin
  ○ Hydralazine
  ○ Isoniazid
  ○ Methysergide
  ○ Penicillin
  ○ Phenylbutazone
  ○ Phenytoin
  ○ Procainamide
▶ Thorax trauma
- Nonpenetrating
- Cardiothoracic surgery
- Cardioversion
- Cardiopulmonary resuscitation
- After sternal puncture
- Invasive cardiologic diagnostic and therapeutic interventions
  ○ Cátheter-or pacemaker induced cardiac perforation
▶ Miscellaneous
- Aortic dissection with hemopericardium
- Perforated esophagus
- Postirradiation
- Associated with atrial septal defect
- Associated with severe chronic anemia

- Chylopericardium
- Acute idiopathic pericarditis

Pericarditis, chronic
▶ Idiopathic
▶ Infections
- Tuberculosis
- Bacterial infections
- Viral
  ○ Coxsackie B3
- Fungal
  ○ Histoplasmosis
  ○ Coccidioidomycosis
- Parasitic diseases
  ○ Echinococcosis
  ○ Amebiasis
▶ Miscellaneous
- Cholesterol pericarditis
- Uremic pericarditis
- Neoplastic pericarditis
- Chylopericardium
- Collagen vascular disease
- After radiation therapy

Perimyocarditis, See Myocarditis → 246, See Pericarditis → 281

Peripheral Arterial Occlusive Disease

Peripheral arterial disease, peripheral vascular disease, arterial insufficiency, (vascular) claudication, Leriche's syndrome.

Causes
▶ Arteriosclerosis
▶ Embolism
- Cardiac sources
  ○ Atrial fibrillation
  ○ Myocardial infarction
  ○ Endocarditis
  ○ Artificial cardiac valve
  ○ Atrial myxoma
- Arterial sources
  ○ Aneurysm

- ○ Arteriosclerosis
- Paradoxical embolus
▶ Thrombosis
- Arteriosclerosis
- Thrombosis of an aneurysm
- Thrombophilia
- Insufficient perfusion
  - ○ Subclavian steal syndrome
  - ○ Long periods of sitting
▶ Trauma
- Penetrating
- Iatrogenic
▶ Hematologic disorders
▶ Connective tissue/vascular diseases
- Takayasu's arteritis
- Raynaud's disease
- Winiwarter-Buerger disease (endangiitis obliterans)
- Progressive systemic sclerosis
- Dermatomyositis
- Systemic lupus erythematosus
- Polyarteritis nodosa
- Rheumatoid arthritis

Risk Factors
▶ Cigarette smoking
▶ Diabetes mellitus
▶ Systolic hypertension
▶ Hypercholesterolemia
▶ Advanced age
▶ Obesity (increased body mass index)

Phosphate

Inorganic phosphorus
85% of phosphate is contained in bones and teeth, 14% in body cells and 1% in the extracellular space. Energy rich phosphates (ATP) supply energy for metabolic reactions.

Reference range
0.95–1.5 mmol/l

Decreased (hypophosphatemia)
▶ Increased renal excretion
- Primary hyperparathyroidism
- Secondary hyperparathyroidism

- Renal tubular defects
- Postrenal transplantation
- ECF volume expansion
- Hyperaldosteronism
- Hypokalemia
- Hypercalcemia
- Hypomagnesemia
- Acidosis (metabolic acidosis)
- Cushing's syndrome
- Drugs
  - ○ Steroid therapy
  - ○ Oral contraceptives
  - ○ Estrogens
  - ○ Diuretics
- Tumor phosphaturia
  - ○ Mesenchymoma
  - ○ Neurofibroma
▶ Decreased intake/absorption, increased nonrenal loss
- Vomitting
- Diarrhea
- Malabsorption
- Cachexia, starvation
- Chronic administration of antacids, phosphate binders
- Hemodialysis
- Inadequate dietary ingestion of phoshorus
▶ Transcellular shift
- Severe respiratory alkalosis
- Metabolic alkalosis
- Catecholamines, androgens
- Hyperthyroidism
- Infusions
  - ○ Glucose
  - ○ Glucagon
  - ○ Bicarbonate
  - ○ Lactate
- Salicylate intoxication
- Sepsis
- Acute gout
- Heat stroke
- Pregnancy
- Myocardial infarction
▶ Vitamin D metabolism disorders

- Vitamin D deficient rickets
- Familial hypophosphatemic rickets
- Vitamin D dependent rickets
- Tumor associated hypophosphatemia
▶ Other mechanisms
- Alcoholism, alcohol withdrawal
- Diabetes mellitus, ketoacidosis
- Hyperinsulinism
- Hepatic disease, hepatic coma
- Hyperalimentation
- Severe burns
- Toxic shock syndrome
- Sepsis

Increased (hyperphosphatemia)
▶ Decreased excretion/increased load
- Increased levels in children and adolescents are physiologic due to elevated bone metabolism
- Acute and chronic renal failure
- Acidosis (lactic acidosis, diabetic ketoacidosis)
- Phosphate administration
  ○ Phosphate
  ○ Phosphate-containing laxatives
  ○ Enemas
- Transfusion of stored blood
- Hemolysis, resolving hematoma
- Rhabdomyolysis
- Tumor lysis syndrome
- Osteolytic metastases
- Vitamin D overdose
- Malignant hyperpyrexia
- Phosphorus burns
▶ Increased renal tubular reabsorption
- Hypoparathyroidism
- Pseudohypoparathyroidism
- Hyperthyroidism
- Volume contraction
- High atmospheric temperature
- Postmenopausal state
- Biphosphonate therapy
- Acromegaly
- Juvenile hypogonadism
- Tumoral calcinosis

Photosensitivity
Abnormal sensitivity to light
Dermatologic
▶ Solar urticaria
▶ Photoallergic reaction
▶ Phototoxic reactin
▶ Polymorphous light eruption
▶ Porphyria cutanea tarda
▶ SLE

Drug-induced
▶ ACE inhibitors
▶ Amiodarone
▶ Antihistamines
▶ Antipsychotics
▶ Benzodiazepines
▶ Calcium channel blockers
▶ Chemotherapeutics
▶ Chloroquine
▶ Chlorpromazine
▶ Dermatologic, topical agents
- Acne vulgaris agents
- Alopecia agents
- Oils, fragrances in perfumes, cosmetics, aftershaves, lipsticks
- Pigments, dyes
- Soap deodorants
- Sunscreen additives
▶ Diuretics
▶ Furosemide
▶ Griseofulvin
▶ Lovastatin
▶ Methyldopa
▶ NSAIDs
▶ Oral hypoglycemics
▶ Quinolones
▶ Phenothiazine
▶ Piroxicam
▶ Quinolones
▶ Sulfonamides
▶ Tegretol
▶ Tetracyclines
▶ Thiazides
▶ Tricyclic antidepressants

Plants (contact)
▶ Agrimony
▶ Ammi majus
▶ Angelica
▶ Bergamot
▶ Buttercup
▶ Carrot
▶ Celery
▶ Citron
▶ Coriander
▶ Dill
▶ Fennel
▶ Fig
▶ Furocoumarins
▶ Goosefoot
▶ Lemon
▶ Lime
▶ Milfoil
▶ Mustard
▶ Parsley
▶ Parsnip
▶ Psoralens
▶ Scurfy-pea
▶ St. John's wort
▶ Yarrow

Phrenic nerve paresis
See Diaphragmatic Dysfunction → 100

PID
See Pelvic Inflammatory Disease → 279

Pituitary Insufficiency
Hypopituitarism
Diminished activity of the anterior lobe of the hypophysis, with inadequate secretion of one or more anterior pituitary hormones due to destruction, displacement, necrosis, surgery, or disconnection from the hypothalamic centers. In anterior pituitary lobe

insufficiency caused by an adenoma, the hormones often fail in the following order: GH, FSH/LH, TSH and finally ACTH.

Causes
▶ Pituitary adenomas
▶ Parasellar tumor/pituitary compression
  • Craniopharyngioma (!)
  • Chromophobe adenoma
  • Meningioma
  • Optic nerve neurinoma
  • Metastases
  • Lymphomas
  • Intracranial carotid branch aneurysm
▶ Ischemic necrosis of the pituitary
  • Sheehan's syndrome (after large postpartum bleeding)
  • Brain trauma
  • Anticoagulant therapy
  • Blood dyscrasias
  • Increased intracranial pressure (→ 213)
  • Tumor
  • Diabetes mellitus
  • Arteritis temporalis
  • Sickle cell anemia
  • Arteriosclerosis
  • Eclampsia
  • Cavernous sinus thrombosis
▶ Head trauma (direct damage)
▶ Empty sella syndrome
▶ Iatrogenic
  • Irradiation of the nasopharynx
  • Irradiation of the sella
  • Surgery
▶ Infiltrative diseases
  • Wegener's granulomatosis
  • Sarcoidosis
▶ Infection
  • Meningitis
  • Tuberculosis
  • Syphilis
  • Malaria
  • Fungal
▶ Drugs
  • Glucocorticoids

O
P

- Anticoagulant therapy
- Sex hormones
▶ Miscellaneous
  - Emotional disorders
  - Changes in body weight
  - Anorexia
  - Bulimia
  - Habitual exercise
  - Autoimmune hypophysitis
  - Hemochromatosis
  - Congestive heart failure (CHF)
  - Renal failure
▶ Idiopathic

Plasma proteins
See Protein in the Serum → 296

Plasminogen

Precursoer of plasmin, that converts fibrin to soluble products. Determine in hyperfibrinolysis, DIC, thrombophilia screening or for monitoring fibrinolytic therapy.

Reference range	
Plasminogen concentration	2.5 mmol/l
Plasminogen activity	70–120%

Plasminogen deficiency
▶ Hereditary
▶ Acquired
  - Physiologic in newborns
  - Fibrinolytic therapy
  - Hyperfibrinolysis
  - Disseminated intravascular coagulation (DIC)
  - Severe liver damages

Increased
▶ Diabetes mellitus
▶ Pregnancy
▶ Oral contraceptives
▶ Paraneoplastic
▶ Acute-phase-reaction

Pleural Effusion

Increased amount of fluid within the pleural cavity.

	Transudate	Exudate
Total protein	< 3 g/l	> 3 g/l
Total protein pleura/ serum protein	< 0.5	> 0.5
Leukocyte count	< 1000/ mm^3	>1000 /mm^3
LDH	< 200 U/l	> 200 U/l
LDH quotient pleura/ serum	< 0.6	> 0.6
Cholesterol	< 55 mg	> 55 mg

Bilateral effusions are usually transudates.

Proof:	
Clinical:	> 200–400 ml (dull note over the effusion)
Radiologic:	> 250 fluid ml
Ultrasound :	> 50 fluid ml

Transudate
Fluid within the pleural cavity, low in protein.
▶ Cardiovascular, pulmonary
  - Congestive heart failure
  - Constrictive pericarditis
  - Vena cava obstruction
  - Pulmonary embolism
  - Pulmonary atelectasis
  - Pneumonia
▶ Hypoalbuminemia (→ 16)
  - Cirrhosis
  - Nephrotic syndrome
  - Malnutrition
  - Malabsorption
  - Exudative enteropathy
  - Chronic inflammation
  - Amyloidosis
▶ Miscellaneous
  - Peritoneal dialysis
  - Hypothyroidism
  - Postpartal

Exudate
Fluid within the pleural cavity, high in protein and white blood cells.
▶ Pulmonary embolism
▶ Infection, inflammation
  • Parapneumonic
    ○ Bacterial
    ○ Viral
    ○ Fungal
  • Tuberculosis
  • Actinomycosis
  • Echinococcosis
  • Pleural empyema
  • Lung abscess
  • Subphrenic
    ○ Pancreatitis
    ○ Cholecystitis
    ○ Liver abscess
    ○ Splenic infarction
    ○ Intraabdominal abscess
▶ Malignancy
  • Pleural mesothelioma
  • Pleural metastases
    ○ Bronchial carcinoma
    ○ Breast carcinoma
    ○ Lymphomas
  • Mediastinal tumor
  • Lymphoma
  • Chronic leukemias
▶ Collagen-vascular disease
  • Rheumatoid arthritis
  • Polyarteritis nodosa
  • Lupus erythematosus
  • Wegener's granulomatosis
  • Sjögren's syndrome
▶ Drugs
  • Bromocriptine
  • Dantrolene
  • Hydralazine
  • Isoniazid
  • Methotrexate
  • Methysergide
  • Nitrofurantoin
  • Procainamide
  • Procarbazine
  • Quinidine
▶ Miscellaneous
  • Asbestosis
  • Sarcoidosis
  • Trauma
  • Dressler's syndrome
  • Post-myocardial infarction
  • Post-cardiotomy
  • Radiation pleuritis
  • Gastrointestinal disease
  • Esophageal perforation
  • Uremia
  • Hypothyroidism
  • Yellow nail syndrome

Pyothorax
Empyema (pus collection) in pleural cavity with bronchopleural fistula.
▶ Infection
  • Pneumonia (!)
  • Lung abscess
  • Subphrenic abscess
  • Tuberculosis
  • Fungal infection
▶ Chest trauma (penetrating wounds)
▶ Spontaneous pneumothorax

Hematothorax
Hemorrhagic effusion, bloody effusion ($>100,000$ cells/mm^2)
▶ Trauma
▶ Pulmonary infarction
▶ Malignancy
  • Pleural mesothelioma
  • Pleural carcinomatosis
  • Malignant lung tumor
  • Leukemia
▶ Infection
  • Tuberculosis
  • Anthrax
▶ Hemorrhagic diathesis

Chylothorax
Presence of lymphatic fluid within the pleural cavity.

O
P

Pneumothorax

Free air in the chest outside the lung with loss of the usually negative intrapleural pressure. Leading to partial or complete collapse of the affected lung.

Causes
▶ Primary spontanous pneumothorax
▶ Traumatic
  • Penetrating trauma
  • Barotrauma
  • Sudden chest compression
  • Blunt abdominal tauma
  • Drug abuse (attempted injection in subclavian/internal jugular vein)
▶ Iatrogenic
▶ Mediastinal emphysema
▶ Lung emphysema
▶ Rupture of cysts/bullae (often congenital)
▶ Honeycomb lung (pulmonary microcysts)
  • Idiopathic
  • Cystic fibrosis
  • Pneumoconiosis
  • Pulmonary tuberous sclerosis
  • Dermatosclerosis
  • Pulmonary lymphangiomatoid granulomatosis
  • Eosinophilic granuloma
  • Marfan's syndrome
▶ Infection
  • Tuberculosis
  • Coccidioidomycosis
  • Bacterial pneumonia with abscess
  • Pneumocystis carinii pneumonia
▶ Miscellaneous
  • Bronchial asthma
  • Sarcoidosis
  • Rheumatoid lung disease
  • Pulmonary infarction with cavitation
  • Pulmonary hemosiderosis
  • Ehlers-Danlos syndrome
  • Pseudoxanthoma elasticum
  • Central bronchial carcinomas
  • Paragonimiasis
  • Hydatid lung disease

Poikilocytosis
See Erythrocyte, Morphology → 132

Pollakisuria
Frequent urge to urinate
Disorders of the bladder
▶ Infection
  • Cystitis
  • Urethritis
  • Prostatitis
▶ Obstruction of the urethra
  • Vesical calculus
  • Prostate hyperplasia
  • Prostate carcinoma
▶ Irritable bladder (psychogenic)
Miscellaneous
▶ Heart failure
▶ Diabetes insipidus
▶ Diabetes mellitus
▶ Hyperhydration (water retention) of various origin
▶ Multiple sclerosis
▶ Endometriosis
▶ Pregnancy
▶ Descensus uteri

Polycythemia
Hyperglobulia, erythrocythemia
Increase above the normal in the number of red cells in the blood.
Pseudopolycythemia
▶ Reduced plasma volume
  • Dehydration
  • Burns
Primary
▶ Polycythemia vera
Secondary
▶ Tissue hypoxia

- Decreased arterial PO_2
  - High altitude exposure
  - Cyanotic congenital heart disease
  - Chronic pulmonary disease
  - Hypoventilation
- Normal arterial PO_2
  - Chronic CO poisoning (smoking)
  - Hemoglobinopathies
  - Cobalt ingestion
▶ Endocrine
  - Cushing´s syndrome
  - Androgen therapy
  - Pheochromocytoma
  - Primary hyperaldosteronism
  - Hyperthyroidism
▶ Renal disorders
  - Renal cysts
  - Renal cell carcinoma
  - Hydronephrosis
▶ Toxins
  - Arsenic
  - Benzol
  - Cobalt
  - Copper
  - Lead
▶ Miscellaneous
  - Liver tumors
  - Lung tumors
  - Uterine leiomyoma
  - Cerebellar hemangioblastoma
  - Acute leukoses
  - Familial erythrocytosis
  - Pregnancy

Polydipsia

Excessive thirst and increased fluid intake of at least 4–5 L/d.

Moderate acute polydipsia (4–5 L/d)
▶ Alcohol (inhibition of ADH secretion)
▶ Diuretics
▶ Osmotic drugs
▶ Extrarenal water loss

Moderate chronic polydipsia (4–5 L/d)
▶ Diabetes mellitus

▶ Conn's syndrome
▶ Chronic renal failure
▶ Hypercalcemia

Excessive persistent polydipsia (6–20 L/d)
▶ Central diabetes insipidus (→ 99)
▶ Nephrogenic diabetes insipidus (→ 99)
▶ Psychogenic polydipsia (→ 289)

Polymenorrhea

Abnormally frequent menstruation of normal quantity and duration with a cycle interval of less than 25 days.

Causes
▶ Bi-phasic cycle
  - With shortened follicle ripening phase
  - With shortened corpus-luteum phase
▶ Anovulatory cycle
▶ Hyperthyroidism

Polyneuropathy, See Paresthesias → 276, See Neuropathy, Peripheral → 258

Polyuria

Urine output > 3 L/d.
Diabetes insipidus
▶ Central diabetes insipidus (→ 99)
▶ Nephrogenic diabetes insipidus (→ 99)
Renal disease
▶ Diuretic phase of acute renal failure
▶ Chronic renal insufficiency
▶ Postobstrctie diuresis
▶ Hypercalcemic nephropathy
▶ Hypokalemic nephropathy
▶ Decreased protein intake
▶ Amyloidosis
▶ Sarcoidosis
▶ Multiple myeloma
Excessive fluid intake
▶ Primary polydipsia
  See Diabetes Insipidus → 99
▶ Iatrogenic (intravenous fluids)

O
P

Osmotic diuresis
▶ Diabetes mellitus, hyperglycemia
▶ Chronic renal failure
▶ After acute renal failure
▶ Mannitol administration
▶ Iodinated contrast dye

Drugs
▶ Alcohol
▶ Clonidine
▶ Diuretics
▶ Gentamicin
▶ Lithium
▶ Methcillin
▶ Phenothiazine
▶ Phenytoine
▶ Radiocontrast
▶ Sulfonylureas
▶ Vinblastine

Popliteal swelling
See Leg Swelling → 220

Porphyrins, Porphobilinogen in the Urine, Porphyria

Porphyrins are of a group of pigments that arise from porphin. Porphyrin protein connections are the basis of hemoglobin, myoglobin and the cytochromes. The biosynthesis of the porphyrins takes place in the bone marrow; catabolism of bile pigments mostly in the liver, bone marrow and spleen. Porphobilinogen (PBG) is a precursor in the biosynthesis of the porphyrins. The determination of porphyrins/PBG in the urine is used for the recognition of hemebiosynthesis impairment. Porphyrias are a group of disorders caused by defects in the synthesis of heme. Porphyrias are divided into acute (abdominal pain,

neuropsychiatric symptoms) and non-acute (photosensitivity) ones.
See δ-Aminolevulinic Acid → 93

Reference range	
Total-porphyrins	< 150 ug/24 h
PBG	< 2 mg/24 h

Common precipitants of porphyrias
▶ Drug ingestion
▶ Alcohol consumption
▶ Endogenous corticosteroids
▶ Exogenous corticosteroids

Increased porphyrins
▶ Hereditary porphyria
  • Erythropoietic porphyria
  • Acute hepatic porphyria
  • Chronic hepatic porphyria
▶ Lead poisoning
▶ Secondary (asymptomatic) porphyria
  • Liver damage
    ○ Fatty liver
    ○ Hepatitis
    ○ Cirrhosis
    ○ Cholestasis
  • Bilirubin transport impairment
    ○ Morbus Meulengracht
    ○ Dubin-Johnson syndrome
    ○ Rotor's syndrome
  • Hematologic
    ○ Anemia
    ○ Leukemias
    ○ Hemoblastosis
    ○ Hemochromatosis
    ○ Hemosiderosis
  • Drugs, toxins
    ○ Alcohol
    ○ Antibiotics
    ○ Chlorated aromatics
    ○ Chlorated biphenyls
    ○ Chloroethylene
    ○ Estrogens
    ○ Heavy metals
    ○ Hexachlorobenzene
    ○ Sedatives
    ○ Sulfonyl ureas

- Infectious diseases
- Neoplasia
- Pregnancy
- Starvation

Protoporphyrin
▶ Increased
- Iron deficiency anemia
- Lead poisoning
- Sideroblastic anemia
- Chronic disease
- Hemolytic anemia
- Erythropoietic protoporphyria

Portal Hypertension

High blood pressure in the portal system, causing obstruction to the portal vein. Most commonly caused by an intrahepatic block due to cirrhosis.

Prehepatic
▶ Portal vein occlusion
- Thrombosis
- Tumor
▶ Splenic vein thrombosis
- Pancreatitis
- Pancreas carcinoma
▶ Congenital abnormalities
▶ Idiopathic tropical splenomegaly
▶ Umbilical sepsis

Intrahepatic
▶ Cirrhosis (→ 78)
▶ Alcoholic hepatitis
▶ Chronic hepatitis
▶ Fatty liver
▶ Fulminant hepatic failure
▶ Hodgkin's lymphoma
▶ Boeck's disease
▶ Wilson's disease
▶ Osteomyelosclerosis
▶ Schistosomiasis
▶ Partial nodular transformation

Posthepatic
▶ Congestive heart failure
▶ Tricuspid insufficiency
▶ Constrictive pericarditis

▶ Inferior vena cava obstruction
▶ Hepatic vein obstruction (Budd-Chiari syndrome)
- Thrombosis
- Endophlebitis obliterans
- Tumor
▶ Cardiomyopathy

Postpartum Hemorrhage

Bleeding from the birth canal > 500 mL after vaginal delivery or > 1000 mL after cesarean delivery.

Types
▶ Primary postpartum hemorrhage during the first 24 hours.
▶ Secondary postpartum hemorrhage after 24 hours.

Causes (Mnemonic 4T's)
▶ Uterine Atony (**tone** diminished)
- Excessive uterine distension
  - Polyhydramnios
  - Multiple gestation
  - Fetal macrosomia
- Multiparity
- Rapid or prolonged labor
- Chorioamnionitis
- Placenta previa
- Abruptio placentae
- Drugs
  - Oxytocin
  - General anesthesia
▶ **Tissue**
- Retained placenta
- Placenta accreta
▶ **Trauma**
- Uterine inversion
- Uterine rupture
- Cervical laceration
- Vaginal hematoma
▶ **Thrombin**
- Disorders of coagulation
- Thrombocytopenia

Postpartum Infection

Postpartum fever

Causes

▶ Endometritis
▶ Postsurgical wound infection
▶ Perineal cellulitis
▶ Mastitis
▶ Respiratory complication (anesthesia)
▶ Retained products of conception
▶ Urinary tract infection (UTI)
▶ Septic pelvic phlebitis

Potassium, See Hyperkalemia → 192,
See Hypokalemia → 202

Potency impairment
See Impotence → 208

PP, See Pancreatic Polypeptide (PP) → 270

Precocious Puberty

Pubertas praecox

Condition in which pubertal changes begin at an unexpectedly early age. In 99% puberty begins between ages of 8 and 14 with girls, and between the ages of 9 and 14.5 with boys. In early sexual development signs of puberty clearly occur before the 8th year in girls and before the 9th year in boys.
True precocious puberty: early adrenarche, with a central cause, gonadotropin dependent. Pseudoprecocious puberty is early puberty without the normal pattern of puberty, e.g. isolated premature pubarche (beginning of pubic hair growth) or isolated premature adrenarche (growth of female glandular tissue).

Causes

▶ Genuine or idiopathic pubertas praecox (True PP is idiopathic in 90% of female cases, and in 50 to 60% of male cases)
▶ Pubertas praecox in
 • Brain tumors (pituitary/hypothalamus)
 • Trauma
 • Radiation
 • Inflammations
 • Recurrent seizure
 • After meningitis
 • Internal hydrocephalus
 • McCune Allbright syndrome
▶ Pseudopubertas praecox
 • Exogenic sexual steroids
 • Endogenous sexual steroids in
  ○ Adrenogenital syndrome
  ○ Hormone producing tumors
   - Ovarian tumors
   - Testicular tumors
   - Adrenal cortex tumors
   - Chorionepithelioma
   - Benign cyst of the ovary
   - Benign cyst of the testicles
 • Albright's syndrome
▶ Pellizzi's syndrome
▶ HCG production
 ○ Hepatomas
 ○ Hepatoblastomas
 ○ Chorion carcinoma

Priapism

Persistent erection of the penis with pain and tenderness.

Drugs

▶ Alprostadil
▶ Antibiotics
▶ Anticoagulants
▶ Antihypertensives
▶ Psychopharmaceutics
▶ Sildenafil

Hematologic

▶ Leukemia
▶ Sickle cell anemia
▶ Pelvic venous thrombosis
▶ Hemodialysis
▶ Local thrombosis

▶ Local hemorrhage

Neurologic
▶ Multiple sclerosis
▶ Cerebral lesion
▶ Spinal cord lesion
▶ Nervi erigentes
▶ Tabes dorsalis

Inflammation
▶ Urethritis
▶ Prostatitis

Local injury
▶ Thrombosis
▶ Hemorrhage
▶ Neoplasm
  • Tumor infiltration
▶ Contusion
▶ Rupture
▶ Urethral lesion
▶ Urethral foreign body

Idiopathic

Progesterone

Progesterone is formed almost exclusively in the corpus luteum. Highest serum levels in the mid-luteal phase (5–8 days after ovulation).

Reference range	
Follicular phase	< 1.4 ng/ml
Luteal phase	5–30 ng/ml
Postmenopausal	< 0.9 ng/ml

Decreased
▶ Ovulation impairment
  • Anovulatory cycle
  • Corpus luteum deficiency syndrome
  • Hyperprolactinemia

Increased
▶ Ovarian tumors
▶ Hydatidiform mole
▶ Adrenal cortex tumors

Prolactin

Glycoprotein that is formed in the anterior lobe of the pituitary. Stimulates the lactogenesis as well as galactopoiesis in humans and maintains postpartal anovulation through sucking-stimulus of the infant. In the last trimester of pregnancy, values can be as high as 300 ng/ml. Prolactin secretion increases through sucking during breast-feeding and through manipulation of the mamilla (Caution: falsely high prolactin values). L-dopa leads to a central inhibition of prolactin secretion. Prolactin values > 200 µg/l are almost always proof of a prolactinoma.

Reference range	
Women	< 15.6 ng/ml (500 µU/ml)
Men	< 12.5 ng/ml (400 µU/ml)

Increased (Hyperprolactinemia)
▶ Physiologic
  • Pregnancy
  • Postpartum
    ○ Nonnursing (four weeks)
    ○ Suckling
  • Stress
  • Exercise
  • Sleep
  • Intercourse, nipple stimulation
  • Food ingestion
▶ Prolactin secreting pituitary tumor
  • Macroprolactinoma (general enlargement of the sella)
  • Microprolactinoma (discrete change of the sella)
▶ Drugs
  • Androgens
  • Antidepressants
  • Antihistaminics
  • Antihypertensives
  • Benzodiazepines
  • Butyrophenones
  • Calcium channel blockers

O
P

- Cimetidine
- Domperidone
- Dopamine antagonists
- Estrogens (in high dosage: therapy of prostate carcinoma)
- Haloperidol
- Hormones
- Imipramine
- Methyldopa
- Metoclopramid
- Neuroleptics
- Opiates
- Phenothiazines
- Reserpine
- Sulpiride
- Thioxanthenes
- TRH
- Vasoactive intestinal peptide
▶ Pituitary stalk damage (impairment of the prolactin inhibiting-hormone-transport to the pituitary)
- Inflammatory, infiltrative, granulomatous diseases
  ○ Sarcoidosis
  ○ Histiocytosis
  ○ Herpes zoster encephalitis
- Trauma, operation
  ○ Stalk section, severance
- Suprasellar tumors (infundibular stalk compression)
  ○ Parasellar tumors
  ○ Tumors in the area of the hypothalamus
  ○ Dermoid cyst
  ○ Lymphomas
  ○ Craniophanyngioma
  ○ Metastatic carcinoma
- Vascular abnormalities
  ○ Aneurysm
▶ Neural stimulation
- Disorders of chest wall and thorax
  ○ Chest wall trauma/surgery
- Major surgery and anesthesia
- Nipple stimulation
- Spine lesion

- Seizures
- Miscellaneous
  - Hypothyroidism with consecutive hypothalamic stimulation
  - Acromegaly
  - Cushing's syndrome
  - Polycystic ovary syndrome
  - MEN type I
  - Chronic renal failure
  - Cirrhosis
  - Hypophysitis
  - Hyperprolactinemia after pituitary interventions
  - Hyperprolactinemia after pituitary radiation
  - Empty sella
  - Idiopathic hyperprolactinemia

Decreased
▶ Pituitary insufficiency (→ 285)
▶ Overdosage of dopamine agonists

Proptosis

Exophthalmos

Protrusion of one or both eyeballs.

Endocrine
▶ Hyperthyroidism
▶ Graves' disease
▶ Hashimoto thyroiditis

Infection
▶ Orbital cellulitis
▶ Mucormycosis
▶ Concurrent sinus disease

Inflammation
▶ Orbital inflammatory syndrome
- Orbital pseudotumor
- Benign orbital inflammation
▶ Myositis of the eye muscles
▶ Myositis of the extraocular eye muscles
▶ Scleritis

Vasculitis
▶ Wegener granulomatosis
▶ Churg-Strauss syndrome

O
P

Orbital vascular disorder
▶ Orbital varix
▶ Carotid–cavernous sinus fistula
▶ Other arteriovenous malformation
▶ Cavernous sinus thrombosis
▶ Aneurysm
▶ Hereditary angioedema

Tumor
▶ Lacrimal tumor
▶ Lymphoma
▶ Leukemia
▶ Meningioma
▶ Glioma
▶ Metastases
  • Breast cancer
  • Lung cancer
  • Prostate cancer
  • Gastrointestinal neoplasm
  • Renal cancer

Trauma
▶ Orbital hemorrhage
  • Traumatic
  • Iatrogenic
▶ Orbital fractures
▶ Facial fractures

Pseudoproptosis (pseudoexophthalmos)
▶ Buphthalmos
▶ Contralateral enophthalmos
▶ Ipsilateral lid retraction
▶ Axial myopia
▶ Contralateral blepharoptosis

Miscellaneous
▶ High-grade myopia
▶ Down syndrome
▶ Dysostosis craniofacialis

Drugs
▶ Thiourazil

Prostate Specific Antigen
PSA
Protein produced by the prostate gland.
PSA in blood is normally minute. Used as
tumor marker for prostate carcinoma.

Reference range	
Total–PSA	< 4.0 µg/l

Increased
▶ Prostate cancer
▶ Benign prostatic hyperplasia (BPH)
▶ Prostatitis
▶ Prostate inflammation
▶ Prostate trauma
▶ Prostate manipulation
▶ Prostatic infarction
▶ Recent sexual activity
▶ Urologic procedures
  • Cystoscopy
  • Palpation of the prostate gland
  • Urinary catheterization

Decreased
▶ Treatment with finasteride

Protein C
Vitamin K dependent inhibitor of the
blood clotting factors V and VIII, that is
synthesized in the liver.
Determination within the course of
screening for thrombophilia, in severe liver
diseases, DIC.

Reference range	
Protein C concentration	0.61–1.32 U/ml
Protein C activity	58–148%

Decreased (protein C deficiency)
▶ Inherited
  • Heterozygous (autosomal dominant)
  • Severe deficiency (autosomal recessive)
▶ Acquired
  • Meningococcal septic shock
  • DIC
  • Liver disease

- Acute inflammation
- Acute thrombosis
- Ill preterm infants
- Drugs
  ◦ Chemotherapeutics
  ◦ L-asparaginase
  ◦ Warfarin

Protein in the Serum

Plasma proteins, serum protein electrophoresis

Proteins in the blood plasma and the interstitial fluid (this group does not include enzymes, hormones, blood clotting factors, and tumor markers). Serum protein level is dependent on protein supply, endogenous protein production and protein loss. Individual fractions can be distinguished in the **serum protein electrophoresis**: Prealbumin, albumin; α1-globulin: lipoprotein (HDL), glycoprotein, antitrypsin; α2-globulin: macroglobulin, haptoglobin, pre-β-lipoprotein; β-globulin: transferrin, β-lipoprotein, complement; γ-globulin: IgA, IgM, IgG.

Increased

▶ Total protein (reference range 60–80 g/l)
- Paraproteinemia → 275
  ◦ Waldenström's macroglobulinemia
  ◦ Multiple myeloma
- Collagen vascular disease
- Sarcoidosis
- Dehydration
- Chronic inflammatory diseases
- Chronic active hepatitis
- Cirrhosis

▶ Prealbumin (reference range 300–350 mg/l)
- Pregnancy

▶ Albumin (reference range 34–46 g/l)
(See Albumin → 16)
- Pregnancy
- Dehydration
- Heart failure

- Hyperbilirubinemia

▶ α1-globulin (reference range 1–5%)
- Acute inflammation
- Tumor
- Nephrotic syndrome
- Inflammation
- Necrotic processes
- Hepatopathy

▶ α2-globulin (reference range 7–13%)
- Acute inflammation
- Haptoglobin (reference range 0.3–1.9 g/l, → 161)
  ◦ Inflammation
  ◦ Myocardial infarction
  ◦ Posthepatic jaundice
  ◦ Tumor
- Ceruloplasmin (→ 72)
- α2-macroglobulin (reference range 2.4–2.9 g/l)
  ◦ Kidney diseases
  ◦ Diabetes
  ◦ Porphyria cutanea tarda

▶ β-globulin (reference range 8–15%)
- β-lipoprotein (reference range of 2–5 g/l)
  ◦ Paraproteinemia
  ◦ Hyperlipidemia
  ◦ Nephrotic syndrome
  ◦ Hypothyroidism
- Transferrin (reference range 2.5–4 g/l) (→ 358)
  ◦ Iron deficiency
  ◦ Oral contraceptives

▶ γ-globulin (reference range 11–22%), gammopathy
- Inflammation, infection, collagenosis
  ◦ Exudative enteropathy
  ◦ HIV infection
  ◦ Dermatomyositis
  ◦ Polyarteritis nodosa
  ◦ Boeck's disease
  ◦ Leishmaniasis
  ◦ Bilharziosis
  ◦ Malaria
- Liver diseases

○ Cirrhosis
○ Chronic hepatitis
• Paraproteinemia
  ○ Multiple myeloma
  ○ Waldenström's syndrome
  ○ Hodgkin's lymphoma
  ○ Lymphatic leukemia
• Reticulosarcoma
• Tumor
• Gaucher's disease
• Cryoglobulinemia
• Mixed connective tissue disease

Decreased
▶ Total protein (reference range of 60–80 g/l)
• Nephrotic syndrome (→ 256)
• Malnutrition
  ○ Starvation
  ○ Anorexia
  ○ GI-tumor
• Maldigestion, malabsorption (→ 233)
  ○ Nontropical sprue
  ○ Celiac sprue
  ○ Disaccharidase deficiency
  ○ Cystic fibrosis
  ○ IgA deficiency
• Protein-loosing enteropathy (→ 126)
• Postoperative
• Hepatopathy
• Hemolytic anemia
• Burns
• Bullous dermatosis
• Chronic inflammation
• Ascites
• Pleural exudate
• Chronic hemodialysis
• Hyperthyroidism
• Overhydration
• Antibody deficiency syndrome
• Analbuminemia
• Pseudohypoproteinemia
  ○ Massive bleeding
  ○ Pregnancy
  ○ Polydipsia
  ○ Infusion therapy

▶ Prealbumin (reference range of 300–350 mg/l)
• Hepatopathy
• Paraproteinemia
• Agammaglobulinemia
▶ Albumin (reference range of 34–46 g/l) (See Albumin → 16)
• Chronic inflammation
• Tumor
• Analbuminemia
• Blood loss
• Burns
• Malnutrition
• Protein loss
• Hepatopathy
• Nephrosis
▶ α1-globulin (reference range 1–5%)
• α_1–antitrypsin deficiency
• Oral contraceptives
• Analphalipoproteinemia
• Hepatopathy
• Protein deficiency
▶ α2-globulin (reference range 7–13%)
• Haptoglobin (reference range 0.3–1.9 g/l, → 161)
  ○ Hepatopathy
  ○ Polycythemia
  ○ Hemolysis
  ○ Ahaptoglobinemia
• Ceruloplasmin (→ 72)
• α2-macroglobulin (reference range 2.4–2.9 g/l)
  ○ Chronic hepatopathy
▶ β-globulin (reference range 8–15%)
• β-lipoprotein (reference range of 2–5 g/l)
  ○ Diabetic coma
  ○ Hepatopathy
  ○ Abetalipoproteinemia
• Transferrin (reference range 2.5–4 g/l)
  ○ Hepatopathy
  ○ Renal disease
  ○ Atransferrinemia
  ○ Neoplastic
  ○ Inflammation

O
P

► γ-globulin (reference range 11–22%)
- Protein deficiency
- Thyrotoxicosis
- Diabetes mellitus
- Cushing's syndrome
- Agammaglobulinemia
- Secondary antibody deficiency syndrome
- Malignant lymphomas
- Nephrotic syndrome
- Uremia
- Nephritis
- Radiation therapy
- Liver diseases
  ○ Hepatitis
  ○ Cirrhosis
  ○ Cholestatic liver diseases
  ○ Liver metastases
- Porphyria cutanea tarda
- Pancreatitis
- Myocardial infarction
- Viral infections
  ○ HIV
  ○ Infectious mononucleosis
- Pneumonia
- Drugs
  ○ Antibiotics
  ○ Antidiabetics
  ○ Antiepileptics
  ○ Halothan
  ○ Thyroid depressants/antithyroid drugs
  ○ Tuberculostatics

Protein S

Vitamin K-dependent antithrombotic protein, functioning as a cofactor of activated protein C.

Decreased (protein S deficiency)
► Genetic defects (hereditary)
► Acquired
- Liver disease
- Vitamin K deficiency
- Antagonism with oral anticoagulants

- Pregnancy
- Sickle cell anemia

Proteinuria

Albuminuria

Presence of urinary protein.
A pathologic albuminuria is an essential hint in the diagnosis of parenchymal inflammatory kidney diseases..

Reference range	
Physiologic protein elimination	< 150 mg protein/24 h
Proteinuria	> 150 mg protein/24 h
Microalbuminuria	< 30 mg albumin/ 24 h

Glomerular proteinuria

Non-selective high molecular weight proteinuria in great amounts: total protein excretion > 3 g/24 h. Albumins and IgG and others (exception: Bence Jones proteinuria)
► Glomerulonephritis
- Minimal change GN
- Membranous GN
- Focal segmental GN
- Membranoproliferative GN
- Mesangioproliferative GN
- Fibrillary glomerulopathy
- Crescentic GN
► Collagen vascular disease, systemic
- Systemic lupus erythematosus
- Sarcoidosis
- Polyarteritis nodosa
- Wegner's granulomatosis
- Henoch-Schönlein purpura
- Other vasculitis
- Mixed cryoglobulinemia
- Kidney amyloidosis
- Grave's disease
- Sickle cell disease
► Neoplastic
- Multiple myeloma
- Lymphomas
- Solid tumors
► Infections

- Hepatitis B and C
- Bacterial
  - Infectious endocarditis
- Toxoplasmosis
- CMV
- EBV
- HIV
- Syphillis
- Malaria
- Helminthic
- Leprosy
- Poststreptococcal glomerulonephritis
▶ Drugs, toxins
- Anticonvulsants
- Captopril
- Gold
- Heavy metals
- Heroin
- NSAIDs
- Penicillamine
▶ Hereditary
- Alport's syndrome
- Sickle cell anemia
- Fabry's disease
- Congenital nephrotic syndrome
- Orthostatic proteinuria
▶ Allergens
▶ Miscellaneous
- Preeclampsia
- Hypothyroidism
- Renal vein thrombosis
- Wegener's granulomatosis
- Nephritis of pregnancy
- Nephrotic syndrome
- Diabetes mellitus

Tubular proteinuria
Mainly LMW proteins occurring
physiologically in the plasma: Total
proteinuria < 2g/24h; Main proteins are
α1 and α2-micro globulins.
- Connatal tubulopathies
▶ Renal tubular acidosis
▶ Hypokalemic nephropathy
▶ Interstitial nephropathy
- Acute renal failure

▶ Toxic nephropathy
- Cadmium

Prerenal and overflow proteinuria
▶ Bence-Jones proteinuria
▶ Increased formation of polyclonal free
   light chains
▶ Myoglobinuria
▶ Hemoglobinuria

**Renal parenchymal and postrenal
proteinuria**
Proteins of the kidneys or the efferent
urinary passages
▶ Local infections
▶ Hemorrhage in the urinary tract
▶ Nephrolithiasis
▶ Prostatitis
▶ Tamm-Horsfall protein

Miscellanous causes for proteinuria
Usually glomerular
▶ Orthostatic proteinuria, idiopathic
   intermittent proteinuria (mostly in
   young men: proteinuria during the day,
   during normal activity, but no
   proteinuria in the urine while at rest)
▶ Unilateral kidney
▶ High fever
▶ Heavy exercise
▶ Heart failure
▶ Tricuspid insufficiency
▶ Constricitive pericarditis
▶ Preeclampsia
▶ Renal vein thrombosis
▶ Massive obesitiy
▶ Chronic pyelonephritis
▶ Arteriolar nephrosclerosis
▶ Malignant hypertension
▶ Acute tubular necrosis
▶ Nephrolithiasis
▶ Renal neoplasm
▶ Polycystic kidney disease
▶ Genitourinary tuberculosis
▶ Allergens
- Poison ivy
- Pollens
▶ Bee or insect stings

Pruritus

Itching sensation on skin. 25 % of patients over 80 years old suffer from pruritus. In chronic pruritus (> 2 weeks) search for basic disease.

Dermatologic
- Dry skin (Xerosis)
- Local infection
  - Bacterial
  - Fungal
  - Varicella, Herpes zoster (preeruptive stage)
- Ectoparasites
  - Scabies
  - Lice
  - Fleas
- Insect bites
- Atopic dermatitis
- Allergic contact dermatitis
- Psoriasis
- Dermatitis herpetiformis
- Lichen planus
- Mycosis fungoides
- Bullous pemphigoid
- Folliculitis
- Sunburn
- Senile pruritus

Liver, bile duct disorder
- Bile duct obstruction
- Hepatocellular jaundice (viral hepatitis)
- Biliary cirrhosis
- Sclerosing cholangitis
- Drug induced cholestasis
- Intrahepatic cholestasis of pregnancy

Hematologic disorders
- Iron deficiency anemia
- Polycythemia vera
- Hodgkin's lymphoma
- Non-Hodgkin's lymphoma
- Leukemia
- Multiple myeloma
- Carcinoid
- Mastocytosis

Neoplasm
- Breast cancer
- Gastric carcinoma
- Prostate carcinoma
- Sarcoma
- CNS carcinoma

Endocrine
- Diabetes mellitus
- Diabetes insipidus
- Hyperthyroidism, myxedema
- Hyper-/ hypoparathyroidism
- Increased estrogen levels
- Gout / hyperuricacidemia
- Porphyria

Drugs
- Alcohol
- Amphetamine
- Antibiotics
- Aspirin
- Barbiturates
- Caffeine
- Cocaine
- Drugs causing cholestasis
  - Anabolics
  - Erythromycin
  - Estrogens
  - Phenothiazines
  - Progesterone
  - Testosterone
  - Tolbutamide
- Gold
- Local anesthetics
- Nicotine
- Nitrofurantoin
- Opiates and their derivates
  - Morphine
  - Butorphanol
- Quinidine
- PUVA (Psoralen + UVA radiation)
- Pyrazolones
- Vitamin B complex
- Subclinical sensitivity to any drug

Exogenic causes
- Cosmetics
- Deodorants

- ► Depilatory cream
- ► Glass wool
- ► Metals
  - • Nickel
  - • Cadmium
  - • Metal dust
- ► Pigments
- ► Preservatives
- ► Soaps
- ► Diseases of the central nervous system
  - • Tabes dorsalis
  - • Thalamus tumor
  - • Multiple sclerosis
- ► Parasites
  - • Ascaris
  - • Echinococcosis
  - • Onchocercosis
  - • Oxyuridae
  - • Schistosomiasis
  - • Trichinosis
  - • Zystirkose
- ► Insects
  - • Wasps
  - • Spiders
  - • Tics
  - • Ants
  - • Moths
  - • Caterpillars
  - • Mosquitoes

Miscellaneous
- ► Severe chronic renal failure (uremic pruritus)
- ► Psychogenic
- ► Idiopathic

Pruritus ani

Anal itching, anal pruritus.

Systemic causes
- ► Diabetes mellitus
- ► Cholestasis
- ► Aplastic anemia
- ► Leukemia
- ► Thyroid disease

Functional, mechanical
- ► Chronic diarrhea
- ► Chronic constipation
- ► Anal fissure
- ► Anal fistula
- ► Tight clothes
- ► Vigorous cleaning
- ► Anal incontinence
- ► Prolapsed hemorrhoids
- ► Rectal prolapse
- ► Anal polyps, carcinoma

Infections
- ► Erythrasma
- ► Candidiasis
- ► Herpes simplex
- ► Human papillomavirus
- ► Pinworms (Enterobius)
- ► Scabies
- ► Perirectal abscess
- ► Sexually transmitted anal ulcer
  - • Gonorrhea
  - • Syphilis

Dermatologic causes
- ► Hemorrhoids
- ► Proctitis
- ► Perianal psoriasis
- ► Seborrheic dermatitis
- ► Intertrigo
- ► Neurodermatitis
- ► Bowen's disease
- ► Atopic dermatitis
- ► Lichen planus
- ► Lichen sclerosis

Exposures
- ► Drugs
  - • Colchicine
  - • Nicotine
  - • Quinidine
- ► Contact dermatitis
  - • Hemorrhoid creams
  - • Soaps
  - • Deodorants
  - • Perfumes
  - • Toilet paper
- ► Food irritants

O
P

- Tomatoes
- Caffeinated beverages
- Beer
- Citrus juices or fruit
- Milk products

Psychogenic

PTH, See Parathyroid Hormone → 275

Ptosis

Drooping upper eyelid due to weakness of the levator palpebrae superioris muscle.

One eyelid
▶ Without additional neurologic failures
- Congenital ptosis
- Ocular myositis (with exophthalmus)
- Isolated denervation of the superior tarsal muscle
▶ With additional peripheral neurologic failures
- Diabetic neuropathy of the oculomotor nerve
- Pancoast tumor (Horner's syndrome)
- Intracranial aneurysm, near the basis
- Traumatic lesion of the oculomotor nerve
- Non-traumatic lesion of the oculomotor nerve
  ○ Parasellar tumors
    - *Dural endothelioma*
    - *Pituitary adenoma*
    - *Erdheim tumor*
    - *Neurofibroma*
    - *Sarcoma*
    - *Oculomotorius neurinoma*
    - *Metastasis*
  ○ Ophthalmoplegic migraine
  ○ Zoster opthalmicus
▶ With supplementary central neurologic failures
- Brain stem infarction
- Brain stem and cervical spinal cord tumor

Both eyelids
▶ Without additional neurologic failures
- Senile ptosis
- Muscle dystrophy
- Dystrophic myotonia (Curschmann's disease)
- Myopathy in
  ○ Dysthyroidism
  ○ Sarcoidosis
  ○ Collagen vascular disease
  ○ Cortisone therapy
- Generalized myositis
▶ With additional peripheral neurologic failures
- Botulism
- Polyradiculitis
- Basal meningitis
- Meningiosis carcinomatosa
▶ With additional central neurologic failures
- Amyotrophic lateral sclerosis
- Spinal muscular atrophy
- Midbrain lesion

Uni- or bilateral strain-dependent ptosis
- Myasthenia gravis

Congenital ptosis – associated with
▶ Weakness of superior rectus muscle (50%)
▶ Marcus Gunn syndrome (5%)
▶ Blepharophimosis (ptosis, telecanthus, epicanthal folds, cicatricial ectropion of lower lid, 5%)

Acquired
▶ Neurogenic
- III nerve palsy
- Horner's syndrome (→ 185)
- Myasthenia gravis
- Chronic progressive external ophthalmoplegia
  ○ Oculopharyngeal dystrophy
- Tabes dorsalis
▶ Myogenic
- Senile
- Myotonic dystrophy

- Mechanical
  - Tumor
  - Scar
  - Vascular abnormality (e.g. haemangioma)
- Trauma
- Botulism

Clinical classification of common causes
▶ With dilated pupil
- Oculomotor nerve palsy
▶ With constricted pupil
- Horner's syndrome
- Tabes dorsalis
▶ With normal pupil
- Congenital
- Myasthenia gravis
- Myotonic dystrophy
- Oculo-pharyngeal dystrophy
- Mitochondrial myopathy
- Thyrotoxic myopathy
- Ocular myopathy
- Botulism

PTT
See Partial Thromboplastin Time → 278

Pubertal Delay
Delayed puberty, pubertas tarda
Delayed adolescence in girls by age 14 and in boys by age 15. Most frequent cause for delayed puberty is a constitutional, non-pathologic delay in growth and puberty.

Causes
▶ Constitutional delay in growth and development
▶ Heavy physical exercise
▶ Chromosomal abnormality
- Turner's syndrome (girls)
- Klinefelter's syndrome (boys)
- Noonan's syndrome
▶ Hypogonadotropic causes
- Multiple tropic hormone deficiency
- Isolated growth hormone (somatotropin) deficiency

- Isolated gonadotropin deficiency (Kallmann's syndrome)
- Prader-Willi syndrome
▶ Iatrogenic
▶ Endocrine
- Hypothyroidism
  - Intracranial lesion
  - Infection of pituitary gland
  - Head injury
- Glucocorticoid excess (Cushing syndrome)
- Hyperprolactinemia
▶ Nutritional
- Anorexia nervosa
- Malnutrition
▶ Miscellaneous
- Malignancy
- Chronic infection
- Inflammatory bowel disease
- Celiac sprue
- Chronic renal failure
- Chronic metabolic disorder
- Cardiac conditions
- Psychogenic
- Brain tumor

Pubertas tarda, See Pubertal Delay → 303

Puberty, See Precocious Puberty → 292, See Pubertal Delay → 303

Pulmonary Edema
Fluid in the lungs usually resulting from mitral stenosis or left ventricular failure.
Elevated microvascular pressure
Due to elevated hydrostatic pressure in the alveolar capillaries
▶ Cardiogenic
- Left heart failure (→ 168)
  - Severe hypertension
  - Coronary heart disease
  - Acute myocardial infarction
  - Aortic and mitral valvular disease

O
P

- ○ Cardiomyopathy
- ○ Arrhythmias
- ○ Pericardial disease
- ○ Myocarditis
- Miscellaneous
  - ○ Acute renal failure
  - ○ Uremia
  - ○ Pulmonary embolism
  - ○ Left-right shunt
  - ○ Pheochromocytoma
▶ Neurogenic pulmonary edema
- Head trauma
- Intracerebral hemorrhage
- Meningoencephalitis
- Postictal
▶ Pulmonary venous obstruction
- Chronic mediastinitis
- Idiopathic venoocclusive disease
- Anomalous pulmonary venous return
- Congenital pulmonary venous stenosis
▶ Decreased plasma oncotic pressure
- Hypoalbuminemia/Albumin deficiency
  - ○ Hepatopathy
  - ○ Renal failure
  - ○ Nephrotic syndrome
  - ○ Burns
- Hyperhydration

Adult respiratory distress syndrome (normal microvascular pressure)
▶ Infections
- Sepsis
- Bacterial toxins
- Toxic shock syndrome
- Pneumonia
  - ○ Bacterial
  - ○ Viral
  - ○ Fungal
  - ○ Mycobacterial
  - ○ P. carinii
  - ○ Legionnaires' disease
  - ○ Aspiration pneumonia
- Malaria
- Miliary tuberculosis
▶ Liquid aspiration
- Gastric content

- (Near-)Drowning
  - ○ Salt water
  - ○ Fresh water
- Alcohol
- Contrast media
▶ Shock (any etiology)
▶ Multiple trauma
- Fat emboli
- Pulmonary contusion
- Massive transfusions
- Burns
▶ Pulmonary embolism (→ 305)
- Thrombus
- Air emboli
- Fatty embolism
- Amniotic fluid embolism
▶ Drugs
- Drug overdose
  - ○ Aspirin
  - ○ Barbiturates
  - ○ Chlordiazepoxide
  - ○ Cocaine
  - ○ Colchicine
  - ○ Ethchlorvinol
  - ○ Narcotics
  - ○ Opiates
  - ○ Propoxyphene
- Drug induced lung injury
  - ○ Amiodarone
  - ○ Nitrofurantoin
  - ○ Paraquat
- Other
  - ○ Dextran
▶ Inhaled toxic gases
- Acid fumes
- Cadmium
- Cl_2
- CO
- Hydrocarbons
- Metallic oxides
- NH_3
- NO_2
- Oxygen (high concentration)
- Ozone
- Phosgene

- Smoke
- SO_2
▶ Pulmonary lymphatic obstruction
  - Fibrotic/inflammatory disease
    ○ Silicosis
  - Lymphangitic carcinomatosis
  - Tumor
  - After lung transplantation
  - Lymphangiography
▶ Hematologic, autoimmune
  - Disseminated intravscular coagulation
  - Blood transfusions
  - Leukemia
  - Thrombocytopenic purpura
  - Goodpasture's syndrome
  - Systemic lupus erythematosus
▶ Physical
  High negative pleural pressure,
  decreased alveolar pressure
  - Postthoracentesis
  - Post-expansion of pneumothorax
  - Acute bronchial asthma
  - High altitude exposure
  - Decompression (diving accident)
  - Hyperbaric treatment over extended period
  - Explosions
  - Complete upper airways obstruction
▶ Miscellaneous
  - Acute pancreatitis
  - Acute radiation pneumonitis
  - Diabetic ketoacidosis
  - Eclampsia
  - After cardiopulmonary bypass
  - Vasoactive substances (histamine)

Pulmonary Embolism

Occlusion of pulmonary arteries,
frequently by detached fragments of
thrombus from a leg or pelvic vein,
commonly when thrombosis has followed
an operation or confinement to bed.
After coronary cardiac disease and CVA,
the most common cardiovascular disease.

Symptoms – DDx
▶ Acute chest pain, angina pectoris → 32
  - Angina pectoris
  - Myocardial infarction
  - Pleuritis
  - Pericarditis
  - Aortic dissection/aneurysm → 32
▶ Acute dyspnea
  - Pneumothorax
  - Pulmonary edema
  - Pneumonia
  - Bronchial asthma
▶ Hemoptysis (→ 175)
  - Bronchial carcinoma
  - Bronchiectasis
  - Tuberculosis
  - Goodpasture's syndrome
    (glomerulonephritis, hemoptyses,
    anti-basement membrane antibodies)
  - Angiodysplasia
  - Hemorrhagic diathesis
  - Mitral stenosis
  - Pulmonary vasculitis
▶ Syncope (massive embolism)
Risk factors
▶ Previous deep vein thrombosis
▶ Obesity
▶ Malignant tumors
  - Pancreatic cancer
▶ Heart failure
▶ Surgery
▶ Bone fractures
▶ Nicotine
▶ Shock
▶ Administration of estrogens, especially
  in combination with nicotine abuse
▶ Trauma
▶ Tumor
▶ Microemboli
▶ Pregnancy
▶ Thrombophilia
▶ Hypertension

O
P

Pulmonary Hypertension

Elevated pressure in the pulmonary circuit.

Idiopathic

Secondary

► Hypoxic vasoconstriction
  • Chronic obstructive pulmonary disease
  • Sleep apnea
  • Alveolar hypoventilation
  • Neuromuscular diseases
    ○ Poliomyelitis
    ○ Myasthenia gravis
    ○ Kyphoscoliosis
  • Interstitial lung disease
  • Bronchiectasis
  • Cystic fibrosis
  • Sarcoidosis
  • Scleroderma
  • High altitude residence
► Obliteration of pulmonary vessels
  • Collagen vascular diseases
  • Pulmonary embolism
    ○ Acute pulmonary embolism
    ○ Chronic proximal pulmonary emboli
  • Infection
    ○ HIV infection
    ○ Schistosomiasis
  • Portal hypertension
  • Drugs, toxins
    ○ Amphetamines
    ○ Chemotherapeutics
    ○ Crack cocaine
    ○ Fenfluramine
    ○ Rapeseed oil
    ○ Tryptophan
  • Sickle cell disease
  • Pulmonary capillary hemangiomatosis
► Volume/pressure overload
  • Atrial septal defect
  • Ventricular septal defect
  • Left atrial hypertension
    ○ Mitral valve dysfunction
    ○ Left ventricular dysfunction
    ○ Systolic/diastolic dysfunction

• Pulmonary venous obstruction
  ○ Mediastinal fibrosis
  ○ Lymphadenopathy
  ○ Pulmonary veno-occlusive disease

Pulmonary Metastases

Tumors metastatic to the lungs

► Breast cancer
► Colon carcinoma
► Prostate cancer
► Renal cell carcinoma
► Hypernephroma
► Thyroid cancer
► Gastric carcinoma
► Cervix carcinoma
► Rectal carcinoma
► Testicular tumor
► Osteosarcoma
► Malignant melanoma
► Pancreas carcinoma
► Lymphomas, leukemias
► Germ cell tumor
► Ovarian cancer

Pulmonary Nodule

Asymptomatic round or oval lesion, surrounded by normal lung.

Main causes

► Bronchial carcinomas
► Metastases
► Granulomas

Solitary pulmonary nodules

► Neoplasm
  • Primary pulmonary neoplasm
    ○ Bronchogenic carcinoma
    ○ Lymphoma
      – *Hodgkin's lymphoma*
      – *Non-Hodgkin's lymphoma*
    ○ Carcinoid
  • Metastatic malignancy
    ○ Prostate cancer
    ○ Gastric cancer
    ○ Malignant melanoma

- ○ Thyroid cancer
- ○ Breast cancer
- ○ Hypernephroma
- ○ Seminoma
- ○ Chorionepithelioma
- ○ Sarcoma
- Multiple myeloma
- Benign tumors
  - ○ Bronchial adenoma
  - ○ Hamartoma
  - ○ Hemangioma
  - ○ Chondroma
  - ○ Neurogenic tumor
  - ○ Bronchial adenoma
- Amyloid
▶ Infections
- Pyogenic pneumonia, lung abscess
- Pneumonia
- Tuberculosis
- Nocardia
- Fungal
  - ○ Histoplasmosis
  - ○ Aspergillosis
  - ○ Coccidiomycosis
  - ○ Cryptococcosis
- Parasites
  - ○ Echinococcus
  - ○ Ascaris
▶ Autoimmune
- Rheumatoid nodule
- Wegener's granulomatosis
▶ Airway causes
- Bronchogenic cyst
- Bronchial atresia
- Infected/fluid filled bulla
▶ Vascular
- Arteriovenous fistula
- Aneurysm of pulmonary artery
- Varicose pulmonary vein
- Pulmonary infarction
▶ Miscellaneous
- Pulmonary sequestration
- Endometriosis
- Localized pleural effusion
- Hematoma (after lung contusion)

- Localized scar
- Lipoid pneumonia
- Mucoid impaction
- Round atelectasis

Multiple pulmonary nodules
▶ Neoplastic
- Hematogenous metastases
  - ○ Prostate cancer
  - ○ Gastric cancer
  - ○ Malignant melanoma
  - ○ Thyroid cancer
  - ○ Breast cancer
  - ○ Hypernephroma
  - ○ Seminoma
  - ○ Chorionepithelioma
  - ○ Sarcoma
- Bronchogenic carcinoma
- Lymphoma
- Histiocytosis X
- Lymphangitic metastases
▶ Granulomatous diseases
- Tuberculosis
  - ○ Miliary tuberculosis
- Histoplasmosis
- Wegner's granulomatosis
▶ Inhalation
- Silicosis
- Asbestosis
▶ Miscellaneous
- Pyogenic abscesses (infective embolisms)
- Echinococcus cysts
- Bronchogenic cysts
- Rheumatoid nodules
- Sarcoidosis
- Varicella pneumonia
- Histiocytosis X
- Lymphangitic metastases

Pulmonary ventilation impairment
See Respiratory Failure → 319

Pulse

Soft pulse
► Reduced cardiac output
  • Heart failure
  • Shock
  • Hypovolemia
  • Myocardial infarction
  • Cardiac tamponade
  • Constrictive pericarditis
  • Perimyocarditis
  • Cardiomyopathy
► Peripheral vasoconstriction
  • Shock
  • Hypovolemia
► Mechanic cause
  • Cardiac valve diseases
    ○ Aortic stenosis
    ○ Mitral stenosis
    ○ Mitral regurgitation
  • Disorders of the aorta
    ○ Aortic arch syndrome
    ○ Stenoses

Hard pulse (pulsus durus)
► Reduced elasticity in the arterial high-pressure system
  • Arteriosclerosis
  • Hypertension
► Elevated stroke volume
  • Heavy exercise
  • Aortic insufficiency
  • Anxiety
► Increased cardiac output
  • Fever
  • Anemia
  • Hyperthyroidism
  • Hyperkinetic heart syndrome
  • Arteriovenous fistula
  • Beriberi
  • Paget's disease

Collapsing pulse (bounding pulse, water-hammer pulse)
► Aortic regurgitation
► Anemia
► Thyrotoxicosis
► Essential hypertension

Paradoxical pulse (pulsus paradoxus)
Inspiratory decrease in arterial pressure
>10 mm Hg
► Cardiac
  • Pericardial effusion
  • Constrictive pericarditis
  • Cardiac tamponade
  • Endocardial fibrosis
  • Myocardial amyloidosis
  • Mitral stenosis (right heart failure)
  • Tricuspid stenosis
► Pulmonary
  • Pulmonary emphysema
  • Severe asthma
  • Obstructive lung disease
  • Pulmonary embolism
► Para-mediastinal effusion
► Scleroderma
► Hypovolemia

Intermittent pulse (pulsus intercidens)
► Arrhythmia
► Extrasystoles

Pulse pressure (→ 308)

Pulse pressure

Difference between systolic and diastolic blood pressure (normal pulse pressure 30–40 mmHg)

High pulse pressure (>40 mmHg)
► Aortic regurgitation (water-hammer)
► Arteriosclerosis of the aorta
► Arteriolosclerosis of renal arteries
► Isolated systolic hypertension
► Hyperthyroidism
► Patent ductus arteriosus
► Arteriovenous fistula
► Cirrhosis
► Beriberi heart
► Aortic coarctation
► Anemia
► Emotional state

Narrowed pulse pressure (<30 mmHg)
► Tachycardia
► Severe aortic stenosis
► Shock
► Constrictive pericarditis
► Pericardial effusion
► Ascites

Pupil diameter, different
See Anisocoria → 35

Purpura

Hematologic
► Platelet disorders
  • Thrombocytopenia (→ 349)
    See Thrombocyte Count → 349
    ○ Drugs
      - Aspirin
      - NSAIDs
      - Thiazides
    ○ Disseminated intravascular coagulation
    ○ Immune thrombocytopenic purpura
    ○ Posttransfusion purpura
  • Platelet dysfunction
  • Thrombocytosis
► Coagulation disorder
  • Factor VIII deficiency
  • Factor IX deficiency
  • Von Willebrand's disease
  • Disseminated intravascular coagulation
  • Liver disease
  • Vitamin K deficiency
  • Hemolytic uremic syndrome

Vascular
► Collagen vascular disease
  • Henoch-Schönlein purpura
  • Polyarteritis nodosa
  • Wegener's granulomatosis
  • Churg-Strauss syndrome
  • Lupus erythematosus
  • Rheumatoid arthritis
  • Sjögren's syndrome

► Lymphoproliferative disorder
  • Hodgkin's lymphoma
► Infections
  • Subacute bacterial endocarditis
  • Septic emboli
  • Meningococcemia
  • Scarlet fever
  • Typhoid
  • Rocky Mountain spotted fever
  • Measles
  • Hepatitis B
  • Echo virus
  • Coxsackie virus
► Drugs
  • Allopurinol
  • Atropine
  • Chloral hydrate
  • Cimetidine
  • Corticosteroids
  • Gold
  • Hydralazine
  • Iodides
  • Ketoconazole
  • Penicillin
  • Phenytoin
  • Propylthiouracil
  • Quinidine
  • Sulfonamides
  • Tetracycline
  • Thiazides
► Trauma
  • Violent coughing
  • Vomiting
  • Strangulation
  • Factitious purpura
  • Religious rituals
  • Child abuse
► Miscellaneous
  • Serum sickness
  • Hereditary hemorrhagic telangiectasia
  • Ehlers-Danlos syndrome (Type IV)
  • Scurvy (vitamin C deficiency)
  • Psychogenic purpura (Gardner-Diamond syndrome)

O
P

PVCs, See Cardiac Dysrhythmias → 62

Pyridoxine Deficiency

Risk factors
▶ Gastrointestinal/hepatic disorders
- Severe malnutrition
- Celiac disease
- Hepatitis
- Extrahepatic biliary obstruction
- Hepatocellular carcinoma

▶ Renal disorders
- Chronic renal failure
- Kidney transplant

▶ Iatrogenic
- Hemodialysis
- Peritoneal dialysis
- Phototherapy for hyperbilirubinemia

▶ Drugs, toxins
- Alcoholism
- Cigarette smoking
- Cycloserine
- D-Penicillamine
- Hydralazine
- Isoniazid
- Mushroom poisoning
- Pyrazinamide

▶ Miscellaneous
- Hyperoxaluria
- High serum alkaline phosphatase
- Catabolic state

▶ Other risk factors
- Advanced age
- Hospitalization
- Pyridoxine-deficient mother
- Pyridoxine-dependent neonatal seizures

Pyuria
Pus in the urine
Causes
▶ Inflammation of the upper urinary tract
- Pyelonephritis
- Interstitial nephritis
- Renal papillary necrosis
- Renal abscess
- Stone

▶ Inflammation of the lower urinary tract
- Cystitis
- Urethritis
- Neoplasm
- Stone
- Vaginitis
- Vulvitis
- Colpitis
- Prostatitis
- Epididymitis

▶ Aseptic pyuria
- Genitourinary tuberculosis
- Stone
- Acute glomerulonephritis
- Analgesic nephritis
- Renal carcinoma
- After chemotherapy

Quick's test
See Thromboplastin time → 352

Rash with fever
See Fever with Rash → 144

Raynaud's Syndrome

Raynaud's disease: periodic states of ischemia caused purely by functional vasoconstriction (angiospasms), with preference for the second to fifth finger. Progression in three phases: paleness, cyanosis, then erythema. Local cold stimuli and emotional stress can cause attacks. Six times more in women than in men. Secondary Raynaud's syndrome: Acral ischemia attacks due to numerous different systemic diseases.

Collagen vascular disease
▶ Lupus erythematosus
▶ Polyarteritis nodosa

- Rheumatoid arthritis
- Wegener's granulomatosis
- Scleroderma
- Dermatomyositis
- Sjörgen's syndrome
- Mixed connective tissue disease

Chronic arterial disease
- Arteriosclerosis obliterans
- Thromboangitis obliterans
- Peripheral embolism

Shoulder girdle syndromes
- Scalenus-anticus syndrome
- Cervical rib
- Costoclavicular syndrome
- Hyperabduction syndrome

Spinal disorders
- Arthrosis of the cervical spine
- Scoliosis

Hematologic
- Cold agglutinins
- Cryoglobulinemia
- Polycythemia vera
- Dysproteinemia (multiple myeloma)
- Leukemia

Neurologic
- Multiple sclerosis
- Poliomyelitis
- Syringomyelia
- Spinal tumor
- Hemiplegia
- Peripheral neuropathy
- Carpal tunnel syndrome
- Thoracic outlet syndrome
- Post-traumatic reflex sympathetic dystrophy

Drugs, toxins
- Arsenic
- Arterenol
- Clonidine
- Cytotoxic drugs
- Ergotamine
- Heavy metals
- Hormonal contraceptives
- Lead
- Propranolol
- Sulfasalazine
- Thallium

Occupational and environmental factors
- After blunt traumas
- After surgery
- Vibrations (pneumatic hammer)
- Percussions (hand strain in typists, pianists etc.)

Miscellaneous
- Arteriovenous fistula
- Cirrhosis
- Axillary vein thrombosis
- Acromegaly
- Hypothyroidism
- Neoplasm

Red cell cast, See Cylindruria → 92

Red Eye

Causes
- Allergic-hyperergic
  - Bacterial toxins
  - Autoantigens (e.g. lens residue)
  - Allergic conjunctivitis
  - Allergic rhinitis
  - Atopic eczema
  - Contact allergies
    - Cosmetics
    - Drugs
      - *Neomycin*
      - *Chloramphenicol*
      - *Erythromycin*
      - *Local anesthetics*
      - *Miotics/mydriatics (atropine)*
      - *Sulfonamides*
      - *Tetracycline*
- Infections
  - EBV
  - Tuberculosis
  - Toxoplasmosis
  - Syphilis
  - Borreliosis
  - Leptospirosis (Weil's disease)

Q
R

- Malaria
- Other bacterial agents
  - Gonococci
  - Chlamydia trachomatis
  - Staphylococci
  - Streptococci
  - Haemophilus
  - Pseudomonas
  - Moraxella
- Other viral agents
  - Adenoviruses
  - Measles
▸ Miscellaneous
  - Keratoconjunctivitis sicca/Sjögren's syndrome
  - Fever
  - Cervical lymphadenopathy
  - Chemical irritants
▸ Hemorrhage (without inflammation)
- Symptomatic
  - Arteriosclerosis
  - Hypertension
  - Hemorrhagic diathesis
  - Anticoagulant therapy
  - Diabetes mellitus
  - Bacterial endocarditis
  - "Red-eye" syndrome in chronic renal failure
  - Osler-Weber-Rendu disease
  - Trauma
  - Coughing/straining
- Local causes
  - Episcleral/conjunctival hamartoma
  - Hemangioma
  - Lymphangioma
- Ciliary and mixed infections
  - Keratitis
  - Corneal erosion
  - Iridocyclitis
    - *Still syndrome*
    - *Bechterew's disease*
  - Acute glaucoma attack
- Idiopathic (in advanced age)

Acute Red Eye
▸ Conjunctivitis (infectious and noninfectious)
▸ Narrow angle glaucoma
▸ Iritis or uveitis
▸ Keratitis
▸ Episcleritis or scleritis
▸ Eyelid abnormalities
- Entropion
- Lagophthalmos with globe exposure
- Trichiasis
- Molluscum contagiosum
▸ Orbital disorders
- Preseptal and orbital cellulitis
- Idiopathic orbital inflammation
  - *Pseudotumor cerebri*

Associated with
▸ Associated with HLA-B27
- Reiter's syndrome
- Bechterew's disease
- Psoriatic arthropathy
- Still syndrome/juvenile rheumatoid arthritis
- Ulcerative colitis
- Crohn's disease
▸ Associated with HLA-B5
- Behçet's syndrome (aphthoid-ulcerative changes in oral and genital mucosa, iritis, erythema nodosum and arthritis)
▸ Associated with arthritis
- Bechterew's disease
- Behçet's syndrome
- Borreliosis
- Chronic inflammatory diseases
- Rheumatoid arthritis
- Whipple's disease
- Psoriatic arthropathy
- Reiter's syndrome
- Sarcoidosis
▸ Associated with diarrhea
- Chronic inflammatory intestinal diseases
- Whipple's disease
- Yersinia/Klebsiella enteritis
▸ Associated with erythema nodosum
- Sarcoidosis

- Psoriatic arthropathy
- Systemic lupus erythematosus
- Crohn's disease
▶ Associated with erythema migrans
- Borreliosis
▶ Associated with genital ulcers
- Behçet's syndrome
- Reiter's syndrome
▶ Associated with cough/dyspnea
- Tuberculosis
- Sarcoidosis
- Malignant tumors
▶ Associated with headaches
- Borreliosis
- Sarcoidosis
- Vogt-Koyanagai syndrome
▶ Associated with oral ulcers
- Behçet's syndrome
▶ Associated with swelling of the salivary glands
- Sarcoidosis

Red face, See Face, Red → 138

Red palms

Causes
▶ Cirrhosis
▶ Other liver disease
▶ Systemic lupus erythematosus
▶ Dermatomyositis
▶ Rheumatoid arthritis
▶ Drug eruption
▶ Viral exanthem
▶ Hemochromatosis
▶ Chronic heart failure
▶ Mitral stenosis
▶ Pulmonary stenosis
▶ Bronchiectasis
▶ Hyperthyroidism
▶ Polycythemia
▶ Pregnancy

Reflexes

Reflex differences
Difference between right and left side
▶ Vascular
- Apoplexy
- Acute subarachnoid bleeding
- Arterial vascular occlusion
▶ Brain tumor
▶ Myelitis
▶ Acute lumbal syndrome
▶ Wallenberg's syndrome
▶ Commotio syndrome

Generalized reflex reduction, missing reflexes (areflexia)
▶ Metabolic, endocrine
- Diabetes mellitus
- Acute hepatic porphyria
- Hypothyroidism
- Hyperaldosteronism (Conn's syndrome)
▶ Electrolyte imbalance
- Hypokalemia
- Hyponatremia
▶ Vitamin deficiency
- Beriberi (vitamin-B_1)
- Subacute combined degeneration of the spinal cord (vitamin B_{12})
▶ Infections
- Tabes dorsalis
- Botulism
▶ Hereditary myopathies
- Dystrophia musculorum progressiva
- Werdning-Hoffmann muscular atrophy
- Neural muscular atrophy (Charcot-Marie-Tooth disease)
- Kugelberg-Welander disease
- Myotonia congenita
▶ Spinal cord lesions
- Tumor
- Trauma
- Circulation disorder
- Inflammation

Q
R

▶ Toxins
- Barbiturates
- Narcotics
- Opiates

▶ Miscellaneous
- Polyneuropathy
- Guillain-Barré syndrome
- Myelitis
- Spinocerebellar heredoataxia
- Brain concussion
- Sarcoidosis
- Adynamia episodica hereditaria
- Familiar areflexia

Failure of individual reflexes
▶ Lesion of the nerve root
▶ Lesion of the peripheral nerve
▶ Posterior horn syndrome
- Circulation disorders
- Tumor
- Syringomyelia
- Poliomyelitis

▶ Arterial vascular occlusion

Hyperreflexia
▶ Neurologic
- Inflammatory processes of CNS
  ○ Meningitis
  ○ Poliomyelitis
  ○ Tetanus
  ○ Rabies
- Degenerative processes of the CNS
  ○ Parkinsonism
  ○ Athetosis
  ○ Amyotrophic lateral sclerosis
  ○ General paralysis
  ○ Spastic spinal paralysis
- Metabolic and toxic processes
  ○ Hereditary metabolic disorders
    - Phenylketonuria
    - Homocystinuria
    - Maple syrup urine disease
  ○ Progressive alcoholic dementia
- Acute brain edema
  ○ Apoplexy
  ○ Intracranial bleeding
- Hyperbaric liquor pressure

  ○ Brain tumor
  ○ Hydrocephalus
  ○ Meningitis
- Multiple sclerosis
- Infantile diplegia

▶ Drugs, toxins
- Alcohol
- Amphetamines
- Caffeine
- Neuroleptic drugs
- Sympathomimetics
- Thyroxine

▶ Hypocalcemia
▶ Hyperthyroidism
▶ Hepatic coma
▶ Autonomic dystonia

Reflux esophagitis, See Esophagitis →
136, See Dysphagia → 110

Renal Cysts
Cystic kidney diseases
Renal cysts occur in one third of people
older than 50 years:

Congenital
▶ Congenital cystic dysplasia (congenital
multicystic kidney disease)

Genetic
▶ Autosomal recessive polycystic kidney
disease
▶ Autosomal dominant polycystic kidney
disease
▶ Nephronophthisis–medullary cystic
kidney disease complex

Acquired
▶ Simple cysts
▶ Acquired renal cystic disease
- Fibrosis
- Oxalate crystals
- Epithelial hyperplasia

Associated with systemic disease
▶ Von Hippel-Lindau syndrome
▶ Tuberous sclerosis

Neoplasm
▶ Renal cell carcinoma

Miscellaneous, DDx
▶ Hemangioma
▶ Hematoma
▶ Dermoid cyst
▶ Abscess
▶ Echinococcal cyst
▶ Tuberculous cavity

Renal Failure, Acute

Acute renal failure, shock kidney.

Sudden partial or complete loss of renal function, resulting in increased serum urea and creatinine (azotemia). Main complaint: decreased urine secretion with oliguria (< 500 ml/d) or anuria (< 100 ml/d). See Renal Failure, Chronic → 317.

Prerenal causes (80%)
▶ Functional oliguria with dehydration
▶ Vascular, ischemic
  • Shock of various origin
  • Hypovolemia
    ∘ Blood losses
      - *Trauma*
      - *Gastrointestinal bleeding*
      - *Metrorrhagias*
      - *Surgery*
    ∘ Water/electrolyte loss
      - *Massive vomiting*
      - *Profuse diarrhea*
      - *Excessive sweating*
      - *Extensive burns*
      - *Diuretic overdose*
      - *Fluid shifts in peritonitis/ pancreatitis*
      - *Addison's disease*
      - *Diabetic coma*
    ∘ Third space
    ∘ Burns
  • Blood pressure drop
    ∘ Myocardial infarction
    ∘ Heart failure
    ∘ Pericardial tamponade
    ∘ Embolism
    ∘ Volume deficiency
    ∘ Pancreatitis
    ∘ Septic shock
    ∘ Major trauma
    ∘ Injury
  • Hepatorenal syndrome
  • Cirrhosis/Ascites
  • Nephrotic syndrome
  • Therapy with ACE inhibitors in existing renal artery stenosis (!)
  • Renal artery stenosis
  • Aortic aneurysm
▶ Blood/muscle pigments
  • Intravascular hemolysis
    ∘ Transfusion reactions
    ∘ Immune reactions
    ∘ Toxins
      - *Fungal, snake, spider venoms*
    ∘ Malaria
  • Hemolytic-uremic syndrome
  • Paroxysmal hemoglobinuria
  • Rhabdomyolysis (→ 322) / myoglobinuria
    ∘ Crush syndrome
    ∘ Burns
    ∘ Myopathies
    ∘ Acute alcoholism
    ∘ Hypokalemia
    ∘ Long-term coma
    ∘ Heatstroke
    ∘ CO poisoning
    ∘ Physical fatigue
▶ Severe sodium and chloride loss
  • Heavy vomiting
  • Diarrhea
  • Diabetic coma
  • Addison's disease
  • Diuretics
▶ Infection, systemic
  • Peritonitis
  • Acute pancreatitis
  • Acute cholecystitis
  • Ileus (→ 206)
  • Pre-eclampsia

▶ Drugs
- Aminoglycosides
- Cefoxitin
- Cephalosporins
- Cephalothin
- Cimetidine
- Diuretics
- Hydantoin
- Methyldopa
- Trimethoprim

Renal causes
▶ Kidney diseases
- Inflammatory nephropathies
  ○ Glomerulonephritis
  ○ Interstitial nephritis
  ○ Pyelonephritis
  ○ Rejection after kidney transplant
- Vascular nephropathies
  ○ Occlusion of the renal arteries/veins
  ○ Arteriosclerosis of the renal arteries/veins
  ○ Bilateral renal cortical necrosis
  ○ Vasculitis
  ○ Malignant hypertension
  ○ Thrombotic thrombocytopenic purpura
  ○ Scleroderma
  ○ Panarteritis
- Hemolytic-uremic syndrome
  ○ Enteropathic hemolyticuremic syndrome with enterohemorrhagic E. coli
  ○ Non-enteropathic uremic syndrome
- Tubulointerstitial renal failure
  ○ Shock kidney
  ○ Drugs
    - *Antibiotics*
    - *Contrast media containing iodine*
    - *Mycotoxins*
    - *NSAIDs*
    - *Sulfonamides*
  ○ Infections
    - *Leptospira*
    - *Legionella*
  ○ Intratubular casts in shock

- *Rhabdomyolysis*
- *Paraproteins in multiple myeloma*
- *Hemoglobinuria*

▶ Intoxication
- Drugs, exogenous toxins
  ○ Aminoglycosides
  ○ Amphotericin B
  ○ Analgesics
  ○ Anesthetics
  ○ Antibiotics
  ○ Aspirin
  ○ Chemicals
  ○ Contrast media
  ○ Drugs
  ○ Metals
  ○ Methoxyflurane
  ○ NSAIDs
  ○ Phenacetin
  ○ Solvents
- Endogenous toxins
  ○ Uric acid
  ○ Oxalate
  ○ Pigments
    - *Hemoglobin*
    - *Myoglobin*
  ○ Hormones
    - *PTH*
  ○ Light chain disease
    - *Multiple myeloma (!)*
- Infection
  ○ Weil's disease
  ○ Pyemia
  ○ Sepsis

Postrenal causes
Drainage disorders of various origin caused by obstruction of the cavities in the urogenital tract.
- Urethral
  ○ Urethral stenosis
  ○ Urethral atresia
  ○ Inflammation
  ○ Stricture
  ○ Trauma
- Ureteral
  ○ Ureteral stricture

- ○ Ureteral stenosis
- ○ Ruptured ureter
- ○ Ureter ansa
- ○ Intrauretral
  - *Clots*
  - *Stones*
  - *Crystal*
  - *Foreign bodies*
  - *Papillae (necrosed)*
  - *Tumor*
  - *Valve formation in the urethra*
  - *Trauma*
- × External compression of the ureter
  - *Tumor (cervical, endometrial, prostatic, sarcoma, ovarian)*
  - *Fibrosis (idiopathic, inflammation, surgery, radiation, inflammatory bowel disease)*
  - *Retroflexion of uterus during pregnancy*
- • Prostatic hypertrophy
- • Prostatitis
- • Bladder
  - ○ Trabeculated bladder
  - ○ Bladder stone
  - ○ Carcinoma
  - ○ Infection
  - ○ Trauma
  - ○ Functional
  - ○ Neuropathie
  - ○ Inflammatory meatus stenosis
  - ○ Sphincter stenosis
  - ○ Drugs
    - *Parasympatholytics*
    - *Ganglionic blockers*
- • Phimosis
- • Accessory vessel
- ▶ Ureteral obstruction with empty bladder
  - • Ureteral stricture
  - • Stone
  - • Blood clot
  - • Lymphoma
- ▶ Urinary retention with full bladder
  - • Bladder stone
  - • Prostatic hypertrophy/ cancer

- • Bladder cancer
- • Displaced urinary catheter
- ▶ Neurologic
  - • Spinal cord tumor
  - • Multiple sclerosis
  - • Neurosyphilis
  - • Syringomyelia
  - • Tabes dorsalis

Renal Failure, Chronic

Irreversible decrease in the glomerular filtrate with progressive loss of functional kidney tissue.
See Renal Failure, Acute → 315

Main causes
- ▶ Chronic glomerulonephritis
- ▶ Diabetic nephropathy
- ▶ Interstitial nephritis
- ▶ Chronic pyelonephritis
- ▶ Polycystic kidneys
- ▶ Vascular kidney damage
  - • Malignant hypertension
  - • Nephrosclerosis
  - • Renal artery stenosis
  - • Renal vein thrombosis
- ▶ Analgesic nephritis
- ▶ Systemic
  - • Vasculitis
  - • Systemic lupus erythematosus
- ▶ Congenital, hereditary
  - • Polycystic disease
  - • Hereditary nephritis
  - • Fabry´s disease
  - • Oxalosis
  - • Cystinosis
  - • Nail-patella syndrome
  - • Congenital nephrotic syndrome

Renal Failure, Reversible

Causes
- ▶ Obstruction
- ▶ Volume depletion
- ▶ Infection of the urinary tract

- Drugs, toxins
- Congestive heart failure
- Hypertension
- Hypercalcemia
- Hypokaliemia

Renin

Proteolytic enzyme formed in the kidneys converting angiotensinogen to angiotensin.

Reference range

	Renin	Renin inactivity
Upright position	4.1–44.7 pg/ml	< 5.6 ng/ml/h
Lying	2.9–27.6 pg/ml	0.2–2.7 ng/ml/h

Increased

- Aldosteronism
  - Primary (Conn's syndrome)
  - Secondary
- Renin secreting tumors
  - Bronchial carcinoma
  - Renal carcinoma
- Drugs
  - Diuretics
  - Estrogens
  - Glucocorticoids
  - Laxatives
  - Minoxidil
  - Oral contraceptives
  - Thiazides
- Renal disease
  - Chronic renal failure
  - Renal artery stenosis
  - Renal hypertension
- Bartter's syndrome
- Pseudo Bartter's syndrome
- Pheocromocytoma
- Cirrhosis
- Heart failure
- Pregnancy
- Reduced plasma volume

Decreased

- Primary hypoaldosteronism (Addison's disease)

- Cushing's syndrome
- Enzymatic defects of the adrenocortical hormone synthesis
  - 11-hydroxylase deficiency
  - 17-hydroxylase deficiency
- Essential hypertension (with low renin level)
- Secondary in diabetes mellitus
- Drugs, toxins
  - Carbenoxolone
  - Clonidine
  - Licorice
  - Propranolol
  - Reserpine
- Increased plasma volume

Respiration, rapid (tachypnea)
See Dyspnea → 112

Respiratory acidosis
See Acidosis, Respiratory → 12

Respiratory alkalosis
See Alkalosis, Respiratory → 19

Respiratory Displacement, Reduced

The respiratory displacement between deepest expiration and deepest inspiration is 4–5 cm.

Reduced

- Pleuritis
- Pleural effusion
- Pleural fibrosis
- Pneumonia
- Pneumothorax
- Bronchial asthma
  - Obstructive emphysema
- Emphysema
  - Blue bloater emphysema
  - Pink puffer emphysema
- Stasis lung
- Silicosis

▶ Pulmonary fibrosis
▶ Diaphragmatic diseases

Respiratory Failure

Hypoventilation

Reduced alveolar ventilation.
See Acidosis, Respiratory → 12
See Dyspnea → 112

Pulmonary disorders
▶ Obstructive lung desease (→ 262)
  • Bronchial asthma
  • COPD
  • Emphysema
  • Foreign body
  • Aspiration
  • Laryngo-/bronchospasm
  • Glottal edema
  • Noxious gases
▶ Restrictive lung desease (→ 320)
▶ Alveolar disorders
  • Bronchial cancer
  • Pneumothorax
  • Pneumonia
  • Pulmonary edema
  • Pleural effusion
  • Atelectasis
  • Foreign body
  • After pulmonary resection
▶ Interstitial disorders
  • Interstitial fibrosis
  • Fibrosing alveolitis
  • Neoplasm
▶ Vascular disorders
  • Pulmonary embolus
  • Arteriovenous fistula
  • Obliterative vasculitis
    ◦ Primary pulmonary hypertension
    ◦ Scleroderma

Pleural and chest wall disorders
  Pleural effusions
  Pleural fibrosis
  Tension pneumothorax
  Flail chest
  Multiple rib fractures

▶ Postthoracotomy
▶ Kyphoscoliosis
Neuromuscular disorders
▶ Guillain-Barré syndrome/Polyradiculitis
▶ Poliomyelitis
▶ Amyotrophic lateral sclerosis
▶ Tetanus
▶ Myasthenia gravis
▶ Muscular dystrophies
▶ Polymyositis/Dermatomyositis
▶ Electrolyte abnormalities
  • Hypokaliemia
  • Hypophosphatemia
Central nervous system disorders
▶ Drug supression of respiratory center
  • Morphine
  • Barbiturates
  • Benzodiazepines
  • Antidepressants
  • Salicylates
  • Drug withdrawal
  • Methylxanthines
    ◦ Theophylline
▶ Cerebral trauma
▶ Infection
  • Viral encephalitis
  • Bulbar poliomyelitis
▶ Vascular disorders
  • Intracranial bleeding
  • Intracranial infarction
  • Shock
▶ Sleep apnea syndrome
▶ Status epilepticus
Miscellaneous
▶ Laryngeal obstruction
▶ Epiglottitis
▶ Congestive heart failure

Respiratory Sounds

Decreased or absent
▶ Pneumothorax
▶ Emphysema
  • Blue bloater emphysema
  • Pink puffer emphysema

Q
R

- ► Pleural effusion
  - Pleural empyema
  - Meigs' syndrome
  - Transudate
  - Exudate
- ► Pleural fibrosis
- ► Pleuritis
- ► Pulmonary stasis
- ► Infiltration
  - Pneumonia
  - Tumor
- ► Asthma
- ► COPD
- ► Atelectasis
- ► Bronchial occlusion
- ► Severe obesity
- ► Diaphragmatic disorders

Restrictive Lung Disease

Reduced lung volume due to alteration in lung parenchyma, disease of pleura, chest wall, or neuromuscular apparatus.
Reduced total lung capacity, vital capacity or resting lung volume.

Parenchymal

- ► Collagen vascular diseases
  - Scleroderma
  - Polymyositis
  - Dermatomyositis
  - Systemic lupus erythematosus
  - Rheumatoid arthritis
  - Ankylosing spondylitis
- ► Drugs, treatments
  - Amiodarone
  - BCNU
  - Bleomycin
  - Cyclophosphamide
  - Dilantin
  - Gold
  - Methotrexate
  - Nitrofurantoin
  - Radiation
- ► Inorganic dust exposure
  - Silicosis

- Asbestosis
- Talc
- Pneumoconiosis
- Berylliosis
- Hard metal fibrosis
- Coal workers pneumoconiosis
- ► Organic dust exposure (hypersensitivity pneumonitis)
  - Farmer's lung
  - Bird fanciers lung
  - Bagassosis
  - Mushroom worker lung
- ► Idiopathic pulmonary fibrosis
  - Interstitial pneumonia
  - Interstitial pneumonitis
- ► Miscellaneous
  - Sarcoidosis
  - Pulmonary histiocytosis X
  - Lymphangioleiomyomatosis
  - Pulmonary vasculitis
  - Alveolar proteinosis
  - Eosinophilic pneumonia
  - Bronchiolitis obliterans organizing pneumonia (BOOP)

Extraparenchymal

- ► Nonmuscular diseases (chest wall)
  - Idiopathic kyphosis
  - Secondary kyphoscoliosis
    ○ Polio
    ○ Muscular dystrophy
  - Fibrothorax
  - Massive pleural effusion
  - Obesity
  - Ankylosing spondylitis
  - Thoracoplasty
- ► Neuromuscular diseases
  - Myopathy
  - Myositis
  - Quadriplegia
  - Phrenic neuropathy
    ○ Infections
    ○ Metabolic

Reticulocytes

Reticulocytes are juvenile red blood cells with a network of precipitated basophilic substance representing residual polyribosomes, and occurring during the process of active blood regeneration. The nucleus will be extruded once RBC has matured. .

Reference range

Newborns/ infants	6-30/1000 (0.6-3%)
Adults	5-20/1000 (0.5-2%)

Increased erythropoiesis

Reticulocyte index >3%

Reticulocyte count >1.5%

▶ Acute blood loss
▶ Acute hemolysis
▶ Hemolytic anemia
▶ Hemoglobinopathy
  • Sickle cell anemia
  • Thalassemia major
▶ Chronic hypoxia
▶ Post-splenectomy
▶ Replacement therapy in
  • Iron deficiency
  • Vitamin B$_{12}$ deficiency
  • Folic acid deficiency
▶ Polycythemia
▶ Erythroblastosis
▶ Zieve's syndrome
▶ Infections
▶ Toxins
  • Lead

Reduced erythropoiesis

Reticulocyte index <1%

Reticulocyte count <0.5%

▶ Aplastic anemia
▶ Panmyelopathy
▶ Bone marrow infiltrate
▶ Bone marrow suppression or failure
  • Sepsis
  • Chemotherapy
  • Radiotherapy
▶ RBC maturation impairment

  • Iron deficiency anemia
  • Vitamin B$_{12}$ deficiency
  • Folate deficiency
  • Sideroblastic anemia
  • Anemia of chronic disease
  • Hypothyroidism
▶ Erythropoietin deficiency
  • Renal failure
▶ Uremia
▶ Blood transfusion
▶ Liver disease
▶ Toxins
  • Chemotherapeutics
  • Chloramphenicol
  • Favistan
  • Radiation

Retinol (Vitamin A)

Fat soluble vitamin mainly found in chicken meat, liver, egg yolk, fish oil, whole milk, butter, and cream. Vitamin A plays an important role in the function of the retinal rods (twilight, night vision). It is also a protective substance for the entire ectoderm and important for the regulation of bone growth. Symptoms of a retinol deficiency include decreased visual acuity, night blindness (→ 259), dry bulbar conjunctiva, dry skin, hyperkeratosis and corneal ulceration.

Decreased

▶ Primary
  • Prolonged dietary deprivation
  • Endemic (southern/eastern Asia)
▶ Secondary
  • Maldigestion
    ○ Cirrhosis
    ○ Obstruction of the bile ducts
    ○ Pancreatic disease
    ○ Cystic fibrosis
    ○ Lipase deficiency
  • Malabsorption
    ○ Celiac disease
    ○ Sprue

Q
R

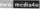

- Crohn's disease
- Ulcerative colitis
- Giardiasis
- Duodenal bypass
- Congenital partial obstruction of the jejunum
- Reduced vitamin A storage/ transport
  - Premature infants
  - Cirrhosis
  - RBP deficiency
  - Nephrotic syndrome
- Protein-energy malnutrition
  - Marasmus
  - Kwashiorkor

Increased
▶ Excessive supply
- Selfmedication
- Vitamin A therapy
  - Psoriasis
  - Acne

Retrosternal pain, See Chest Pain → 72, See Angina → 32

Rhabdomyolysis

Acute, fulminating, potentially fatal breakdown of muscle fibers with leakage of toxic cellular contents into the systemic circulation.

Causes
▶ Limb ischemia
▶ Hypoxia
▶ Trauma
- Significant blunt trauma (crush injury)
- High voltage electrical injury
- Extensive burns
- Near drowning
- Prolonged immobilization
- Snake bites
- Spider bites
▶ Heat injury
- Hyperthermia
- Hypothermia
- Heat stroke

- Malignant hyperthermia
- Neuroleptic malignant syndrome
▶ Excessive muscular activity
- Sporadic strenuous exercise (marathons)
- Overexertion
  - Deconditioned athletes
- Impaired heat dissipation
  - Heavy or occlusive sports equipment
  - Humid, warm environment
- Systemic disorders
  - Status epilepticus
  - Status asthmaticus
  - Severe dystonia
  - Acute psychosis
▶ Infection
- Viral
  - Influenza virus A
  - Influenza virus B
  - HIV
  - Herpes viruses (EBV, CMV, HSV)
- Bacterial
  - Legionella
  - Salmonella
  - Streptococcus
▶ Endocrine
- Thyroid disease
- Diabetic ketoacidosis
▶ Metabolic
- Hyponatremia
- Hypernatremia
- Hypokalemia
- Hypophosphatemia
- Hypothyroidism
- Hyperthyroidism
- Diabetic ketoacidosis
- Nonketotic hyperosmolar diabetic coma
▶ Drugs, toxins
- Alcohol (alcoholic myopathy)
- Aminocaproic acid
- Amphetamine
- Amphotericin B
- Anesthetics
- Antihistamines

- Barbiturates
- Caffeine
- Carbon monoxide poisoning (!!)
- Cocaine
- Colchicine
- Corticosteroids
- Cyclic antidepressants
- Cyclosporine
- Ecstacy
- Erythromycin
- Ethanol
- Fibric acid derivatives
  ○ Bezafibrate
  ○ Clofibrate
  ○ Fenofibrate
  ○ Gemfibrozil
- Hemlock herbs
- Heroin
- HMG-CoA reductase inhibitors
- Isopropanol
- Itraconazole
- Lovastatin
- LSD (Lysergic acid diethylamide)
- Methadone
- Methanol
- Neuroleptics
- Phencyclidine (PCP)
- Propofol
- Quinine
- Salicylates
- Selective serotonin reuptake inhibitors
- Simvastatin
- Theophylline
- Toluene
- Zidovudine
▶ Connective tissue diseases
  - Polymyositis
  - Dermatomyositis
- Miscellaneous
  - Enzyme deficiencies
    ○ Carbohydrate metabolism
    ○ Lipid metabolism
  - Myopathies
  - Sickle cell anemia

Rheumatoid Factor

Antibodies in the serum of people with rheumatoid arthritis, reacting with antigenic determinants or immunoglobulins.

Reference range
< 30 IU/ml

Positive
▶ In normal persons
  Only relevant if present with symptoms
▶ Rheumatoid arthritis
▶ Autoimmune disease
  - Juvenile rheumatoid arthritis
  - Sjögren's syndrome
  - Systemic lupus erythematosus
  - Scleroderma
  - Polymyositis
  - Dermatomyositis
  - Cryoglobulinemia
  - Mixed connective tissue disease
  - Behçet's syndrome
▶ Infections
  - Bacterial endocarditis
  - Mononucleosis
  - Osteomyelitis
  - Hepatitis (acute and chronic)
  - Tuberculosis
  - Syphilis
  - After vaccination
▶ Lung diseases
  - Bronchitis
  - Asthma
  - Anthracosis
  - Asbestosis
  - Sarcoidosis
  - Diffuse interstitial pulmonary fibrosis
▶ Other diseases
  - Cirrhosis
  - Myocardial infarction
  - Neoplasm
  - Cryoglobulinemia

Right axis deviation
See ECG, Cardiac Axis → 116

Right bundle-branch block
See Cardiac Dysrhythmias → 62

Right-ventricular failure
See Heart Failure, Acute → 167
See Heart Failure, Chronic → 168

Salivary Gland Tumor
Neoplasm of the sailvary gland.
Benign
▶ Pleomorphic adenoma (mixed tumor)
▶ Monomorphic adenoma
▶ Warthin tumor (papillary cystadenoma)
▶ Sebaceous tumors
▶ Benign lymphoepithelial lesion
Malignant
▶ Mucoepidermoid carcinoma
▶ Malignant mixed tumor
▶ Squamous cell carcinoma
▶ Adenoid cystic carcinoma
▶ Adenocarcinoma

Salivary Glands, Enlargement
Unilateral enlargement
▶ Bacterial infection
▶ Chronic sialadenitis
▶ Obstruction of the salivary passages
▶ Salivary gland tumor
  • Benign
    ○ Pleomorphic adenoma (mixed tumor)
    ○ Monomorphic adenoma
    ○ Warthin's tumor
  • Malignant
    ○ Mucoepidermoid carcinoma
    ○ Adenoid cystic carcinoma
Bilateral enlargement
▶ Viral infections

  • EBV
  • Mumps
  • CMV
  • HIV
  • Coxsackie
▶ Sjögren's syndrome (→ 332)
▶ Amyloidosis
▶ Granulomatous diseases
  • Sarcoidosis
  • Tuberculosis
  • Lepra
▶ Hyperlipidemia
▶ Cirrhosis
▶ Acromegaly
▶ Anorexia

Salpingitis
See Pelvic Inflammatory Disease → 279

Schistocytes
See Erythrocyte, Morphology → 132

Sciatica
Relapsing, often acute pain in the lower back and hip radiating down the back of the thigh into the leg.
Skeletal
▶ Spinal stenosis
▶ Irritation of the spinal nerve root
  • Protruding disc
  • Herniated disc
▶ Spondylarthritis
  • Spondylarthritis deformans
  • Infections
    ○ Chlamydia
    ○ Yersinia
  • Concomitant inflammation in
    ○ Chronic inflammatory diseases
    ○ Whipple's disease
    ○ Sprue
▶ Spondylolisthesis
▶ Tumor
  • Osteosarcoma

- Multiple myeloma
- Metastases
▸ Paget's disease
▸ Osteoporosis
▸ Osteomalacia
▸ Secondary hyperparathyroidism
▸ (Stress) fracture
▸ Osteomyelitis
▸ Periostitis
▸ Neurofibromatosis
▸ Scheuermann's disease
▸ Chondrocalcinosis
▸ Renal osteopathy

Neurologic
▸ Spinal lesions
▸ Prolapsed disk
▸ Pinched nerves
▸ Radicular lesions (L4, L5, S1-S3)
▸ Radicular syndrome
- Borrelia radiculitis
▸ Lesion of the lumbosacral plexus
▸ Lesion of the peripheral nerves (ischial nerve, peroneal nerve)
- Mechanical effects
- Tumors of the nerves
- Toxins
- Drugs
- Incorrect injection
▸ Polyneuropathy
- Diabetes mellitus
▸ Sciatica as main or partial symptom of other neurologic disorders
- Intraspinal tumor
- Herpes zoster
- Jacksonian epilepsy
- Tabes dorsalis
- Multiple sclerosis
- McArdle's disease
- Sudeck's disease
- Encephalitis
- Meningitis
- Brachial plexus neuritis
- Anorectal spasm (episodic pain in the rectal area)
▸ Burning feet syndrome

- Hernias
- Coccygodynia (severe pain in the coccygeal region)

Joint-related
▸ Arthritis
▸ Arthrosis
▸ Periarthropathy
▸ Bursitis

Disorders of the muscles
▸ Fibromyalgia
▸ Myogelosis
▸ Scleroderma
▸ Dermatomyositis
▸ Piriformis syndrome

Vascular
▸ Leriche's syndrome
▸ Arteriosclerosis
▸ Abdominal aneurysm
▸ Acute deep vein thrombosis
▸ Arterial thrombosis
▸ Arterial embolism
▸ Varicosis
▸ Polyarteritis nodosa
▸ Hematoma
- Thrombophilia
- Anticoagulants
▸ Thrombophlebitis
▸ Post-thrombotic syndrome
▸ Acute lymphangitis
▸ Vasculitis
▸ Obliterating endarteritis
▸ Sudeck's atrophy
▸ Raynaud's syndrome
▸ Erythema nodosum
▸ Anterior tibial compartment syndrome

Miscellaneous
▸ Tumor
- Pancreatic cancer
- Prostate cancer
- Bladder cancer
- Retroperitoneal tumors
▸ Pelvic infections
- Cystitis
- Prostatitis

S

▶ Diseases of the urogenital system
  • Pyelonephritis
  • Urolithiasis
▶ Diseases of the gastrointestinal system
  • Diverticulitis
▶ Retroperitoneal fibrosis
▶ Abscess
▶ Gout
▶ Porphyria
▶ Infectious diseases

Sclera, Blue

Associated systemic disorders
▶ Osteogenesis imperfecta
▶ Marfan syndrome
▶ Ehlers-Danlos syndrome
▶ Crouzon syndrome (craniofacial dysostosis)
▶ Pagets disease (Pseudoxanthoma elasticum)
▶ Alkaptonuria
▶ Iron deficiency anemia
▶ Pectus excavatum
▶ Other rachitic skeletal defects

Associated eye disorders
▶ Myopia
▶ Scleral staphyloma
▶ Scleral ectasia
▶ Enlarged globe
▶ Infantile glaucoma
▶ Keratoconus

Sclera, Yellow

Causes
▶ Scleral icterus (See Bilirubin → 51)
  • Hepatopathy (→ 226)
    ○ Infectious hepatitis
    ○ Toxic hepatitis
  • Obstructiion of the bile ducts (→ 75)
  • Congenital non-hemolytic jaundice
    ○ Crigler-Najjar syndrome
    ○ Meulengracht's disease
    ○ Dubin-Johnson syndrome
  • Hemolytic jaundice
▶ Vitamin B_{12} deficiency (→ 378)
  • Pernicious anemia
▶ Vitamin A deficiency (→ 321)
▶ Quinacrine (discoloration near limbus)
▶ Yellow subscleral fat (in the area farthest from the limbus)

Scleritis, See Red Eye → 311

Scoliosis
Abnormal curvature of the spine. Spine curves to the side and each vertebrae also twists on the next one.

Nonstructural scoliosis
Temporary condition
▶ Leg length discrepancy (→ 219)
▶ Muscle spasms
▶ Local inflammation
▶ Appendicitis

Structural scolioisis
▶ Idiopathic (85%; appears in a previously straight spine, of unknown cause)
  • Infantile (0-3 years)
  • Juvenile (4 years to puberty)
  • Adolescent (puberty to epiphyseal closure)
▶ Skeletal dysplasia
  • Failure of formation (hemivertebrae)
  • Failure of segmentation (unilateral bar)
  • Mixed
▶ Neuromsucular
  • Neuropathic
    ○ Upper motor neuron lesions
      - Cerebral palsy
      - Syringomyelia
      - Spinal cord trauma
    ○ Lower motor neuron lesions.
      - Poliomyelitis
      - Spinal muscular atrophy
    ○ Dysautonomia (Riley-Day syndrome)
  • Myopathic
    ○ Arthrogryposis

- Muscular dystrophy
  - Other forms of myopathy
  - Friedreich's ataxia
▶ Congenital
  • Marfan's syndrome
  • Ehlers-Danlos syndrome
  • Neurofibromatosis (Von Recklinghausen's disease)
  • Morquio's disease
  • Amyoplasia congenita
  • Various types of dwarfism
  • Scheuermann's disease
  • Homocystinuria
  • Chondrodysplasia
  • Osteogenesis imperfecta
▶ Rheumatic
  • Rheumatoid arthritis
  • Still's disease
  • Bechterew's disease
  • Other rheumatic diseases of the spine
▶ Trauma
  • Fracture
  • Dislocation
  • Irradiation
  • Postoperative
  • Burns
▶ Metabolic
  • Osteoporosis (→ 266)
  • Osteomalacia
  • Rickets
▶ Neoplasm
  • Benign tumors
  • Malignant tumors
    - Multiple myeloma
    - Metastasis
▶ Infection
  • Tuberculosis of the spine
  • Salmonella infection of the spine
  • Brucella infection of the spine
▶ Hysterical

Scotoma

Isolated area within the visual field, in which vision is absent or depressed. Varying size and shape.

Central scotoma
▶ Macular degeneration (age related)
▶ Optic neuritis
▶ Ischemic optic neuropathy
▶ Macular hole
▶ Idiopathic central serous chorioretinopathy
▶ Leber's hereditary optic atrophy
▶ Achromatopsia

Peripheral scotoma
▶ Chronic glaucoma
▶ Pigmental degeneration
▶ Siderosis retinae
▶ Paraneoplastic retonopathy

Scintillating scotoma
▶ Migraine

Scrotal Pain

Torsion
▶ Testicular torsion
▶ Torsion of testicular appendage
▶ Torsion of spermatocele
▶ Torsion of cavernous lymphangioma

Vascular
▶ Infarction
▶ Thrombosis of the pampiniform plexus
▶ Thrombosis of the testicular artery
▶ Local hemorrhage
▶ Varicocele
▶ Polyarteritis nodosa
▶ Henoch-Schönlein purpura

Hernias
▶ Inguinal hernia
▶ Strangulated inguinal hernia
▶ Scrotal hernia

Trauma
▶ Blunt trauma
▶ Penetrating injury

S

Cystic lesions
► Hydrocele
► Gonocele
► Hematozele
► Dermoid cyst (children)

Inflammation, infection
► Epididymitis
► Orchitis (e.g. Mumps)
► Deferentitis
► Scrotal abscess
► Infective gangrene (Fournier's disease)
► Scrotal parasitosis
  • Lice
  • Scabies
► Cysticercosis
► Tick bite
► Venomous bite
► Contact dermatitis

Referred pain
► Pancreatitis
► Diverticulitis
► Acute appendicitis
► Lumbar radiculopathy

Neoplasm
► Seminoma
► Teratoma
► Chorion carcinoma
► Leydig cell tumors
► Sertoli call tumors
► Lymphomas
► Rhabdomyoblastoma
► Metastases

Familial mediterranean fever
See Priapism → 292

Scrotal Swelling

Causes
► Hydrocele
► Vascular disorders
  • Varicocele
  • Torsion of testis
  • Torsion of epididymis
  • Torsion of spermatic cord
  • Twisted echinococcus cyst

  • Polyarteritis nodosa
  • Henoch-Schönlein purpura
  • Thrombosis of spermatic veins
  • Infarction
  • Congestive heart failure
  • Lymphedema
► Neoplasm
  • Seminoma
  • Teratoma
  • Chorion carcinoma
  • Leydig cell tumor
  • Sertoli cell tumor
  • Lymphomas
  • Metastases
► Infection, inflammation
  • Orchitis
  • Acute epididymitis
  • Folliculitis
  • Scrotal abscess
  • Scrotal gangrene
  • Scrotal parasitosis
► Trauma
  • Trauma
  • Injury
  • Postoperative
► Hernia
  • Inguinal
  • Scrotal
► Spermatocele
► Sebaceous cyst
► Insect bite
► Drugs

Selenium

Selenium may reduce cancer risk.

Reference range

20 µg/dl

Decreased
► Malnutrition
► Parenteral nutrition
► Cirrhosis
► Muscular dystrophy
► Cardiomyopathy

Increased
▶ Uncontrolled self-medication
▶ Occupational intoxication
  • Electrical industry
  • Porcelain industry
  • Glass industry

Serum protein electrophoresis
See Protein in the Serum → 296

Sexual development, late,
See Pubertal Delay → 303

Sexual development, premature,
See Precocious Puberty → 292

Sexually Transmitted Diseases
STD
Genital ulcers
▶ Painful ulcers
  • Genital herpes (HSV)
  • Chancroid (Haemophilus ducreyi)
▶ Non-Painful ulcers
  • Granuloma inguinale
    (Calymmatobacterium granulomatis)
  • Lymphogranuloma venereum
    (Chlamydia trachomatis)
  • Syphilis (early, Treponema pallidum)
Non-ulcerative
▶ Non-gonococcal urethritis
▶ Pelvic inflammatory disease (→ 279)
▶ Gonorrhea (Neisseria gonorrhoeae)
▶ Chlamydia
▶ Syphilis (secondary, tertiary)
▶ Genital warts (Condylomata acuminata,
  HPV = Human Papillomavirus)
▶ HIV
▶ Hepatitis A, B, C
▶ Cytomegalovirus infection
▶ Pediculosis pubis (pubic louse)
▶ Scabies (Sarcoptes scabiei var. hominis)

Shock
Acute or subacute beginning, increasingly generalized circulatory collapse, characterized by microcirculation impairment.
Hypovolemic shock
▶ Hemorrhage
  • Upper and lower intestinal hemorrhage
  • Retroperitoneal and endoperitoneal hemorrhage
  • Soft tissue hemorrhage (fractures)
  • Hematothorax
  • Pneumonorrhagia
▶ Plasma losses
  • Peritonitis
  • Ascites
  • Pancreatitis
  • Skin diseases
    ○ Burns
    ○ Generalized dermatitis
  • Drainage of large effusions
▶ Water and electrolyte losses
  • Gastrointestinal fluid loss
    ○ Vomiting
    ○ Diarrhea
  • Renal fluid loss
    ○ Diabetes mellitus
    ○ Diabetes insipidus
    ○ Diuretics
    ○ Diuretic phase of acute renal failure
  • Excessive sweating without appropriate water supply
  • Ileus (→ 206)
Cardiogenic shock
▶ Myopathic processes
  • Acute myocardial infarction
  • Papillary muscle rupture/ ventricle septum rupture
  • Ventricular wall aneurysms
  • Decompensated cardiac vitium
  • Endocarditis
  • Myocarditis

- Dilated or restrictive cardiomyopathy
▶ Obstructive cardiac lesions
  - Critical valvular stenosis
  - Sever valvular insufficency
  - Hypertrophic cardiomayopathy
  - Atrial myxoma
  - Intracardiac or valvular thrombus
▶ Pericardial disease
  - Cardiac tamponade
  - Constrictive pericarditis
▶ Aortic lesion
  - Rupture
  - Acute dissection
▶ Occlusion of the vena cava
▶ Cardiac dysrhythmia
  ○ Braddysrhythmias
    - *Sinus bradycardia*
    - *High-degree AV block*
    - *Junctional rhythm*
  ○ Tachydysrhythmias
    - *Ventricular tachycardia*
    - *Atrial fibrillation with rapid ventricular response*
  ○ Asystole

Vascular obstructive shock
▶ Tension pneumothorax
▶ Massive pulmonary embolism
▶ Excessive positive pressure ventilation

Endocrine shock
▶ Hyperglycemia
  - Ketoacidotic coma
  - Hyperosmolar coma
▶ Hypoglycemia
  - Insulinoma
  - Iatrogenic
▶ Addisonian crisis
▶ Pheochromocytoma
▶ Hypothyroid coma
▶ Hyperthyroid coma
▶ Coma in hypo-/ hyperparathyroidism
▶ Pituary failure

Vasogenic shock
▶ Septic shock
  - Acute infections
    ○ After diagnostic and surgical

interventions
    ○ Open wounds
    ○ Burns
  - Chronic inflammation of the gastrointestinal tract and the bile ducts
  - Pneumonia
  - Chronic inflammation of the tonsils
  - Bladder /vein indwelling catheter
  - Artificial respiration
  - Systemic diseases with suppression of the immune system
  - Treatment with corticosteroids and chemotherapeutics

Anaphylactic shock
- Drugs
- Infusion of colloidal volume replacement solutions
- Contrast media
- Injection of sera
- Blood transfusions
- Insect bites

Neurogenic shock
- Cranio cerebral trauma
- Cerebrovascular insult
- Paraplegia
- Spinal anesthesia
- Severe pain
- Intoxication through drugs with central depressing effects

Miscellaneous
▶ Severe acidosis or alkalosis
▶ Hypo-/Hyperthermia
  - Hepatic failure

Shock, cardiogenic, See Shock → 329

Shock syndrome, toxic
See Toxic Shock Syndrome → 357

Shoulder, Frozen
Adhesive capsulitis, periarthritis humeroscapularis adhesiva
Painful limitation of motion in the shoulder due to inflammatory thickening of the capsule. Common cause of stiffness in the shoulder.
Causes
▶ Idiopathic
▶ Metabolic, endocrine
  • Diabetes mellitus
  • Hyperthyroidism
  • Hypertriglyceridemia
▶ Trauma, injury
  • Brachial plexus injury
  • Cervical spinal cord injury
▶ Neurologic
  • Cerebrovascular accident with upper extremity paresis
  • Parkinson disease
▶ Repetitive movements of the upper extremities
▶ After active glenohumeral synovitis
▶ Inflammatory, rheumatologic
  • Rheumatic fever
  • Rheumatoid arthritis
  • Still's disease
  • Felty's syndrome
  • Reiter's disease
  • Caplan's syndrome
  • Postoperative immobilization of the shoulder

Shoulder Pain
Musculoskeletal
▶ Shoulder impingement syndrome
▶ Rotator cuff tear
▶ Fracture
  • Clavicle
  • Scapula
  • Humeral
▶ Shoulder degenerative joint disease

  • Acromioclavicular joint
  • Glenohumeral joint
▶ Shoulder instability
  • Shoulder subluxation
  • Recurrent anterior shoulder dislocation
  • Recurrent posterior shoulder dislocation
▶ Adhesive capsulitis (shoulder, frozen)
▶ Acromioclavicular joint separation
▶ Biceps tendonitis
▶ Tear of long head of biceps
▶ Diffuse shoulder strain
Abdominal (referred pain)
▶ Abdominal trauma
  • Ruptured spleen
  • Liver injury
  • Pancreas injury
  • Kidney injury
▶ Peptic ulcer disease with perforation
▶ Subphrenic abscess
▶ Diaphragmatic pleurisy
▶ Acute pancreatitis
▶ Appendicitis (with peritonitis)
▶ Liver abscess
▶ Cholelithiasis
▶ Perihepatic inflammation (Fitz-Hugh-Curtis syndrome)
Thoracic
▶ Cardiac
  • Pericarditis
  • Myocardial infarction
▶ Pulmonary
  • Carcinoma
  • Pneumonia
  • Abscess
▶ Pancoast tumor
▶ Hiatal hernia
Neoplasm
▶ Malignancy
  • Thyroid
  • Breast
  • Lung
  • Kidney
  • Hodgkin's lymphoma

- Prostate
- Bone metasteses
  - Multiple myeloma

Miscellaneous
► Paget's disease
► Herpes zoster
► Brachial neuritis
► Cervical disc syndrome
► Shoulder-Band syndrome
► Carpal tunnel

SIADH
Syndrome of inappropriate secretion of antidiuretic hormone
Continued secretion of antidiuretic hormone despite low serum osmolality and expanded extracellular volume.

Neoplasm
► Lung carcinoma
► Bronchial adenoma
► Pancreas carcinoma
► Duodenum carcinoma
► Carcinoid
► Ewing's sarcoma
► Ovary carcinoma
► Mesothelioma
► Thymoma

Head trauma

Infections
► Bacterial, viral pneumonia
► Lung abscess
► Brain abscess
► Lung cavitation (aspergillosis)
► Tuberculosis
► Meningitis
► Encephalitis
► AIDS

Vascular
► Stroke
► Cavernosus sinus thrombosis

Neurologic
► Guillain-Barré syndrome/Polyradiculitis
► Multiple sclerosis
► Delirium tremens
► Amyotropic lateral sclerosis
► Hydrocephalus
► Psychosis
► Peripheral neuropathy

Congenital
► Agenesis corpus callosum
► Midline defects

Metabolic
► Acute intermittent porphyria

Pulmonary
► Asthma
► Pneumothorax
► Positive pressure respiration

Drugs
► Carbamazepine
► Chlorpropamide
► Cyclophosphamide
► DDAVP
► Monoamine oxidase inhibitors
► Narcotics
► Nicotine
► Oxytocin
► Phenothiazines
► SSRIs
► Tricyclic antidepressants
► Vasopressin
► Vincristine

Sicca Syndrome
Sjögren's syndrome
Syndrome of keratoconjunctivitis sicca, dry mouth (See Xerostomia → 384), dryness of mucous membranes, telangiectasia, and bilateral parotid enlargement (See Salivary Glands, Enlargement → 324).

Associated with
► Autoimmune disorders
  • Rheumatoid arthritis
  • Scleroderma
  • Polymyositis
  • Polyarteritis nodosa
  • Hashimoto thyroiditis

- Chronic hepatobiliary cirrhosis
- Lymphocytic interstitial pneumonitis
- Thrombocytopenic purpura
- Hypergammaglobulinemia
- Waldenström's macroglobulinemia
- Progressive systemic sclerosis
- Dermatomyositis
- Interstitial nephritis
▸ Hepatopathy
- Hepatitis
- Primary biliary cirrhosis

Sickle cells
See Erythrocyte, Morphology → 132

Single Stranded DNA Antibody
Anti-ssDNA
See Autoantibodies in Connective Tissue Diseases → 47
Positive in
▸ Systemic lupus erythematosus
▸ Mixed connective tissue disorders (MCTD)
▸ Sjögren's syndrome
▸ Scleroderma
▸ Polymositis

Sinus bradycardia
See Cardiac Dysrhythmias → 62

Sinus tachycardia
See Cardiac Dysrhythmias → 62

Sjögren's syndrome
See Sicca Syndrome → 332

Skin Changes, Skin Lesions
Cutaneous changes
See Drug Eruptions → 105
Paleness, white skin
▸ Generalized
- Albinism

- Anemia
- Pituitary insufficiency
- Chronic renal failure
▸ Localized
- Vitiligo
- Raynaud's syndrome
Dry skin
▸ Hypothyroidism
▸ Atopic
▸ Chronic renal failure
Red skin (Erythema)
▸ Generalized
- Fever
- Polycythemia
- Urticaria
- Viral exanthems
- Cushing's disease
- Hypertension
- Alcohol abuse
- Diabetes mellitus
- Carcinoid syndrome
- Mitral facies
▸ Localized
- Inflammation
- Infection
- Raynaud's syndrome
Yellow skin
▸ Generalized
- Liver disease
- Chronic renal disease
- Anemia
- Hypothyroidism
- Carotene (in vegetable)
- Drugs
▸ Localized
- Resolving hematoma
- Infection
- Peripheral vascular insufficiency
Blue skin
▸ Lips, mouth, nail beds
- Cardiovascular disease
- Pumonary disease
- Raynaud's syndrome

S

Brown skin
▶ Generalized
  • Pituitary disease
  • Adrenal disease
  • Liver disease
▶ Localized
  • Nevi
  • Neurofibromatosis

Thin skin
▶ Cushing's disease

Thick skin
▶ Dermatosclerosis
▶ Acromegaly
▶ Hypothyroidism

Spider nevi
▶ Hepatopathy (→ 226)

Bleeding
See Purpura → 309

Pustules
▶ Acne vulgaris
▶ Rosacea
▶ Bacterial folliculitis
▶ Fungal folliculitis
▶ Candidiasis

Pustule-like lesions (white papules)
▶ Milia
▶ Keratosis pilaris
▶ Molluscum contagiosum

Bullous
▶ Pemphigus vulgaris
▶ Bullous pemphigoid
▶ Pemphigus foliaceus
▶ Paraneoplastic pemphigus
▶ Cicatricial pemphigoid
▶ Erythema multiforme (Stevens-Johnson syndrome)
▶ Dermatitis herpetiformis
▶ Herpes gestationis
▶ Impetigo
▶ Erosive lichen planus
▶ Porphyria cutanea tarda
▶ Linear IgA bullous dermatosis
▶ Epidermolysis bullosa acquisita

Skin Crepitation

Crepitations can be described as a noise similar to the rustling of a paper bag heard on chest auscultation.

Causes
▶ Cutaneous emphysema
  • Lung trauma
  • Rib fracture
  • Thorax fracture
  • Central venous catheter placement
▶ Mediastinal emphysema
▶ Boerhaave's syndrome
▶ Gas gangrene

Sleep disorders, See Insomnia → 212,
See Hypersomnia → 194,
See Narcolepsy → 252

Smell Loss, Smell Aberrations

Hyposmia, anosmia, olfactory anesthesia/dysesthesia, olfactory dysfunction
Loss or impairment of the sense of smell.
See Parosmia → 277

Most common causes
▶ Nasal, sinus disease
▶ Viral upper respiratory infection (URIs)
▶ Idiopathic
▶ Head trauma

Conductive defects
▶ Inflammation
  • Viral upper respiratory infection
  • Rhinitis
    ○ Allergic
    ○ Acute
    ○ Toxic (e.g. cocaine)
    ○ Chronic
  • Chronic sinusitis (progressive mucosal disease)
  • Infection
    ○ Influenza
    ○ Viral hepatitis

- Bronchial asthma
- Sarcoidosis
- Wegener granulomatosis
▶ Tumor
  - Nasal polyposis
  - Inverting papilloma
  - Malignancies
▶ Trauma
  - Septal deviation
  - Accumulation of blood
  - Accumulation of cerebrospinal fluid
▶ Developmental abnormalities
  - Encephalocele
  - Dermoid cyst
  - Septal deviation
▶ Iatrogenic
  - Laryngectomy
  - Tracheotomy

Central, sensorineural defects
▶ Inflammation
  - Viral infection
  - Sarcoidosis
  - Multiple sclerosis
▶ Congenital
  - Kallman syndrome
▶ Nutritional deficiencies
  - Vitamin A
  - Vitamin B_{12}
  - Thiamine
  - Zinc
▶ Endocrine, metabolic
  - Diabetes mellitus
  - Hypothyroidism
  - Hypoadrenalism
  - Cushing's syndrome
▶ Normal aging
▶ Neurologic
  - Head trauma
  - Subarachnoid hemorrhage
  - Brain surgery
  - Frontal brain tumor
    ○ Meningeoma
  - Frontal lobe aneurysm
  - Multiple sclerosis
  - Parkinson's disease

- Alzheimer's disease
▶ Drugs, toxins
  - Alcohol
  - Aminoglycosides
  - Formaldehyde
  - Nasal sprays
  - Nicotine
  - Organic solvents
  - Zinc sulfate (direct application)
▶ Miscellaneous
  - Renal failure
  - Hepatitis

Smooth Muscle Antibody

Normal: negative
Positive
▶ Titer >1:80
  - Chronic active hepatitis
▶ Titer <1:80
  - Primary biliary cirrhosis
  - Epstein–Barr virus infection (EBV)
  - Cytomegalovirus infection (CMV)

Snoring

Rough, rattling, inspiratory noises made on inspiration during sleep by vibration of the soft palate and the uvula.
Intrinsic factors
▶ Structural
  - Small jaw
  - Enlarged tongue
  - Thick and long soft palate
  - Enlarged tonsils
  - Enlarged adenoids
  - Loose and easily collapsible side walls in the portion of the upper airway directly behind the soft palate
  - Thickening of the muscles in front of spinal column
  - Nasal septum deviation
  - Small nasal valves
  - Decreased lung volumes
    ○ Obesity

S

- ○ Chest deformity
- ▶ Inflammation
  - Sinusitis
  - Tonsillitis
  - Hyperplasia of the tonsils
  - Bronchitis
  - Eustachian tube infection
- ▶ Neuromuscular
  - Insensitivity to higher than normal concentrations of carbon dioxide in the blood
  - Weakness due to problems with nerves and/or muscles
- ▶ Endocrine
  - Hypothyroidism
  - Gigantism
- ▶ Allergies
- ▶ Sleep apnea

Extrinsic factors
- ▶ Smoking
- ▶ Inhalation of other irritants
- ▶ Chronic exposure to allergens
- ▶ Alcohol abuse
- ▶ Sedatives

Associated factors
- ▶ Obesity
- ▶ Lack of fitness
- ▶ Aging
- ▶ Loss of general muscle tone

Sodium

Sodium is the essential electrolyte in the extracellular space (ECS), as potassium is in the intracellular space. Sodium and its anions provide more than 90% of the osmotic pressure in the plasma. Due to the free water flow through the cell membrane, the volume of ECS is directly dependent on the total concentration of sodium in the serum. Through the free water flow, changes of the serum sodium (SS) indirectly cause changes in osmolality and volume in the intracellular space (ICS) (dehydration). Usually the SS is held within very tight limits by the organism.

Reference range

135-145 mmol/l
See Hyponatremia → 203
See Hypernatremia → 193

Somatotropic hormone
See Growth Hormone → 159

Sore Throat

Pharyngitis
Infection
- ▶ Bacterial infection
  - Group A Streptococci
  - Pneumococcus
  - Staphylococcus aureus
  - Haemophilus influenzae
  - Moraxella catarrhalis
  - Other Streptococci
  - Neisseria gonorrhoeae
  - Chlamydia pneumoniae
  - Klebsiella
  - Moraxella
  - Mycoplasma
  - Corynebacterium diphtheriae
  - Mycobacterium
  - Tonsillitis
  - Tonsil abscess
  - Ludwig's angina
- ▶ Viruses
  - Rhinovirus
  - Coronavirus
  - Adenovirus
  - Influenza
  - Parainfluenza
  - Epstein-Barr virus (Mononucleosis)
  - Coxsackievirus
  - Cytomegalovirus (CMV)
  - Herpes simplex virus (HSV)
  - Respiratory syncytial virus (RSV)
  - Mumps
  - Rabies

▶ Fungal
  • Candida albicans
  • Rhinosporidium
  • Cryptococcus
  • Histoplasma
  • Blastomyces
  • Paracoccidioides

Other inflammation, infection
▶ Laryngitis
▶ Thyroiditis
▶ Retropharyngeal abscess
▶ Tracheobronchitis
▶ Cervical phlegmon
▶ Stomatitis (contact stomatitis)
▶ Epiglottitis
▶ Allergic rhinitis
▶ Sinusitis

Malignancy
▶ Leukemia
▶ Lymphoma
▶ Squamous cell carcinoma
▶ Tonsil carcinoma

Autoimmune, allergic reaction
▶ Behçet's syndrome
▶ Reiter's syndrome
▶ Kawasaki's disease
▶ Erythema multiforme
▶ Pemphigus

Chemical, physical
▶ Smoke
▶ Environmental pollutants (smog)
▶ Gastroesophageal reflux
▶ Chemical burns
▶ Caustic ingestion
▶ Drug related (e.g. Aspirin)
▶ Thermal injury (Hot foods or liquids)
▶ Toxins

Iatrogenic
▶ Tonsillectomy
▶ Airway management during surgery
▶ Chemotherapy
▶ Radiation

Trauma
▶ Accidents

▶ Child abuse
▶ Scrape from bone fragment

Speech disturbance, See Aphasia → 39

Sperm, See Azoospermia, Oligospermia → 48, See Impotence → 208

Spherocytes
See Erythrocyte, Morphology → 132

Spinal Tumors
Tumors of the spine, spinal neoplasms
Benign primary
▶ Osteoid osteoma
▶ Eosinophilic granuloma
▶ Aneurysmal bone cyst
▶ Osteoblastoma
Malignant primary
▶ Sarcoma
▶ Multiple myeloma
Metastatic tumors of the spine
▶ Breast cancer
▶ Lung cancer
▶ Renal cancer
▶ Prostate cancer
▶ Thyroid cancer
▶ Lymphoma

Splenomegaly
Abnormal enlargement of the spleen.
Immune hyperplasia
▶ Infections
  • AIDS
  • Bacterial septicemia
  • Brucellosis
  • Congenital syphilis
  • Cytomegalovirus
  • Epstein-Barr virus infection
  • Ehrlichiosis
  • Fungal infections
  • Histoplasmosis

S

- Infectious endocarditis
- Infectious mononucleosis
- Leishmaniasis (Kala-azar)
- Malaria
- Q fever
- Schistosomiasis
- Splenic abscess
- Subacute bacterial endocarditis
- Syphilis
- Toxoplasmosis
- Trypanosomiasis
- Tuberculosis
- Typhoid fever/ parathyphoid
- Viral hepatitis
- Weil's disease
► Autoimmune
  - Angioimmunoblastic lymphadenopathy
  - Castleman's syndrome
  - Collagen vascular diseases
  - Drugs
    ◦ Interleukin-2
  - Felty's syndrome (splenomegaly with rheumatoid arthritis and leukopenia)
  - Immune hemolytic anemias
  - Immune neutropenias
  - Immune thrombocytemias
  - Rheumatoid arthritis
  - Sarcoidosis
  - Serum sickness
  - Still's disease (juvenile form of rheumatoid arthritis)
  - Systemic lupus erythematosus
  - Thyrotoxicosis (benign lymphoid hypertrophy)

Reticuloendothelial system hyperplasia
► Hemolytic anemia
  - Autoimmune hemolytic anemia
  - Hereditary spherocytosis
  - Hemoglobinopathy
  - Early sickle cell anemia
  - Ovalucytosis
► Nutritional anemias
► Thalassemia major
► Paroxysmal nocturnal hemoglobinuria

► Idiopathic thrombocytopenic purpura (Werlhof's disease)

Extramedullary hematopoesis
► Myelofibrosis
► Bone marrow damage
  - Radiation
  - Toxins
► Bone marrow infiltration
  - Gaucher's disease
  - Leukemias
  - Tumors

Increased splenic or portal blood flow
► Cirrhosis
► Vein obstruction
  - Hepatic vein obstruction
  - Portal vein obstruction
    ◦ Intrahepatic
    ◦ Extrahepatic
  - Splenic vein obstruction
► Cavernous transformation of the portal vein
► Splenic artery aneurysm
► Heart disorder
  - Congestive heart failure
  - Constrictive pericarditis
► Myeloid metaplasia
► Vinyl chloride
► Hepatic infection
  - Hepatic echinococcosis
  - Hepatic schistosomiasis
► Portal hypertension

Infiltration of the spleen
► Depositions
  - Gaucher's disease
  - Niemann-Pick disease
  - Amyloidosis
  - Tangier disease
  - Letterer-Siwe disease
  - Hurler's syndrome (mucopolysaccharidoses)
  - Hyperlipidemias
► Cellular infiltration
  - Leukemias
    ◦ Acute
    ◦ Chronic

- ○ Lymphoid
- ○ Myeloid
- ○ Monocytic
- Lymphomas
  - ○ Hodgkin's lymphomas
  - ○ Non-Hodgkin's lymphoma
- Myeloproliferative syndrome s
  - ○ Chronic myelocytic leukemia
  - ○ Polycythemia very
  - ○ Idiopathic thrombocythemia
  - ○ Osteomyelosclerosis
- Metastatic tumors (melanoma)
- Eosinophilic granuloma
- Angiosarcomas
- Hemangiomas
- Lymphangiomas
- Fibromas
- Lympho-reticulosarkoma
- Hamartomas
- Splenic cysts
- Histiocytosis

Miscellaneous
▶ FUO (fever of unknown origin) with splenomegaly
▶ Idiopathic splenomegaly
▶ Iron-deficiency anemia

Sputum
Expectoration
Mucus or mucopurulent matter, expectorated in diseases of the air passages.
Bloody sputum
▶ Blood streaked sputum
- Upper respiratory inflammation
  - ○ Nose
  - ○ Nasopharynx
  - ○ Gums
  - ○ Larynx
  - ○ Severe coughing (→ 87)
- Trauma
▶ Pink sputum
- Pneumonia
- Pulmonary edema

▶ Heavy bleeding
See Hemoptysis → 175
Purulent
Yellow, green or dirty gray.
▶ Small amounts
- Upper respiratory disease
  - ○ Acute sinusitis
  - ○ Allergic rhinitis
  - ○ Chronic bronchitis
- Pneumonia
- Tuberculosis
  - ○ Cavity
- Lung abscess
▶ Large amounts
- Lung abscess
- Bronchiectasis
- Bronchopleural fistula
Rusty sputum
▶ Pneumococcal pneumonia
Sputum with feculent odor
▶ Anaerobic infection
▶ Bronchiectasis
Viscous-glassy
▶ Acute bronchitis
▶ Pertussis
▶ Bronchial asthma
- Curschmann's spirals (twisted masses of mucus in the sputum in asthma)
▶ Pulmonary eosinophilia
Watery
▶ Aspiration
▶ Fistula

Steatorrhea
Fatty stool
Excretion of unabsorbed lipids with the stool. Steatorrhea is regarded as a screening test for malassimilation → 233 (maldigestion and malabsorption).
Exocrine pancreatic insufficiency See Pancreatic Insufficiency, Exocrine → 269
▶ Chronic pancreatitis
▶ Pancreas tumor

Lack of conjugated bile acids
► Obstructive icterus
► Cholestasis
► Liver parenchyma damage
► Ileectomy
► Bacterial colonization of the thin bowel in stasis syndrome

Thin bowel disorders
► After intestinal surgery (small intestine)
► Resection
► Intestinal fistula
► Diseases of the ileum with reduced gall resorption
► Whipple's disease
► Amyloidosis in the area of the intestine
► Chronic inflammatory bowel diseases
► Intestinal lymphangiectasis
► Celiac sprue
► Tropical sprue
► Occlusion of the mesenteric lymph vessels
► Intestinal lymphomas
► After radiation therapy

Drugs
► Orlistat (with dietary restrictions)

Infection
► Tuberculosis
► Parasites

Endocrine
► Diabetes mellitus
► Hyperthyroidism
► Carcinoid
► Hyperparathyroidism
► Gastrinoma
► Verner-Morrison syndrome

Miscellaneous
► Abetalipoproteinemia
► Cystic fibrosis
► Mastocytosis
► Food allergy
► Acanthocytosis
► Dermatosclerosis
► Idiopathic

Stippling, basophil
See Erythrocyte, Morphology → 132

Stones, See Nephrolithiasis → 255,
See Urolithiasis → 371

Strabismus

Manifest lack of parallelism of the visual axes of the eyes. See Heterophoria → 181

Nonparalytic (concomitant) strabismus
► Refractive anomaly
  • Hyperopia (especially in esotropia)
► Anatomical
  • Abnormality of the orbita
  • Malformation of the lateral muscles
► Fusion disorder
► Anisometropia
► Congenital ptosis
► Retinopathy of prematurity
► Toxoplasmosis
► CNS impairment

Paralytic (nonconcomitant) strabismus
► Neurogenic
  • Congenital nuclear aplasia
  • Cerebral circulation disorders
  • Hemorrhage
  • Encephalomyelitis
  • Neoplasm
  • Syphilis
  • Multiple sclerosis
► Myogenic
  • Myositis
  • Mechanical
    ◦ Blow-out fracture

Stress Fracture

Fracture resulting from force on a bony structure during use as opposed to one resulting from exogenous trauma.

Causes, risk factors
► Extrinsic
  • Excess training

- Increases in intensity, frequency
- Cigarette smoking
- Inadequate nutrition
  - Calories
  - Calcium
- Worn-out shoes
- Changes in training surface
- Musculoskeletal disorder
- Over pronators or supinators
- Hallux valgus
- Genu varum
- Genu valgus
- Leg length discrepancy
- External hip rotation
- Osteoarthritis
- Osteoporosis
  - Senile
  - Acromegaly
  - Diabetes mellitus
  - Cushing's syndrome
  - Long-term glucocorticoid therapy
  - Menopause
  - Long inactivity through immobilization
- Osteomalacia
- Osteogenesis imperfecta
- Juvenile bone cyst
- Joint replacement
- Rheumatoid arthritis
- Pyrophosphate arthropathy
- Tendonitis
- Muscle fatigue
- Muscle strain
- Herniated intervertebral disc
- Infections
- Chronic osteomyelitis
- Subacute osteomyelitis
- Neoplasm
- Primary benign bone neoplasm
  - Osteoid osteoma
  - Osteoblastoma
  - Eosinophilic granuloma
- Primary malignant bone neoplasm
  - Osteosarcoma
- Metastatic neoplasm
  - Breast cancer
  - Prostate cancer
  - Multiple myeloma
- ▶ Nerve compression syndromes
  - Tarsal tunnel syndrome
  - Carpal tunnel syndrome
  - Ulnar tunnel syndrome
- ▶ Miscellaneous
  - Genetic predisposition
  - Systemic lupus erythematosus
  - Renal disease
  - Hormonal irregularities
  - Hyperparathyroidism
  - Hypertrophic pulmonary osteoarthropathy
  - Reticular cell proliferation
    - Hand-Schüller-Christian disease
    - Gaucher's disease

Stress incontinence
See Urinary Incontinence → 365

Striae Distensae
Striae atrophica, stretch marks
Common skin dermatosis with linear dermal scars accompanied by epidermal atrophy, mostly due to continuous and progressive stretching.
Causes
- ▶ Pregnancy
- ▶ Puberty
- ▶ Lactation
- ▶ Weight lifting
- ▶ Obesity
- ▶ Cirrhosis
- ▶ Cushing's syndrome
- ▶ Ehlers-Danlos syndrome
- ▶ Drugs
  - ACTH
  - Estrogens
  - Glucocorticoids
  - Progesterone
  - Topical corticosteroid overuse
- ▶ Infection

S

- Influenza
- Paratyphoid
- Scarlet fever
- Tuberculosis
- Typhoid fever

Stridor

A high-pitched respiratory sound due to constriction or obstruction of the upper airways. See Stridor in Children → 342

Inspiratory stridor
Stenosis in the upper airways

▶ Congenital
- Choanal atresia
- Maxillo-facial dysplasia
- Vascular anomalies (e.g vascular ring)
- Laryngeal or tracheal abnormalities
- Laryngomalacia
- Tracheomalacia (expiratory stridor)
- Bronchomalacia (expiratory stridor)

▶ Inflammation
- Laryngo-tracheo bronchitis (Croup)
- Epiglottitis
- Bacterial tracheitis
- Tonsillitis
- Peritonsillar abscess
- Retropharyngeal abscess
- Diphtheria

▶ Tumor
- Laryngeal papillomas
- Hemangioma
- Larynx carcinoma
- Vocal cord cancer
- Nasal polyp
- Enlarged tonsils or adenoids

▶ Compression
- Nasal septum deviation
- Aortic aneurysm
- Goiter
- Mediastinal tumor
- Neck or face swelling

▶ Neurologic
- Vocal cord paralysis
- Aspiration

- Nerve paresis

▶ Trauma, injury
- Foreign body aspiration
- Facial fracture
- Mandibular fracture
- Laryngeal fracture
- Subglottic stenosis
- Inhalation injury (smoke)
- Scar stenosis

▶ Iatrogenic
- Neck surgery
- Prolonged intubation (breathing tube)
- After radiaton
- Diagnostic tests
  ○ Bronchoscopy
  ○ Laryngoscopy

▶ Allergy
- Spasmodic croup
- Angioneurotic edema

▶ Miscellaneous
- Laryngospasm in tetany
- Secretions (sputum)

Expiratory stridor
Stenosis in trachea, bronchi
- Bronchitis
- Bronchial asthma
- Emphysema
- Foreign body aspiration
- Compression of the bronchi due to lymph node enlargement

Inspiratory and expiratory stridor
- Tracheobronchitis
- Pneumonia
- Pneumothorax
- Tumor infiltration
- Pleura processes

Stridor in Children

See Stridor → 342

Acute stridor
▶ Laryngotracheobronchitis (croup)
▶ Aspiration of foreign body
- Nuts
- Hot dogs

- Popcorn
▶ Bacterial tracheitis
▶ Retropharyngeal abscess
▶ Peritonsillar abscess
▶ Acute spasmodic laryngitis (Croup)
▶ Allergic reaction
▶ Epiglottitis

Chronic stridor
▶ Laryngomalacia
▶ Subglottic stenosis
▶ Vocal cord dysfunction
▶ Laryngeal webs
▶ Laryngeal cysts
▶ Laryngeal hemangiomas
  - Glottic
  - Subglottic
▶ Laryngeal papillomas
▶ Tracheomalacia
▶ Tracheal stenosis
▶ Extrinsic causes
  - Vascular rings
  - Double aortic arch
▶ Choanal atresia

Stroke
See Cerebrovascular Accident → 71

Struma, See Goiter → 156

Subarachnoid hemorrhage
See Bleeding, Intracranial → 56

Sudden Death

Death within 60 minutes after onset of symptoms, usually without warning symptoms. Usually result of coronary heart disease (80%).

Cardiac
▶ Coronary artery disease
  - After myocardial infarction (most frequent cause of death)
  - Coronary sclerosis
  - Spasms

- Embolism
- Arteritis
▶ Valvular heart disease
  - Aortic stenosis
  - Mitral valve prolapse
  - Rupture of the papillary muscles
▶ Myocardial disease
  - Cardiomyopathy (10 %)
  - Myocarditis
  - Ventricle rupture
▶ Aute cardiac tamponade
▶ Stokes-Adams syndrome
▶ Cardiac arrhythmias
  - Preexcitation syndromes
    ○ Wolff-Parkinson-White
  - Complete atrioventricular block
  - Prolonged Q-T interval syndrome
  - Arrhythmogenic right-ventricular dysplasia
▶ Drugs
  - Antidysrhythmic drugs
  - β2 stimulators
  - Digitalis
  - Drug abuse
    ○ Cocaine
  - Tricyclic antidepressants

Pulmonary
▶ Pulmonary embolism
▶ Status asthmaticus
▶ Tension pneumothorax
▶ Asphyxia
▶ Hypoxia
▶ Hypercapnia

Metabolic
▶ Hypokalemia
▶ Hyperkalemia
▶ Hypercalcemia
▶ Thyrotoxicosis

Miscellaneous
▶ Dissecting aneurysm of the aorta
▶ Apoplexy
▶ Shock of every genesis
▶ SIDS
▶ Pickwickian syndrome

Superior Vena Cava Syndrome
Superior vena cava obstruction
Obstruction of the superior vena cava with edema and engorgement of the vessels of face, neck, and arms, also causing nonproductive cough and dyspnea.

Malignancy
▶ Bronchogenic carcinoma (80%)
▶ Malignant lymphoma (15%)
▶ Metastases
  • Breast carcinoma
  • Testicular seminoma

Benign disease
▶ Mediastinal disorder
  • Idiopathic mediastinal fibrosis
  • Histoplasmosis
  • Actinomycosis
  • Tuberculosis
  • Syphilis
▶ Vena cava thrombosis
  • Idiopathic
  • Behçet's syndrome
  • Polycythemia vera
  • Paroxysmal nocturnal hemoglobinuria
  • Long-term venous catheter
  • Shunts
  • Pacemakers
▶ Benign mediastinal tumor
  • Aortic aneurysm
  • Dermoid tumor
  • Retrosternal goiter
  • Sarcoidosis
▶ Cardiac
  • Right ventricular failure
  • Constrictive pericarditis
  • Pericardial tamponade

Syncope
Fainting, faintness
Sudden, reversible loss of consciousness and postural tone due to diminished cerebral blood flow.

Circulatory causes
▶ Inadequate vasoconstriction
  • Orthostatic reaction
  • Vagovasal syncope
  • Autonomic insufficiency
  • Sympathectomy
    ○ Drugs (see below)
    ○ Surgery
  • Carotid sinus syndrome
  • Hyperbradykininemia
▶ Hypovolemia
  • Blood loss
  • Addison's disease
▶ Mechanical reduction of venous return
  • Valsalva maneuver
  • Cough
  • Micturition
  • Defecation
  • Atrial myxoma
  • Valve thrombus
▶ Reduced cardiac output
  • Arrhythmias
    ○ Bradyarrhythmias
      - *Atrioventricular block*
      - *Ventricular asystole*
      - *Sinus bradycardia*
      - *Sick sinus syndrome*
    ○ Tachyarrhythmias
      - *Supraventricular tachycardia*
      - *Ventricular tachycardia*
    ○ Pacemaker malfunction
  • Reducesd left ventricular outflow
    ○ Aortic stenosis

- Hypertrophic subaortic stenosis
- Reducesd pulmonary flow
  - Pulmonary stenosis
  - Pulmonary embolism
  - Pulmonary hypertension
- Myocardial infarction
- Cardiac tamponade
- Carotid sinus hypersensitivity
- Heart failure
▶ Other vascular causes
- Subclavian steal syndrome
- Aortic dissection
- Arteriosclerosis of the carotid
- Arteriosclerosis of cerebral vessels
- Transient ischemic attacks (TIA)
- Hypertensive encephalopathy (diffuse spasms of cerebral vessels)
- Takayasu's arteritis
- Cervical spine abnormalities

Miscellaneous
- Anemia
- Heat
- Hyperventilation
- Hypoglycemia
- Hypoxia

Drugs
- Adriamycin
- Alphablockers
- Antiarrhythmics
- Antihypertensives
- Barbiturates
- Betablockers
- Digitalis
- Diuretics
- Hydralazine
- Nitrates
- Ophthalmic betablockers
- Opiates
- Phenothiazines
- Recreational drugs
  - Alcohol
  - Ecstasy
  - Methamphetamine
- Sedatives
- Tricyclic antidepressants

Neurologic, psychologic DDx
- Seizures
- Emotional impairment
- Anxiety
- Hysteric attacks

Syndrome of inappropriate secretion of antidiuretic hormone, See SIADH → 332

T_3, See Thyroxin (T_4) → 354
See Hyperthyroidism → 196
See Hypothyroidism → 206

T_4, See Thyroxin (T_4) → 354
See Hyperthyroidism → 196
See Hypothyroidism → 206

Tachycardia
See Cardiac Dysrhythmias → 62

Tachypnea, See Dyspnea → 112

Target cells
See Erythrocyte, Morphology → 132

Tarry stool
See Gastrointestinal Bleeding → 152

Taste Loss, Taste Aberrations

Ageusia/dysgeusia, gustatory anesthesia/dysesthesia, gustatory dysfunction
Loss or impairment of the sense of taste.

Causes
▶ Primary defects in olfaction (smell disorder alters flavor)
▶ Upper respiratory tract infection
▶ Central lesion
  - Head trauma
  - Tumor
▶ Idiopathic

- Normal aging
- Disorders of the oral cavity
  - Oral infection, inflammation
    - Viral infection
      - *Influenza*
    - Bacterial infection
    - Fungal infection
    - Parasitic infection
  - Poor oral hygiene
  - Dentures or other palatal prostheses
  - Malignancies
  - Radiation-induced mucositis
- Surgery
  - Laryngectomy
  - Resection of the tongue
  - Resection of portions of the oral cavity
  - Otologic surgery
    - Stretching of chorda tympani nerve
- Nutritional deficiencies
  - Vitamin B$_{12}$
  - Zinc
  - Copper
  - Nickel
  - Anorexia
  - Malabsorption
  - Increased urinary losses
- Endocrine, metabolic
  - Diabetes mellitus
  - Hypogonadism
  - Cushing's syndrome
  - Hypothyroidism
  - Pseudohypoparathyroidism
  - Menstruation (hormonal changes)
  - Pregnancy (hormonal changes)
- Heredity
  - Disability to taste bitter (phenylthiourea)
  - Familial dysautonomia (e.g. Riley-Day syndrome)
- Neurologic
  - Head trauma
  - Multiple sclerosis
  - Bell's palsy (facial paralysis)
  - Herpes zoster infection of the geniculate ganglion
  - Cholesteatoma
  - Thalamic lesions
  - Uncal lesions
- Psychiatric
  - Depression
- Drugs, toxins
  - Alcohol
  - Allopurinol
  - Antirheumatics
  - Azetazolamide
  - Captopril
  - Clofibrate
  - Hot beverages
  - L-dopa
  - Lithium
  - Metronidazole
  - Smoking
  - Tetracycline
  - Tricyclic antidepressants
- Miscellaneous
  - Cancer
  - Lichen planus
  - Erythema multiforme
  - Aglycogeusia
  - Sjögren syndrome
  - Renal failure (uremia)
  - Cirrhosis
  - Hepatitis
  - Pregnancy
  - Geographic tongue

TBG

Thyroxin binding globulin
Normal range: 14–28 ng/l (240–480 nmol/l)
Increased
- Newborns
- Pregnancy
- Hepatitis
  - Acute hepatitis
  - Chronic active hepatitis
- Biliary cirrhosis
- Infection
- Metabolic, endocrine

- Acute intermittent porphyria
- Hypothyroidism
- Familial hyperthyroxinemia
- Estrogen producing tumors
▶ Drugs
- Estrogen therapy
- Heroin
- Methadone
- Oral contraceptives
- Perphenazine
- Tamoxifen

Decreased
▶ Chronic liver disease
▶ Obstructive biliary disease
▶ Cirrhosis
▶ Nephrotic syndrome
▶ Cachexia
▶ Malnutrition
▶ Severe systemic illness
▶ Metabolic, endocrine
- Acromegaly
- Hyperthyroidism
- Cushing's disease
- Androgen producing tumor
▶ Surgical stress
▶ Drugs
- Anabolic steroids
- Androgens
- Glucocorticoids (large doses)
- L-asparaginase
- Lithium
- Salicylates
- Thyroid depressants

Telangiectasia

Abnormally dilated blood vessels,
especially seen in the skin.
Causes
▶ Herditary
- Hereditary hemorrhagic telangiectasia
  (Rendu-Osler-Weber syndrome)
- Ataxia-telangiectasia
- Xeroderma pigmentosa
- Bloom syndrome

- Fabry's disease
- Klippel-Trenaunay-Weber syndrome
- Sturge-Weber disease
- Cutis marmorata telangiectatica
  congenita
▶ Physical
- Long-term sun exposure (face)
- Burns
- Radiation dermatitis
▶ Endocrine
- Chronic liver disease
  ○ Cirrhosis (alcoholism)
- Female hormones
  ○ Estrogen, progesterone therapy
  ○ Pregnancy
- Topical corticosteroid therapy
- Hyperthyroidism
- Diabetes mellitus
▶ Collagen-vascular disease
- Lupus erythematosus
- Dermatomyositis
- Rheumatoid arthritis
▶ Cardiovascular disorders
- Chronic lung disease
- Chronic heart disease
- Chronic-venous insufficiency
- Hypertension
▶ Neoplastic disease
- Breast cancer
- Bile duct carcinoma
- Carcinoid syndrome
▶ Dermatologic
- Spider angioma
- Nevus flammeus
  ○ Port-wine stain
- Rosacea

Testicular dysfunction
See Hypogonadism → 200
See Impotence → 208

Testosterone

Most potent naturally occurring androgen, produced under gonadotropin stimulation mainly by the interstitial cells of the testes.

Total testosterone	
Prepuberty, boys	0.05-0.2 ng/ml
Puberty, boys	0.8-1.8 ng/ml
Men	3-10 ng/ml
Sexually mature women	< 1 ng/ml
Post-menopause	0.08-0.35 ng/ml

Increased
▶ Men
- Exogenic testosterone supply
- Tumors producing testosterone
  - Leydig cell tumor
  - Androblastoma
  - Adrenal carcinoma
- Androgen resistance
  - Androgen receptor defect

▶ Women
- Tumors producing testosterone
  - Ovarian tumor
  - Adrenal carcinoma
- Adrenal hyperplasia
- Cushing's syndrome
- Adrenogenital syndrome

Decreased
▶ Men
- Primary (hypergonadotropic) hypogonadism
  - Klinefelter's syndrome
  - Cryptorchism
- Secondary (hypogonadotropic) hypogonadism
- Malnutrition
- Anorexia
- Heavy exercise
- Cirrhosis
- Drugs
  - Anabolic steroids
  - Artificial androgens

▶ Women
- Gonadal insufficiency
  - Prepuberty
  - Post-menopause
- Adrenal insufficiency
  - Addison's disease
  - After adrenectomy
- Drugs
  - Contraceptives
  - Estrogens
- Malnutrition
- Anorexia
- Cirrhosis

Tetany

Syndrome with muscle twitches, cramps, and carpopedal spasm.
See Trousseau's sign → 361
See Chvostek's Sign → 77

Main causes
▶ Hypoparathyroidism
▶ Hyperventilation
▶ Hypocalcemia
▶ Hypomagnesemia

Normocalcemic tetany
▶ Hyperventilation
▶ Recurring vomiting
▶ Long-term saluretic medication
▶ Hypomagnesemia
- Malnutrition
  - Anorexia nervosa
  - Cachexia
- Malabsorption syndrome
- Lactation
- Pregnancy
- Cirrhosis
- Alcoholism
- Pancreatitis
- Nephropathy
▶ Conn's syndrome
▶ Zollinger-Ellison syndrome
▶ Hyperkalemic tetany
- Renal failure
- Hemolytic crisis

- Addisonian crisis
- Diabetic precoma
- Burns
- Uncontrolled intravenous potassium supply
▶ Drugs, toxins
  - Adrenaline
  - Caffeine
  - Carbon monoxide
  - Ergotamine
  - Guanidine
  - Lead
  - Morphine
  - Nicotine
  - Phosphorus
▶ Brain disorder
  - Brain injury
  - Brain tumor
  - Encephalitis
  - Encephalomalacia
  - Psychogenic

Hypocalcemic tetany (→ 348)
▶ Hypoparathyroidism
  - Postoperative
  - Idiopathic
    ◦ Hypoplasia, aplasia
    ◦ Autoantibodies
▶ Pseudohypoparathyroidism
▶ Lack of active vitamin D
  - Insufficient supply
  - Lack of sun exposure
  - Anticonvulsants
  - Insufficient endogenous production
▶ Miscellaneous
  - Maldigestion, malabsorption
  - Renal failure
  - Pancreatitis
  - After multiple transfusions
  - Intoxication
    ◦ Fluorides
    ◦ Oxalic acid
  - Rickets, osteomalacia (healing phase)

TG, See Thyroglobulin (TG) → 353

TgAb

Antithyroglobulin Antibody (TgAb), ATA
Antibody against thyroglobulin.

Reference range	
Women	< 100 IU/ml
Men	< 60 IU/ml

Increased
▶ Hashimoto's thyroiditis
▶ Grave's disease
▶ Primary myeloma
▶ Postpartal thyroiditis
▶ DsQuervain's thyroiditis

Thenar muscle atrophy

Causes
▶ Carpal tunnel syndrome
▶ Median nerve paralysis
▶ Duchenne-type muscular atrophy
▶ ALS
▶ Syringomyelia

Thiamin, See Vitamin B1 → 377

Thirst, See Polydipsia → 289

Thrombocyte Count

Thrombocytopenia, thrombocytosis
Thrombocytes (platelets) are built by megakaryocytes in the bone marrow, and are anuclear, disc-shaped blood components. Their main function is maintenance of homeostasis. Through the effects of miscellaneous substances (collagens, immunocomplexes, fibrinogenase) they aggregate, degranulate and release platelet factors that induce blood coagulation in the endogenous system, and form a thrombus.

Reference range	
Adults	140-440 x 10^3/µl

Children	150–300 x 10³/µl
Newborns	100–200 x 10³/µl

Increased (Thrombocytosis)

▶ Primary thrombocytosis
  (Myeloproliferative syndromes)
  • Polycythemia vera
  • Polycythemia
  • Essential thrombocythemia
  • Chronic myelogenous leukemia
  • Osteomyelofibrosis
  • Agnogenic myeloid metaplasia with
    myelofibrosis
▶ Secondary thrombocytosis
  • Acute infection
  • Neoplasm
  • Splenectomy
  • Chronic inflammation
    ○ Collagen vascular disease
      - Rheumatoid arthritis
      - Rheumatic fever
      - Wegener's granulomatosis
      - Other vasculitis
    ○ Infection
      - Tuberculosis
      - Osteomyelitis
    ○ Sarcoidosis
    ○ Crohn's disease
    ○ Ulcerative colitis
  • Iron deficiency
  • Trauma
  • Acute hemorrhage
  • Hemolytic anemia
  • Cirrhosis
  • Rebound-phenomenon
    ○ Recovery from thrombocytopenia
    ○ Alcohol withdrawal
    ○ Myelosuppressive therapy
    ○ Vitamin B_{12} therapy
    ○ Heavy exercise
    ○ Surgery
  • Drugs
    ○ Norepinephrine
    ○ Vincristine

Decreased (Thrombocytopenia)

< 130.000 mm³, critical < 10.000 mm³)
▶ Reduced thrombopoiesis (reduced
  megakaryocyte number)
  • Bone marrow hypoplasia/ -aplasia
    ○ Chemicals and drugs
      - Chemotherapy
      - Thiazides
      - Estrogens
      - Alcohol
      - Interferon
    ○ Radiation
    ○ Infections
      - HIV
      - Influenza
      - Rubella
      - Infectious mononucleosis
      - Dengue fever
      - Viral hepatitis
      - Tuberculosis
      - Malaria
      - Coli sepsis
      - Meningococcemia
  • Bone marrow infiltration, hematologic
    disorders
    ○ Leukemia
    ○ Lymphoma
    ○ Multiple myeloma
    ○ Aplastic anemia
    ○ Osteomyelofibrosis
    ○ Metastastatic infiltration
    ○ Infection
      - Tuberculosis
      - Others
    ○ Osteoporosis
  • Myelopathy
    ○ Fanconi's syndrome (hereditary
      impairment of the amino acid
      metabolism with cystine storage in
      miscellaneous organs, rachitic
      microplasia and nephropathy)
    ○ Amegakaryocytosis
  • Missing stimulation
  • Thrombopoietin deficiency
▶ Maturation impairment (normal or

elevated megakaryocyte count)
- Vitamin B_{12} deficiency
- Folic acid deficiency
- Iron (rare)
- Hereditary impairment
  - Wiskott-Aldrich syndrome
  - May-Hegglin anomaly
▶ Antibodies
- Autoantibodies
- Idiopathic thrombocytopenia (Werlhoff's disease)
- Hemolytic anemia
- Lymphoreticular impairment
- Systemic lupus erythematosus
- Drug-induced
  - Acetazolamide
  - α-methyldopa
  - Apronalid
  - Arsenic
  - Aspirin
  - Barbiturates
  - Captopril
  - Chloro thiazide
  - Chloroquine
  - Chlorthalidone
  - Diazoxid
  - Digitoxin
  - Diphenyl hydantoin
  - Gold
  - Heparin
  - Insecticides
  - Interferon
  - Meprobamate
  - Mercury
  - Phenylbutazone
  - Potassium iodide
  - Quinidine
  - Quinine
  - Rifampicin
  - Sedatives
  - Streptomycin
  - Sulfonamides
  - Thiourea
- Alloantibodies
  - Histo-incompatibility (fetus–mother)

  - Transfusion result
▶ Miscellaneous
- After thrombopenia
- Parainfectious
  - Measles
  - Mumps
  - Varicella
  - Mononucleosis
  - Cytomegalic disease
  - Epstein-Barr
- Disseminated intravascular coagulation
- Hemorrhage (loss)
- Thrombotic thrombocytopenic purpura (Moschcowitz' disease)
- Hemolytic-uremic syndrome
- Cyclic thrombocytopenia
- Paroxysmal nocturnal hemoglobinuria
- Damage in connection with posthetic heart valves
▶ Distribution impairment
- Splenomegaly
- Hypothermia (anesthesia)

Thrombophilia

Thrombocytosis, thrombosis, hypercoagulability, hypercoagulable state

Increased occurrence of arterial and venous vascular occlusions.
Thrombocytosis (> 400000 thrombocytes/mm^3 blood).

Risk factors for thrombosis
▶ Prior deep venous thrombosi
▶ Surgery or trauma of pelvis or lower extremities
▶ Surgery with > 30 minutes general anesthesia
▶ Immobilzation
▶ Malignant tumors
▶ Advanced age
▶ Pregnancy
▶ Estrogen therapy
▶ Obesity

T

- ▶ Nicotine abuse
- ▶ Nephrotic syndrome
- ▶ Antiphospholipid antibody syndrome
- ▶ Inflammatory bowel disease
- ▶ Erythrocythemia
- ▶ Idiopathic thrombocythemia
- ▶ Paroxysmal nightly hemoglobinuria

Thrombophilia with thrombophile family history without thrombocytosis (hereditary thrombophilia)
- ▶ APC resistance/factor V leiden mutation
- ▶ Prothrombin variant
- ▶ Homocystinuria
- ▶ Lupus anticoagulant (kardiolipin antibodies/ autoimmune disease)
- ▶ Antithrombin III deficiency
- ▶ Protein C deficiency
- ▶ Protein S deficiency
- ▶ Hageman factor deficiency
- ▶ Plasminogen deficiency
- ▶ Dysfibrinogenemia
- ▶ Sticky platelet syndrome
- ▶ Thrombomodulin defects
- ▶ Increased histidine rich glycoprotein
- ▶ Antiphospholipid antibody syndrome
- ▶ Heparin cofactor II deficiency
- ▶ α2-plasminogen-inhibitor excess
- ▶ Plasminogen-activator deficiency
- ▶ Plasminogen-activator-inhibitor excess

Thrombophilia in predisposing systemic diseases (acquired thrombophilia)
- ▶ Without thrombocytosis
  - • Surgical interventions
  - • Bacterial and viral infections
  - • Neoplastic diseases, especially:
    - ○ Lung cancer
    - ○ Pancreas carcinoma
    - ○ Gastric carcinoma
    - ○ Colon carcinoma
    - ○ Ovar/ uterus carcinoma
    - ○ Prostate carcinoma
  - • Drugs
    - ○ Chemotherapeutics
    - ○ Diuretics
    - ○ Corticosteroids
    - ○ Oral contraceptives
  - • Cardial diseases
    - ○ Myocardial infarction
    - ○ Cardiac valve defect
    - ○ Prosthetic heart valve
    - ○ Myocardial infarction
  - • Vasculopathy
    - ○ Primary and secondary varicose conditions
    - ○ Status varicosus
    - ○ Degenerative and inflammatory vasculopathies
    - ○ Vein compression syndrome
  - • Hyperviscosity syndrome
    - ○ Hyperglobulia
    - ○ Paraproteinemia
    - ○ Diuretics
  - • Systemic lupus erythematosus
- ▶ With thrombocytosis increased thrombocyte count (→ 349)

Thromboplastin time

Quick's test

Concerns the factors of the exogenic coagulation system. If platelet count, bleeding time and thrombin time are normal, an increased thromboplastin time suggests a reduction of the vitamin K-dependent factors II, V, VII, X.
See Disseminated Intravascular Coagulation → 104
See Partial Thromboplastin Time → 278

Reference ranges:
70-120% of the norm.
Therapeutic ranges during warfarin therapy are different according to indication: e.g., 20-35% of the norm and/or INR: 2.0-3.0

Increased thromboplastin time

- ▶ Drugs
  - • Allopurinol
  - • Anabolic steroids
  - • Antacids
  - • Antibiotics
  - • Butazolidin

- Chloral Hydrate
- Diphenylhydantoin
- Estrogens
- Heparin
- Phenylbutazone
- Quinidine
- Salicylates
- Sulfonamides
- Warfarin
▶ Factor II, V, VII, X deficiency
  - Liver diseases (cirrhosis)
  - Congenital factor deficiency
  - Antibodies (SLE)
▶ Vitamin K deficiency
  - Malabsorption syndroms
  - Broad-spectrum antibiotic therapy
  - Cholestatic jaundice
  - Dietary deficiency
  - Hemorrhagic diseases of the newborn
  - Therapy with vitamin K antagonists
▶ Disseminated intravascular coagulation
▶ Fibrinolitic states
▶ Congenital deficiency of one or more clotting factors
▶ Fibrinogen disorder
  - Afibrinogenemia
  - Hypofibrinogenemia
  - Dysfibrinogenemia
  - von Willebrand´s disease
  - Lupus anticoagulant
  - Hemophilia A
  - Hemophilia B
  - Excess AT III
  - Vitamin A intoxication

Decreased thromboplastin time
Vitamin K supplementation
Thrombophlebitis
Drugs
  - Diphenhydramin
  - Estrogens
  - Gluthetimide
  - Griseofulvin

Thyroglobulin (TG)

Thyroid hormone-containing protein, stored in the colloid within the thyroid follicles. Used in monitoring recurrence of papillary and follicular carcinoma. After successful total thyroidectomy, thyroglobulin level should be low or undetectable.

Reference range
2–70 µg/l

Increased
▶ Malignant diseases
  - Papillar thyroid carcinoma
  - Follicular thyroid carcinoma
  - Metastases of thyroid carcinoma
▶ Miscellaneous
  - Grave's disease
  - Thyroiditis
    ○ Hashimoto thyroiditis
  - Goiter
    ○ Euthyroid goiter
    ○ Nodular goiter
  - Autonomous adenoma
  - T_3-medication
  - Follicle necrosis
  - Reactive overproduction
    ○ Traumatic thyroid gland damage
    ○ Radioactive iodine therapy

Thyroid disorders
See Hyperthyroidism → 196
See Hypothyroidism → 206

Thyroid enlargement, See Goiter → 156

Thyroid stimulating hormone
See TSH → 362

Thyroiditis

Inflammation of the thyroid gland with heterogenous etiologies.

Classification

▶ **Hashimoto's thyroiditis** (chronic lymphocytic thyroiditis)
▶ **Subacute thyroiditis** (subacute granulomatous thyroiditis, De Quervain's thyroiditis
▶ **Silent thyroiditis** (subacute lymphocytic thyroiditis, painless thyroiditis, postpartum thyroiditis, pregnancy associated thyroiditis)
▶ **Suppurative thyroiditis** (acute thyroiditis, bacterial thyroiditis, microbial thyroiditis)
▶ **Riedel's thyroiditis** (invasive fibrous thyroiditis)

Thyroxin (T$_4$)

Reference range
5–12 µg/dl (65–155 nmol/l)
See Hyperthyroidism → 196
See Hypothyroidism → 206

Thyroxin binding globulin
See TBG → 346

Tinnitus

Noises in the ears

Objective (others may also hear it)

▶ Muscular
  • Palatal myoclonus
  • Stapedius spasm
▶ Patulous eustachian tube
▶ Vascular
  • AV shunts
    ○ Glomus tympanicum/jugulare tumor
  • Arteriovenous malformation
  • Arterial bruits
    ○ Aberrant carotid artery
    ○ Carotid stenosis
    ○ Persistent stapedial artery
  • Venous hums (alter by pressing on lateral neck)
    ○ Hypertension
    ○ Hyperthyroidism
    ○ Hypothyroidism
    ○ High jugular bulb

Subjective (only patient hears it)

▶ Otologic
  • Noise induced hearing loss
  • Presbyacusis (hearing loss due to aging)
  • Otitis media with effusion
  • Mastoiditis
  • Otosclerosis
  • Meniere disease
  • Cerumen
  • Foreign body against tympanic membrane
▶ Drugs
  • Alcohol
  • Aminoglycosides
  • Antibiotics
  • Antidepressants
  • Aspirin
  • Diuretics
  • Heavy metals
  • Heavy smoking
  • Indomethacin
  • Omeprazole (i.v.)
  • Quinine
▶ Metabolic, endocrine
  • Vitamin A deficiency
  • Vitamin B deficiency
  • Hyperlipidemia
  • Hypothyroidism
  • Hyperthyroidism
  • Diabetes mellitus
▶ Neoplasm
  • Acoustic neuroma
  • Brain tumor
    ○ Temporal lobe tumor (bilateral tinnitus)
  • Nasopharyngeal cancer
  • Glomus tumor
▶ Neurologic
  • Head trauma
  • Multiple sclerosis
  • Meningitis

- Epilepsy
- After spinal anesthesia
► Causes in the dental/jaw area
  - Faulty jaw position
  - Extractions
  - Bruxism
  - Tooth abnormalities
► Psychic
  - Anxiety
  - Depression
  - Hallucinations
► Miscellaneous
  - Cervical spine diseases
    ○ Cervical osteochondrosis
  - Cardiovascular
    ○ Hypertension
    ○ Cardiac dysrhythmias
  - Anemia

Classification according to type of sound heard
► Pulsatile tinnitus (related to blood flow)
  - Hypertension
  - Abnormal blood vessels,Aneurysm
  - Glomus tumor
  - Mastoiditis
  - Acute otitis media
  - Anemia
  - Hyperthyroidism
  - Pregnancy
► Whistling, rumblingtinnitus
  - Ménière's disease
  - Otosclerosis
  - External auditory canal obstruction
  - Middle ear diseases
► Hissing, wheezing tinnitus
  - Circulation disorder
  - Inner ear diseases
  - Diseases of the statoacoustic nerve
    ○ Acoustic neurinoma
    ○ Acoustic trauma
    ○ Anemia
    ○ Polycythemia
► Clicking tinnitus
    ○ jaw joint misalignment (TMJ) problems or muscles of the ear or

throat "twitching."

Tissue polypeptide antigen
See TPA → 358

Tongue, Coated

Infections
► Candidiasis
► Streptococcal tonsillitis/ scarlet fever
► Diphtheria
► Meningitis
► Infectious mononucleosis

Gastrointestinal
► Starvation
► Acute gastritis
► Acute enteritis
► Chronic hepatic failure

Tongue, large, See Tongue Swelling → 356

Tongue Pain

Glossalgia, glossodynia
Burning or painful tongue

Without lesions
► Burning mouth syndrome
► Smoking
► Non-specific glossitis
► Menopausal glossitis
► Heavy metal poisoning

With deep lesion
► Sialolithiasis
  - Submaxillary gland
  - Sublingual gland
► Foreign body
► Lingual muscle disorder
  - Myositis
  - Neoplasm
► Trichinosis
► Periostitis (hyoid bone)

With localized superficial lesions
► Tongue biting
► Lingual frenulum trauma

T

- Dental ulcer
- Prosthesis incompatibility
- Foreign body
- Ranula
- Epithelioma
- Carcinoma
- Tuberculosis ulcer
- Herpes simplex stomatitis
- Vincent's stomatitis
- Leukoplakia
- Thrush (candida albicans)

Systemic disease
- Atrophic glossitis (→ 155)
- Vitamin deficiencies
  - Niacin deficiency (pellagra)
  - Vitamin B_2 deficiency (riboflavin)
  - Vitamin C deficiency (scurvy)
- Drugs, toxins
  - Antibiotics
  - Chemotherapeutics
  - Heavy metals
  - Phenytoin
  - Sulfonamides
- Leukemia
- Collagen vascular disease
  - Sjögren's syndrome
- Lichen planus
- Scarlet fever
- Celiac sprue
- Cystic fibrosis
- Diabetes mellitus
- Uremia
- Psychic

Tongue, Red

Inflammation, infection
- Scarlet fever
- Chronic enterocolitis
- Celiac disease (sensitivity to gluten)

Deficiencies
- Folic acid deficiency
- Vitamin B_{12} deficiency
  - Pernicious anemia
- Niacin deficiency (pellagra)

- Iron deficiency anemia
  - Plummer-Vinson syndrome

Miscellaneous
- Diabetes mellitus
- Cirrhosis
- Gastrointestinal tumor

Tongue Swelling

Macroglossia
Enlargement of the tongue

Transient swelling
- Inflammation
  - Glossitis
  - Wasp sting
  - Stomatitis
  - Neck cellulitis
- Angioneurotic edema (Quincke's edema)
- Venous stasis
- Hematoma
- Infection
  - Abscess
  - Actinomycosis
  - Leprosy
  - Streptococcal infection
  - Syphilis, stage III

Persistent swelling
- Down's syndrome
- Hypothyroidism
- Acromegaly
- Amyloidosis
- Lymphangioma
- Tongue cancer
- Leukemia
- Hemangioma
- Neurofibromatosis
- Tumor of the pituitary gland
- Hurler-Pfaundler syndrome
- Acanthosis nigricans
- Pellagra
- Pernicious anemia
- Beckwith-Wiedemann syndrome

Tooth Loss
Premature loss of teeth

Trauma
► Accident
► Radiation

Infection, inflammation
► Periodontitis
► Tuberculosis
► Syphilis
► Leptospirosis
► Cholera

Neoplasm
► Lymphoma
► Leukemia
► Local tumor
  • Neuroectodermal tumor
  • Central giant cell granuloma
  • Fibrous dysplasia
  • Sarcoma

Hematologic
► Agranulocytosis
► Leukemia
► Reticulosis

Endocrine
► Acromegaly
► Hypopituitarism
► Diabetes mellitus
► Primary hyperparathyroidism

Drugs, toxins
► Butazolidin
► Chemotherapeutics
► Chloramphenicol
► Mercury
► Phosphorus
► Pyrazolone

Hereditary
► Acatalasia
► Chediak-Higashi syndrome
► Chronic neutropenia
► Cyclic neutropenia
► Dentin dysplasia
► Hypophosphatasia
► Hypophosphatemic vitamin D resistant rickets
► Lesch-Nyhan syndrome
► Papillon-Lefèvre syndrome

Miscellaneous
► Acrodynia
► Histiocytosis X
► Hand-Schüller-Christian syndrome
► Odontodysplasia
► Osteomyelitis
► Periodontitis
► Trisomy 21 (Down's syndrome)
► Vitamin C deficiency
► Psychotic patients

Total-CK, See Creatine Kinase (CK) → 88

Total protein
See Protein in the Serum → 296

Toxic Shock Syndrome
Inflammatory response syndrome mediated by bacterial toxins characterized by shock and multiple organ dysfunction. With fever, rash, hypotension, constitutional symptoms, and multiorgan involvement.

Causes
► Coagulase-positive staphylococci (Staphylococcus aureus)
► Group A beta-hemolytic streptococci (Streptococcus pyogenes)

Risk factors
► Absence of protective immunity
► Menstruation (superabsorbent tampons)
► Wound infection (postoperative)
► Childbirth (postpartum toxic shock)
► Nasal packing
► Infections
  • Common bacterial infections
  • Influenza A
  • Varicella
  • HIV

T

▸ Chronic cardiac disease
▸ Chronic pulmonary disease
▸ Diabetes mellitus
▸ NSAIDs

TPA

TPA (tissue polypeptide antigen) occurs in cell membranes of almost all epithelial cells. TPA has a high sensitivity in all malignant tumors. and can be used as an unspecific tumor marker.

Reference range

TPA	< 80 U/l

Increased

▸ Benign diseases
  • Lung disease
  • Urogenital disease
  • Gastrointestinal disease
  • Hepatitis
  • Cirrhosis
  • Pregnancy (third trimester)
▸ Malignant diseases
  • Almost all malignant tumors (combined with other tumor markers)
  • Bronchial carcinoma
  • Breast cancer
  • Urinary bladder carcinoma
  • Stomach carcinoma
  • Colon carcinoma
  • Rectal carcinoma

Transferrin Saturation

Transferrin is capable of associating reversibly with iron and acting therefore as an iron-transporting protein. Transferrin saturation (%)= 100 x serum iron (ug/dl) / TIBC (ug/dl) is only diagnostically relevant in conjunction with iron and ferritin levels.

Reference range

Transferrin	250–450 mg/dl
Transferrin saturation	15–45%

Increased transferrin saturation

▸ Iron overloading
  • Hemochromatosis
  • Hemoglobinopathy
  • Hemolytic anemia
  • Ineffective erythropoiesis
  • Frequent blood transfusions
▸ Iron utilization impairment/ hemolysis
  • Anemia (hemolytic, sideroblastic, megaloblastic)
  • Hemoglobinopathy
  • Porphyria
  • Lead intoxication
▸ Starvation
▸ Nephrotic syndrome
▸ Cirrhosis

Decreased transferrin saturation

▸ Iron deficiency anemia
▸ Iron distribution disorder
  • Chronic infection
  • Chronic inflammations
  • Advanced malignancy
  • Liver parenchyma damage
  • Collagen-Vascular disease
  • Uremia
  • Third trimester of pregnancy

Transudate, See Pleural Effusion → 286

Tremor

Involuntary, fast consecutive rhythmic twitches. Passive tremor: present in relaxed posture; in extrapyramidal impairment intention tremor: present during precise motions; cerebellar impairment.

CNS disorders

▸ Parkinson's disease
▸ CNS trauma
▸ General paralysis
▸ Multiple sclerosis
▸ Arteriosclerosis of cerebral vessels
▸ Brain tumor (cerebellum)
▸ Brain abscess

- Friedreich's ataxia
- Wilson's disease
- HIV infection

Intoxication
- Alcohol
- Arsenic
- Caffeine
- Carbon monoxide
- Copper
- Cyanide
- Lead
- Manganese
- Mercury
- Nicotine
- Phosphorus

Drug induced
- Alcohol
- Alpha-methyldopa
- Amphetamines
- Antidepressants
- Antiphlogistics
- Ciclosporin
- Corticosteroids
- Drug withdrawal
- Lithium
- Methotrexate
- Neuroleptics
- Phenytoin
- Reserpine
- Sympathomimetics
- Theophylline derivates
- Thyroxin
- Tiaprid
- Valproic acid

Endocrine, metabolic
- Hepatic failure ("flapping tremor")
- Hyperthyroidism
- Hypoparathyroidism
- Hypoglycemia
- Pheochromocytoma
- Preeclampsia
- Phenylketonuria
- Delirium tremens
- Electrolyte disturbance

Miscellaneous
- Physiologic tremor
  - Pain
  - Psychogenic tremor
  - Cold
  - Fatigue
- Peripheral neuropathy
- Essential tremor
- Senile tremor

Tricuspid Insufficiency

- Rheumatic heart disease
- Endocarditis
- Myocardial infarction
- Trauma
- Pulmonary hypertension
- Ebstein´s anomaly
- Pulmonary artery catheter (Swan-Ganz)
- Carcinoid
- Rheumaoid arthritis
- Radiation
- Prolapse

Trigeminal Neuralgia
Tic douloureux
Severe, paroxysmal pain in one or more branches of the trigeminal nerve. Often induced by touching trigger points in or about the mouth. Sometimes with contractions of the mimic facial muscles (tic douloureux), redness of the face, tears and sweating.

Causes
- Idiopathic (usually women > 50 J.)
- Blood vessels (compressing the trigeminal nerve root)
  - Superior cerebellar artery
  - Anterior inferior cerebellar artery
  - Posterior inferior cerebellar artery
  - Vertebral artery
  - Basilar artery
  - Other arteries
  - Veins

T

- Multiple sclerosis (demyelinization of the nerve)
- Brain tumor (pressure on the trigeminal nerve)
- Physical damage to the nerve
  - Dental disease, procedures
  - Surgical procedures
  - Injury to the face
  - Orbital disease
  - Shingles (varicella zoster virus)
  - Other infections
- Chronic meningeal inflammation
- Ischemic cerebrovascular disorders
  - Basilar artery
  - Thrombosis
  - Aneurysm
- Temporal arteritis

DDx
- Cluster headache
- Glossopharyngeal neuralgia
- Postherpetic neuralgia
- Dental infection
- Temperomandibular joint syndrome
- Multiple sclerosis
- Acoustic neuroma
- Vascular malformation

Triglycerides

See Hypercholesterolemia → 188
See Coronary Risk Factor → 66
See LDL Cholesterol → 218
See HDL Cholesterol → 162

Triglycerides (TGs) consist of three fatty acids bound to glycerol. They have physiologic significance especially as an energy supply. Endogenic TGs are mostly synthesized in liver, kidney and heart muscle and reach the blood as VLDL. Exogenic TGs are taken up with the food and reach the blood as chylomicrons.

Together with cholesterol, TGs form the basis for the lipid metabolism assessment. Values > 200 mg/dl indicate a risk factor for arteriosclerosis just like hypercholesterolemia.
In about 20 % of cases very high triglyceride levels (> 1000 mg/dl) are the cause of an acute pancreatitis.

Reference range

< 160 mg/dl (< 1.8 mmol/l)

Increased (hypertriglyceridemia)
- Primary hypertriglyceridemia
  - Hyperlipidemia type IIb/IV/V
- Secondary hypertriglyceridemia
  - Systemic diseases
    ○ Diabetes mellitus
    ○ Chronic renal failure
    ○ Nephrotic syndrome
    ○ Hypothyroidism
    ○ Hypertension
    ○ Myocardial infarction
    ○ Gout
    ○ Liver diseases
      - Obstructive jaundice
      - Bile duct stenosis
      - Alcoholic cirrhosis
    ○ Cushing's syndrome
    ○ Systemic lupus erythematosus
    ○ Glycogen storage disease
    ○ Malignant lymphoma
    ○ Multiple myeloma
  - Drugs
    ○ Anabolic steroids
    ○ Betablockers
    ○ Estrogens
    ○ Glucocorticoids
    ○ Oral contraceptives
    ○ Thiazides
  - Miscellaneous
    ○ Obesity
    ○ Alcohol abuse
    ○ High-carbohydrate diet
    ○ Pregnancy

Decreased
► Cachexia
► Burns
► Exudative enteropathy
► Malabsorption syndrome
► Malnutrition
► Hyperthyroidism
► Abetalipoproteinemia

Triiodothyronine (T₃)

Reference range
70–180 ng/dl (1.1–2.79 nmol/l)

Increased
► T_3-therapy
► Isolated T_3-hyperthyroidism

Decreased
► Impaired T_4 to T_3 conversion
  • Systemic illness
  • Fasting
  • Surgery (stress)
  • Drugs
    ○ Amiodarone
    ○ Glucocorticoids
    ○ Prednisone
    ○ Propranolol
    ○ Propylthiouracil
    ○ Radiocontrast
  • Idiopathic

Troponin I and Cardiac Troponin T

Troponin T and Troponine I are serum cardiac markers highly sensitive for detecting myocardial infarction. The troponin T concentration correlates with the infarction size. It increases 3–4 hours after onset of the pain.

Reference range

Cardiac TnT	< 0.2 µg/l
Cardiac TnI	< 0.1 µg/l

Troponin T
► High sensitivity: 94% of myocardial infarctions
► Low specificity: 22% have unstable angina

Troponin I
► High sensitivity: 100% of myocardial infarctions
► Low specificity: 36% have unstable angina.

Increased
► Myocardial infarction
► Unstable angina
► Chronic renal failure (Troponine T)

Trousseau's sign

Occurrence of carpopedal spasm with paresthesia when the upper arm is compressed.

In latent tetany (→ 348)

Trypsin

Proteolytic enzyme formed in the small intestine from trypsinogen by the action of enteropeptidase. Proteinase that hydrolyzes peptides, amides, esters, etc..

Reference range (Serum)
15–65 ng/ml

Increased
► Acute pancreatitis
► Chronic pancreatitis
► Pancreatic cancer
► Cystic fibrosis
► Abnormal pancreatic production

Decreased
► Pancreatic insufficiency
► Chronic pancreatitis

TSH

Thyroid-stimulating hormone, thyrotropin, thyrotrophin, thyrotropic hormone

Hormone produced by the anterior lobe of the hypophysis, stimulating growth and function of the thyroid gland. Controlling iodine uptake in the thyroid gland, synthesis of the thyroid hormones and hormone secretion. TSH secretion is regulated through TRH (thyrotropin releasing hormone).

Reference range
0.3–3.5 mU/l

Increased TSH
► Endemic goiter
► Hypothyroidism (with and without goiter)
► Secondary hyperthyroidism
  • Pituitary tumor
  • Thyroid hormone resistance
► Autoimmune thyroiditis with hypothyroid metabolic status (Hashimoto's thyroiditis)
► Suppressive therapy
  • Thyroid depressants
  • Radioactive iodine therapy
  • Thyroidectomy
► Drugs
  • Amphetamine
  • Chlorpromazine
  • Domperidone
  • Haloperidol
  • Iodous substances
  • Metoclopramide

Decreased
► Hyperthyroidism
► Autoimmune thyroiditis (with hyperthyroidism)
  • Grave's disease
  • Initially in de Quervain's thyroiditis
  • Initially in Hashimoto's thyroiditis
► Secondary hypothyroidism
  • Pituitary insufficiency
► Drugs
  • Bromocriptine
  • Diphenylhydantoin
  • Dopamine
  • Estrogens
  • Glucocorticoids
  • Levodopa
  • Pyridoxine
  • Somatostatin
► Acute illness
► Hyponatremia
► Malnutrition

TSH Receptor Antibody

Antithyroid antibody, thyroid stimulating immunoglobulin

Binds and activates TSH receptor in thyroid.

Reference range
< 14 IU/ml

Increased
► Grave's disease
► Ophthalmopathy without hyperthyroidism
► Hypothyroidism through blocking antibodies

Tubulointerstitial Diseases of the Kidney

Renal diseases that involve tubules and/or the interstitium of the kidney and spare the glomeruli.

Drugs, toxins
► Allopurinol
► Alpha-interferon
► Antibiotics
  • Cephalosporins
  • Cotrimoxazole
  • Erythromycin
  • Ethambutol
  • Penicillins
  • Quinolones

- Sulfonamides
- Tetracycline
- Vancomycin
▶ Cimetidine
▶ Cyclosporine
▶ Diuretics
  - Thiazides
  - Furosemide
▶ Heavy metals
  - Lead
  - Cadmium
  - Mercury
▶ Lithium
▶ NSAIDs (analgesic nephropathy)
▶ Phenytoin
▶ Rifampin
▶ Tacrolimus

Metabolic toxins
▶ Acute uric acid nephropathy
▶ Gouty nephropathy
▶ Hypercalcemic nephropathy
▶ Hypokalemic nephropathy
▶ Cystinosis
▶ Hyperoxaluria
▶ Fabry's disease

Urinary tract disorders
▶ Chronic urinary tract obstruction
▶ Vesicoureteral reflux
▶ Nephrolithiasis

Infections
▶ Acute pyelonephritis
▶ Chronic pyelonephritis
▶ Bacterial (with obstruction or reflux)
▶ Viral
  - Cytomegalovirus (CMV)
  - Hantavirus
  - HIV
  - Hepatitis B
▶ Fungal
  - Histoplasmosis
▶ Parasitic
  - Leishmania
  - Toxoplasmosis

Immune disorder
▶ Hypersensitivity nephropathy (drugs)
▶ Sjögren syndrome
▶ Amyloidosis
▶ Transplant nephropathy
▶ HIV-associated nephropathy
▶ Primary glomerulopathies
▶ Sarcoidosis
▶ Lupus
▶ Goodpasture syndrome
▶ Vasculitis
  - ANCA-associated vasculitis
  - Wegener granulomatosis

Neoplasm
▶ Lymphoma
▶ Leukemia
▶ Multiple myeloma

Vascular
▶ Arteriolar nephrosclerosis
▶ Atheroembolic disease
▶ Sickle cell nephropathy
▶ Acute tubular necrosis
▶ Medullary sponge kidney
▶ Polycystic kidney disease

Hereditary
▶ Alport syndrome
▶ Medullary cystic disease

Miscellaneous
▶ Radiation nephritis
▶ Balkan endemic nephropathy
▶ Chinese herb nephropathy

Tumor marker, See CA-19-9 → 60, See CA-125 → 60, See CEA → 70, See NSE → 260, See Prostate Specific Antigen → 295, See TPA → 358

U wave, See ECG, U–, Delta Wave → 122

Ulcerations, genital
See Genital Ulcer → 154

Ulcer disease
See Peptic Ulcer Disease → 279

Ulcer on the penis
See Genital Ulcer → 154

Underweight, See Weight Loss → 382

Unequal pulse

Between arms
▶ Aortic arch syndrome (subclavian steal syndrome)
▶ Takayasu's syndrome
▶ Thoracic outlet syndrome
▶ Arterial thromboses and emboli
▶ Thoracic aortic aneurysm
▶ Dissecting aneurysm
▶ Aortic stenosis
▶ Patent ductus arteriosus
▶ Subclavian artery abnormality/stenosis
▶ Stenosis of the brachiocephalic trunk
▶ Syphilis
▶ Vasculitis
▶ Hemiplegia

Between arms and legs
▶ Aortic isthmus stenosis (hypertension in the arms and hypotension in the legs)

Unstable angina pectoris
See Angina → 32

Upper eyelid, drooping, See Ptosis → 302

Urea

Blood urea

Chief end product of of the protein and amino acid metabolism, formed in the liver and excreted in normal adult human urine (about 32 g/d). Increases if renal function is absent. Serum creatinine (→ 89) is a better measure of renal function.

Reference range	
Men	23–44 mg/dl
Women	13–40 mg/dl

Increased
▶ Drugs
  • Aminoglycosides
  • Corticosteroids
  • Diuretics
  • Lithium
▶ Dehydration (→ 93)
▶ Gastrointestinal bleeding (→ 152)
▶ Decreased renal blood flow
  • Shock
  • Congestive heart failure
  • Myocardial infarction
▶ Renal disease
  • Glomerulonephritis
  • Pyelonephritis
  • Diabetic nephropathy
▶ Urinary tract obstruction

Decreased
▶ Liver disease
▶ Overhydration
▶ Poor nutrition
▶ Pregnancy (third trimester)

Urge incontinence
See Urinary Incontinence → 365

Uric Acid

The uric acid pool of the organism is approx. 1 g. The synthesis of uric acid needed for the break-down of purines occurs only in tissues with xanthine oxidase, mainly liver and small intestine. Uric acid elimination occurs about 80 % in the kidney and about 20 % in the intestines. Complications of hyperuricemia are acute gouty arthritis, chronic soft part- and/or bone tophi, nephrolithiasis and acute uric acid nephropathy.

Reference range (in serum)	
Men	2.5–8.0 mg/dl
Women	1.5–6.0 mg/dl
Uric acid elimination	0.25–0.75 g/24 h

Increased (hyperuricemia)
▶ Primary overproduction
- Idiopathic
- HPRT deficiency (Hypoxanthine-guanine phosphoribosyl-transferase)
  ○ Lesch-Nyhan syndrome
  ○ Kelley-Seegmiller syndrome
- Increased PRPP-synthetase-activity (Phosphoribosylpyrophosphate)

▶ Secondary overproduction
- Food rich in purines
- Food rich in fruit sugar
- Infusions of sorbite or xylitol
- Chemotherapeutic therapy
- Hemolytic diseases
- Hemoglobinopathies
- Myeloproliferative syndromes
- Multiple myeloma
- Lymphoma
- Rhabdomyolysis
- Psoriasis
- Starvation
- Hyperuricemia after kidney or heart transplantation and cyclosporine therapy

▶ Decreased renal excretion
- Chronic renal failure
- Consumption of alcohol
- Diabetes insipidus
- Hypertension
- Ketoacidosis
  ○ Diabetic
  ○ Starvation
- Lactic acidosis
- Lead nephropathy
- Hyperparathyroidism
- Hypercalcemia

- Drugs
  ○ Diuretics (except spironolactone)
  ○ Salicylates (< 3 g/d)
  ○ Cyclosporine A
  ○ L-dopa
  ○ Omeprazol
  ○ Ethambutol
  ○ Pyrazinamide
  ○ Nicotinic acid

▶ Miscellaneous
- Cytorrhexis
  ○ Tumor
  ○ Chemotherapy
- Hypercholesterolemia type II
- Respiratory acidosis
- Sarcoidosis
- Hypoparathyroidism
- Hypo-/Hyperthyroidism
- Paget´s disease
- Acromegaly
- Glykogen storage disease
- Down syndrome

Uric acid stones, See Uric Acid → 364,
See Urolithiasis → 371,
See Nephrolithiasis → 255

Urinary Incontinence
Inability to prevent the discharge of urine. Involuntary urine discharge. Prevalence increases with age. Most frequent causes are stress incontinence, urge incontinence, reflex incontinence and overflow incontinence. Risk factors: advanced age, female sex, prostate hyperplasia, multipara, dementia, diabetes, multiple sclerosis and apoplexy.

Stress incontinence
Caused by malfunction of the urethral sphincter, so that urine leaks from the bladder when intra-abdominal pressure increases (coughing, lifting, laughing).
▶ Multiparity
▶ Pregnancy

- Postpartum
- Obstetric/gynecologic surgery
- Obesity
- Pelvic surgery
- Bladder tumor
- Prostate surgery
- Neuropathic bladder dysfunction

Urge incontinence
Bladder contractions preceded by a strong urge to void, overwhelming the ability of the cerebral centers to inhibit them.
- Idiopathic
- Infection, inflammation, irritiation
  - Cystitis
  - Urethritis
  - UTI
  - Chemical or mechanical bladder irritation
  - Stones
- Tumor
  - Bladder papilloma
  - Bladder carcinoma
- Outlet obstruction
- Vesicovaginal fistula
- Neurologic
  - Stroke
  - Multiple sclerosis
  - Brain tumor
  - Dementia
  - Parkinson disease
  - Tension or anxiety

Overflow incontinence
Bladder overdistention with urinary retention.
- Obstruction
  - Pelvic tumors
  - Benign prostatic hypertrophy
  - Prostate carcinoma
  - Urethral stricture
  - Bladder neck stricture
- Neurologic
  - Diabetes mellitus
  - Vitamin B_{12} deficiency
  - Herniated intervertebral disc
  - Multiple sclerosis

- Drugs
  - Anticholinergics
  - Calcium channel blockers

Low pressure urethra
Sphincteric atony
- Trauma
- Surgery

Risk factors for urinary incontinence
- Age
- Sex (women > men)
- Pregnancy
- Childbirth
- Breast-feeding
- Obesity
- Menopause
- Smoking
- Prostate enlargement
- Prostate surgery
- Pelvic muscle weakness
- Pelvic surgery
- Hysterectomy
- Hormone replacement therapy
- Radiation therapy to the pelvis
- Diabetes mellitus
- Parkinson's disease
- Back injury
- Cerebral vascular accident
- Dementia

DDx
- Delirium
- Infection, inflammation
  - UTI
  - Cystitis
  - Vaginitis
  - Bladder carcinoma-in-situ
- Atrophic urethritis/vaginitis
- Drugs
  - Antipsychotics
  - Diuretics
  - Hypnotics
  - Muscle relaxants
  - Sedatives
  - Sympathetic blockers
- Polyuria
  - Diabetes mellitus

- Stool impaction
- Restricted mobility
- Psychologic

Urinary retention
See Urinary Tract Obstruction → 367

Urinary tract infection (UTI)
See Dysuria → 114

Urinary Tract Obstruction

Drainage disorders of various origin caused by obstruction of the cavities in the urogenital tract.

Urethral
- Congenital
  - Urethral stenosis
  - Urethral atresia
  - Web
- Urethral valves
- Urethral stricture
- Inflammation
- Trauma

Bladder neck
- Benign prostatic hypertrophy (BPH)
- Prostatitis
- Carcinoma
  - Prostate
  - Bladder
- Infection
- Inflammation
- Trauma
- Trabeculated bladder
- Bladder stone
- Neurologic, functional
  - Autonomic neuropathy
  - Spinal cord injury
  - Spinal cord tumor
  - Trauma
  - Multiple sclerosis
  - Neurosyphilis
  - Syringomyelia
  - Tabes dorsalis

- Drugs
  - Parasympatholytics
  - Ganglionic blocking drugs

Ureteral
- Ureteral-pelvic junction stricture
- Ureteral stenosis
- Intraureteral
  - Clots
  - Crystals
  - Stones
  - Foreign bodies
  - Papillae (necrosed)
  - Tumor
  - Trauma
  - Edema from retrograde pyelography
- Extraureteral
  - Endometriosis
  - Retroperitoneal tumor
    - Prostate cancer
    - Bladder cancer
    - Cervical cancer
    - Endometrial cancer
    - Ovarian cancer
    - Lymphoma
    - Sarcoma
  - Retroperitoneal fibrosis
  - Pregnancy
  - Aneurysm
  - Aberrant vessel
  - Thrombosis
  - Accidental surgical ligation

Urination problems,
See Urinary Incontinence → 365,
See Urinary Tract Obstruction → 367

U
V

Urine Appearance and Color

Urine-quality	Possible causes
Yellow	Vit. B$_{12}$-intake
Yellow-red	Laxatives
Orange	Rifampicin, nitrofurantoin
Dark	Alcaptonuria, porphyria
Milky	Lymphatic fistulas
Opaque	Bacteria, cells
Smelly	Urinary infection
Red / pink	Hematuria, hemoglobinuria
Dark	Concentrated, hemoglobinuria
Yellowish-brown	in jaundice with overflow of bile
Pale	Polyuria, chronic renal failure
Foamy	Proteinuria
With sediment	Precipitation of urate salts
Cloudy	Pus, tissue parts
With intestinal contents	Intestinal fistulas

Urine Calcium

Increased (Hypercalciuria)
Urinary excretion > 250 mg/24 hr of calcium for women or > 275–300 mg/24 hr for men while on a regular, unrestricted diet.

▶ Primary hyperparathyroidism
▶ Hypervitaminosis D
▶ Bone metastases
▶ Multiple myeloma
▶ Increased calcium intake
▶ Steroids
▶ Prolonged immobilization
▶ Sarcoidosis
▶ Paget's disease
▶ Idiopathic hypercalciuria
▶ Renal tubular acidosis

Decreased (Hypocalciuria)
▶ Hypoparathyroidism
▶ Pseudohypoparathyroidism
▶ Vitamin D deficiency
▶ Vitamin D-resistant rickets
▶ Diet low in calcium
▶ Drugs
  • Oral contraceptives
  • Potassium citrate therapy
  • Thiazide diuretics
▶ Familial hypocalciuric hypercalcemia
▶ Renal osteodystrophy

Urine Catecholamines

Generic term for norepinephrine, noradrenaline as well as dopamine. Metanephrine, normetanephrine, and homovanillic acid are formed during catabolism of catecholamines. Indications are impaired adrenal medulla function, pheochromocytoma, neuroblastoma and relapsing hypoglycemia. Vanillylmandelic acid is the major urinary metabolite of adrenal and sympathetic catecholamines (epinephrine, norepinephrine).

Upper reference range in the urine (24h urine)	
Norepinephrine	23–105 µg/24 h
Dopamine	190–450 µg/24 h
Metanephrine	74–297 µg/24 h
Normetanephrine	105–354 µg/24 h
Vanillic acid	3.3–6.5 mg/24 h

Reference range Vanillylmandelic Acid
17–33 µmol/l (3.3–6.5 mg/24 h)

Increased
▶ Pheochromocytoma
▶ Multiple endocrine neoplasia, type 2
▶ Von Hippel-Lindau syndrome
▶ Neuroblastoma
▶ Ganglioma
▶ Stress
▶ Drugs
  • Alpha$_1$ blockers
  • Betablockers

- Calcium antagonists
- Labetolol
- MAO inhibitors
- Methyldopa
- Nitroglycerin
- Sodium nitroprusside
- Theophylline
- Miscellaneous
- Postoperative
- Myocardial infarction
- Hypoglycemia
- Nicotine
- Caffein
- Exogenic catecholamines
  - Nose drops
  - Eye drops
  - Cough drops

Decreased
▶ Drugs
- ACE inhibitors
- β2 sympathomimetics
- Chronic therapy with calcium antagonists

Urine Osmolality

The examination of the urine osmolality is important for the clarification of increased urine volume (See Polyuria → 289). Indicated in the examination of renal concentration defects, diabetes insipidus, osmotic diuresis and water diuresis . The human antidiuretic hormone (ADH) is arginine-vasopressin (AVP). The release of AVP is regulated by the increase of the osmolality in the plasma or by a reduction of the intravascular volume (extracellular volume). AVP causes a reduction (antidiuresis) of water excretion. In plasma osmolality of < 280 mosmol/kg H_2O the AVP release is small, in plasma osmolality of > 290 mosmol/kg H_2O release is increased to maximum levels.

Reference range

Osmolality in the plasma:	285-295 mosmol/kg H_2O
Osmolality in the urine:	50-1400 mosmol/kg H_2O

Increased urine osmolality
▶ Syndrome of inappropriate antidiuretic hormone secretion (SIADH)
▶ Acidosis
▶ Shock
▶ Hypernatremia
▶ Hepatic cirrhosis
▶ Congestive heart failure
▶ Addison's disease

Decreased urine osmolality (hyposthenuria)
▶ Diabetes insipidus
▶ Hypercalcemia
▶ Drinking excess water
▶ Renal tubular necrosis
▶ Aldosteronism
▶ Hypokalemia

Urine osmolality in renal diseases
Urine osmolality does not increase above 400-500 mosmol/kg H_2O
▶ Nephrogenic diabetes
▶ Glomerulonephritis
▶ Chronic pyelonephritis
▶ Chronic interstitial nephritis
▶ Polycystic kidneys
▶ Amyloidosis
▶ Lithium damage

Urine osmolality in polyuria
See Polyuria → 289
▶ Osmotic diuresis (urine osmolality > 400 mosmol/kg H_2O)
- Diabetes mellitus, hyperglycemia
- Chronic renal failure
- After acute renal failure
- Na^+Cl^-
- Drugs
  - Mannitol
  - Radiocontrast
▶ Water diuresis (urine osmolality < 150 mosmol/kg H_2O)

U
V

- Drinking excess water
- Primary polydipsia
- Diabetes insipidus (→ 99)

Syndrome of inappropriate antidiuretic hormone secretion (SIADH)
See SIADH → 332
No polyuria. Despite hyponatremia the osmolality of the urine is higher than the plasma osmolality. Clinical picture mainly caused through water intoxication and hyponatremia.

Urine pH

Reference range

5.5–7.0

Increased, alkalic pH

- Vegetarian diet
- Bacteriuria
- Kidney diseases
  - Renal failure
  - Renal tubular acidosis
  - Cystic kidney
  - Hydronephrosis
  - Pyelonephritis
- Metabolic, respiratory alkalosis
- Aldosteronism
  - Hyperkalemia
- Drugs
  - Acetazolamide
  - Antibiotics
  - Sodium acetate
  - Sodium bicarbonate
  - Sodium lactate

Decreased, sour pH

- Metabolic, respiratory acidosis
- Diabetes mellitus
- Increased protein catabolism
  - Starvation
  - Fever
  - Malignant tumor
  - Thyrotoxicosis
  - Burns
- Diarrhea (hypokalemia)
- Proximal-tubular acidosis

- Renal tubular acidosis type II
- Fanconi's syndrome
- Amyloidosis
- Lupus erythematosus
- Hypochloremic alkalosis (massive vomiting)
- Protein-rich diet
- Drugs
  - Methenamine mandelate
  - Methionine
  - Ammonium chloride
  - Arginine-/lysine hydrochloride

Urine sediment, See Crystalluria → 90

Urobilinogen

Natural breakdown product and intestinal metabolite of bilirubin (heme, → 51). Excreted in the urine as a pigment giving it a varying orange-red coloration

Reference range

1–3.5 mg/24 h

Increased

- Impaired liver uptake and excretion
  - Hepatitis
    - Viral hepatitis
    - Toxic hepatitis
    - Drug-induced hepatitis
  - Liver disease
    - Cirrhosis
    - Liver metastases
    - Liver infarction
    - Toxic liver damage
    - Congested liver
  - Hemolytic jaundice
  - Biliary tract obstruction
- Hemolysis (excess pigment formation)
  - Hemolytic anemia
  - Intravascular hemolysis
- Hemoglobinuria
- Pernicious anemia
- Polycythemia

Urolithiasis

Nephrolithiasis, renal calculi, kidney stones

See Nephrolithiasis → 255

Types of stones
- Calcium nephrolithiasis (75%)
- Uric acid nephrolithiasis (10-15%)
- Struvite (15-20%)
- Cystine (1%)
- Drug-induced (1%)
  - Indinavir
  - Triamterene

See Nephrolithiasis → 255

Causes
- Supersaturation of stone-forming compounds in urine
  - Hypercalciuria (most common)
  - Hyperoxaluria
  - Hyperuricosuria
- Inadequate amounts of inhibitors of stone formation
  - Hypomagnesiuria
  - Hypocitraturia
  - Low urine volume
- Chemical or physical stimuli in urine, that promote stone formation
  - Low urine pH: uric acid and cysteine are less soluble in acid urine
  - High urine pH: struvite and calcium phosphate are less soluble in alkaline urine
  - Presence of nidus for crystal precipitation
- High urinary sodium
- Other factors
  - Developmental abnormalities of the urinary tract
  - Urinary obstruction
  - Urinary stasis
  - Infection with urea-splitting microorganisms

Urticaria

Hives

Eruption of itching wheals, due to hypersensitivity to foods, drugs, foci of infection, physical agent or psychic stimuli. See Anaphylaxis → 27

Acute generalized urticaria
- Infections
  - Pharyngitis
  - GI infections
  - Genitourinary infections
  - Respiratory infections
  - Fungal infections
    - Dermatophytosis
  - Malaria
  - Amebiasis
  - Hepatitis
  - Mononucleosis
  - Coxsackievirus
  - Mycoplasmal infection
  - Infestations
    - Scabies
  - HIV
  - Parasitic infections
    - Ascariasis
    - Strongyloidiasis
    - Schistosomiasis
    - Trichinosis
- Foods
  - Shellfish
  - Fish
  - Eggs
  - Cheese
  - Chocolate
  - Nuts
  - Berries
  - Tomatoes
- Drugs, toxins, environmental factors
  - Chemicals
  - Codeine
  - Danders
  - Dust
  - Latex (!)

U
V

- Mold
- NSAIDS
- Penicillins
- Plants
- Pollens
- Salicylates
- Sulfonamides
▶ Exposure to cold or heat
▶ Emotional stress
▶ Exercise
▶ Pregnancy
  - Pruritic urticarial papules and plaques of pregnancy (PUPPP)

Chronic urticaria
▶ Cholinergic urticaria
  - Emotional stress
  - Heat
  - Exercise
▶ Systemic disease
  - Hyperthyroidism
  - SLE
  - Rheumatoid arthritis
  - Polymyositis
  - Amyloidosis
  - Polycythemia vera
  - Carcinoma
  - Lymphoma
▶ Pregnancy
▶ Cold urticaria
  - Cryoglobulinemia
  - Cryofibrinogenemia
  - Syphilis
  - Connective tissue disorder
▶ Urticaria pigmentosa

Recurrent urticaria
▶ Sun exposure (solar urticaria)
▶ Exercise (cholinergic urticaria)
▶ Emotional stress
▶ Physical stress
▶ Water (aquagenic urticaria)

Uveitis, See Red Eye → 311

Vaginal Discharge
Secretion from the vagina, vaginitis.
See Sexually Transmitted Diseases → 329

Infection
▶ Primary infection
  - Candidiasis
  - Trichomoniasis
  - Gonorrhea
  - Syphilis
  - HSV
  - Human papilloma virus
  - Chlamydia
  - HIV
  - Molluscum contagiosum
  - Sexually transmitted disease
  - Scabies
  - Granuloma inguinale
  - Pityriasis
  - Parasites
    ○ Threadworms
  - Protozoa
    ○ Amoebae
▶ Secondary infection
  - Systemic diseases
    ○ Infection
    ○ Anemia

Non-infectious causes
▶ Hypersecretion of the cervix
  - Chronic alkalization of the vagina
  - Diseases of the parametrium
  - Ectopy
  - Pelvipathia
  - Vegetative dystonia
▶ Ovarial insufficiency
  - Transient ovarial insufficiency during
    ○ Sexual maturity
    ○ Menopause
    ○ Puberty
▶ Atrophy
  - Prepubertal
  - Postmenopausal
▶ Excretions
  - Vesicovaginal fistula

- Rectovaginal fistula
▶ Serosanguinous discharge
  - Carcinoma (in vagina, cervix, endometrium or Fallopian tubes)
  - Necrotic polyp
    ◦ Fibroid polyp
    ◦ Cervical polyp
▶ Endocrine
  - Diabetes mellitus
▶ Foreign body
  - Any small object in a child
  - Intrauterine contraceptive device (IUCD)
  - Inserted foreign bodies (sexual practices)
  - Forgotten tampon
  - Incompatibility with intravaginal anticonceptives
▶ Chemicals
  - Anticonceptive drugs
  - Douches
  - Foams
▶ Miscellaneous
  - Exfoliation
  - Salpingitis
  - Hydrosalpinx
  - Corpus carcinoma
  - Endometritis
  - Descensus uteri

Drugs
▶ Antibiotics
▶ Estrogen-containing drugs

Miscellaneous
▶ Irradiation of the reproductive tract
▶ Sexual excitement (normal discharge)
▶ Emotional stress (normal discharge)
▶ During ovulation

Valve diseases, See Aortic Insufficiency → 38, See Aortic Stenosis → 39, See Mitral Valve Diseases → 242

Vasculitis

Large-sized vessel vasculitis
▶ Temporal arteritis
▶ Takayasu's arteritis

Medium-sized vessel vasculitis
▶ Polyarteritis nodosa
▶ Kawasaki disease

Small-sized vessel vasculitis
▶ Wegener's granulomatosis
▶ Churg-Strauss syndrome
▶ Microscopic polyangiitis (MPA)
▶ Henoch-Schönlein purpura
▶ Essential cryoglobulinemic vasculitis
▶ Cutaneous leukocytoclastic vasculitis

Vasoactive intestinal polypeptide
See VIP → 376

Vasogenic shock, See Shock → 329

Vasopressin (ADH, See Diabetes Insipidus → 99, See SIADH → 332

Venous thrombosis
See Thrombophilia → 351

Ventilation disorder
See Lung Disease → 228

Ventricular hypertrophy
See Hypertrophy of the Heart → 196

Vertigo
Generic term for subjective impairment of the orientation of the body in space, featured by nystagmus, nausea, vomiting and ataxia.

Central causes
▶ Vertebro-basilar insufficiency and thromboembolism

- Lateral medullary syndrome
- Subclavian steal syndrome
- Basilar migraine
▶ Central
  - CVA
  - Tumor
    ◦ Acoustic neuroma
  - Drugs
  - Aging
▶ Metabolic disorders
▶ Decreased proprioception
  - Alcoholism
  - Vitamin B_{12} deficiency
  - Diabetes mellitus
  - Visual deficit
▶ Inflammation
▶ Autoimmune disease
▶ Tertiary syphilis
▶ Vascular
  - Arteriosclerosis
  - Hypertension
  - Anemia
  - Atrial fibrillation
  - Postural hypotension
  - Syncope
▶ Brain tumour
  - Ependymoma
  - Metastasis
▶ Aura of epileptic attack
▶ Multiple sclerosis
▶ Syringobulbia

Peripheral causes
▶ Otitis
  - Serous otitis media
  - Chronic otitis media
  - Otitis externa
▶ Cholesteatoma
▶ Mastoiditis
▶ Trauma
  - Temporal bone fracture
  - Labyrinthine concussion
▶ Meniere's disease
▶ Serous labyrinthitis
▶ Infectious labyrinthitis
  - Viral labyrinthitis

- Bacterial labyrinthitis (rare)
▶ Vestibular neuronitis
▶ Benign paroxysmal positional vertigo
▶ Perilymphatic fistula
▶ Cervicogenic vertigo
▶ Cervical spondylosis

Vertigo associated with auditory symptoms
▶ Meniere's disease
▶ Acute labyrinthitis
▶ Perilymphatic fistula
▶ Ototoxic drugs
  - Aminoglycosides
▶ Cholesteatoma
▶ Acoustic neuroma
▶ Ramsay-Hunt syndrome

Vertigo associated with deafness
▶ Meniere's disease
▶ Labyrinthitis
▶ Labyrinthine trauma
▶ Acoustic neuroma
▶ Acute cochleo-vestibular dysfunction
▶ Syphilis

Drugs
▶ Anticonvulsants
  - Phenobarbital
  - Primidone
▶ Antihypertensives
▶ Diuretics
▶ Sedative

Vertigo attacks
▶ Vertigo attacks without ear symptoms
  - Relapsing, acute vestibulopathy (= acoustic nerve crisis, monosymptomatic Ménière's disease)
  - Benign paroxysmal positional vertigo
  - Orthostatic vertigo
▶ Vertigo attacks with ear symptoms
  - Ménière's disease

Vertigo with sudden onset and slow improvement
▶ Single acute vestibulopathy (= neuronopathia vestibularis, neuronitis vestibularis)

- ▶ Labyrinth apoplexy
- ▶ Brain stem injury

Chronic fluctuating vertigo
- ▶ Cervicogenic vertigo (= vertebral vertigo)
- ▶ Circulation-caused vertigo
- ▶ Relapsing labyrinthic circulation disorders (= vertebralis-basilaris insufficiency)
- ▶ Lesions of the vestibulocochlear nerve (cerebellopontine angle tumor)
  - • Acoustic neurinoma
- ▶ Multiple sclerosis
- ▶ Basal meningitis
- ▶ Infections
  - • Measles
  - • Typhoid fever
- ▶ Drugs, toxins
  - • Amidobenzene
  - • Antibiotics
  - • Barbiturates
  - • Chemotherapeutics
  - • Chloride
  - • CO
  - • Cyan
  - • Lead
  - • Mercury
  - • Nitrobenzene
  - • Phosgene
  - • Phosphorus
  - • Quinine
  - • Salicylates
- ▶ Endogenous intoxication
  - • Uremia
  - • Diabetes mellitus

Intermittent, fluctuating vertigo
- ▶ Car sickness
- ▶ Height vertigo
- ▶ Phobic vertigo

Other vertigo forms
- ▶ Cardiac diseases
  - • Cardiac dysrhythmia
  - • Cardiac valve stenosis
  - • Heart failure
- ▶ Hematologic diseases

- • Anemia
- • Hyperglobulia
- • Hypoxia
- ▶ Epilepsy
- ▶ Vigilance impairment

Permanent vertigo with abating symptomatic complex
- ▶ Neuritis vestibularis
- ▶ Traumatic labyrinth damage
- ▶ Labyrinth apoplexy
- ▶ Vertebrobasilar insufficiency
- ▶ Subclavian-steal syndrome
- ▶ Ocular vertigo
- ▶ Cervical vertigo
- ▶ Intoxications
- ▶ Kinetosis
- ▶ Advanced age
- ▶ Pychosogenic

Rotatory vertigo
- ▶ Ménière's disease
- ▶ Multiple sclerosis
- ▶ Vertebrobasilar insufficiency
- ▶ Labyrinthitis
- ▶ Trauma
- ▶ Wallenberg's syndrome
- ▶ Spondylosis cervicalis
- ▶ Vestibular neuronitis
- ▶ Cerebellopontine angle tumor
- ▶ Head trauma with labyrinth involvement
- ▶ Occlusion of labyrinth vessels
- ▶ Semicircular duct fistula
- ▶ Von Hippel-Lindau disease
- ▶ Traumatic cervical cord-brainstem syndrome
- ▶ Epidemic vertigo
- ▶ Tumor
- ▶ Drugs
  - • Alcohol
  - • Antibiotics
  - • Anticonvulsants
  - • Hypnotics

U
V

Vesicular breathing
See Breathing, Vesicular → 59

Vigilance impairment, See Coma → 79,
See Confusion → 81

VIP

Vasoactive intestinal polypeptide
Peptide found throughout the body, but in
highest concentration in the nervous
system and the gastrointestinal tract.
Increasing rates of glycogenolysis and
water and electrolyte secretion from the
pancreas and gut. Stimulating bile flow.
Inhibiting gastrin and gastric acid
secretion.

Reference range
< 30 pg/ml
Increased
▶ VIP-secreting tumors (VIPoma) leading
to Verner-Morrison syndrome (WDHA
syndrome) with watery diarrhea,
hypokalemia and achlorhydria

Virilism, See Hirsutism → 182

Vision, Blurred

**Vision impairment, diminished eyesight,
decreased vision, impaired vision**
Loss of sharpness of vision with a loss of
ability to see small details.
See Vision Loss, Acute → 376
Causes
▶ Presbyopia
▶ Cataracts
▶ Glaucoma
▶ Diabetic retinopathy
▶ Macular degeneration
▶ Infection, inflammation (keratitis) or
injury of the cornea with scarring or
perforation

• Trachoma
▶ Infections of the retina
  • Viruses (e.g. HIV)
  • Fungi
  • Parasites
▶ Periphlebitis retinae
▶ Floaters (tiny particles the vitreous)
▶ Fatigue
▶ Prolonged exposure to the outdoors
▶ Drugs
  • Anticholinergics
  • Antihistamines
  • Chloroquine
  • Clomiphene
  • Cycloplegic
  • Ethambutol
  • Glycosides
  • Guanethidine
  • Indomethacin
  • Methanol
  • Phenothiazines
  • Phenylbutazone
  • Quinine sulfate
  • Reserpine
  • Thiazide diuretics
▶ Neurologic disorders
  • Migraine (ophthalmic migraine
    without headache)
  • Chiasma syndrome
  • Multiple sclerosis
▶ Congenital disorders

Vision, double, See Diplopia → 103

Vision Loss, Acute

Amaurosis, sudden loss of vision, vision
loss, acute blindness
Trauma
▶ Chemical burns
▶ Injuries
  • Bungie cords
  • Fishing hooks
  • Racket ball
  • Fireworks

- Others
▶ After eye surgery

Ocular tumor
▶ Melanoma
▶ Retinoblastoma
▶ Optic glioma

Vascular
▶ Acute retinal artery occlusion (Amaurosis fugax)
  • Central retinal artery occlusion
  • Branch occlusion
▶ Retinal vein occlusion
  • Central retinal vein occlusion
  • Branch occlusion
▶ Temporal arteritis (giant cell arteritis)
▶ Ischemic cerebral insult
▶ Carotid insufficiency
▶ Cardiac arrhythmias

Other eye disorders
▶ Glaucoma
▶ Iritis
▶ Keratitis
▶ Corneal ulcer
▶ Optic neuritis (papillitis)
  • Multiple sclerosis
▶ Vitreous hemorrhage
▶ Retinal detachment
▶ Macular degeneration
▶ Retinitis pigmentosa

Drugs, toxins
▶ Ergotamine
▶ Lead (!)
▶ Methyl alcohol
▶ Quinine
▶ Thallium

Neurologic
▶ Increase of the intracranial pressure
▶ Migraine
▶ Focal epileptic attack
▶ Hysteria

Miscellaneous
Diabetes mellitus
Hypertension
Vitamin A deficiency

▶ Tay-Sachs disease
▶ Chlamydial conjunctivitis (trachoma)

Vision Loss, Chronic

Causes
▶ Cataract
▶ Macular degeneration
▶ Refractive errror
▶ Open-angle glaucoma
▶ Cerebral neoplasm

Vital Capacity

Maximal volume expelled after maximal inspiration. Normal adult 3000-5000 mL.

Decreased
▶ Restrictive lung desease (→ 320)

Vitamin A, See Retinol (Vitamin A) → 321

Vitamin B₁
Thiamin, antiberiberi vitamin, antineuritic vitamin

Thiamin is a water-soluble vitamin contained in milk and yeast. It is essential for growth. A deficiency is associated with beriberi and Wernicke-Korsakoff's syndrome. Wernicke-Korsakoff syndrome describes thiamine deficiency causing major organic brain disease, particularly in Western countries. There is a gradual transition between the reversible deficits of Wernicke's encephalopathy and the irreversible damage of Korsakoff's psychosis.

Reference range according to laboratory

lower limit : 15-45 µg/l
upper limit: 50-90 µg/l

Decreased
▶ Insufficient supply
  • One-sided nutrition (alcoholics)
▶ Increased demand
  • Strong physical work

U
V

- Pregnancy
- Lactation
▶ Malabsorption
▶ Maldigestion
▶ Dialysis
▶ Diuresis
- High carbohydrate intake

Increased
▶ Leukemia
▶ Hodgkin's lymphoma
▶ Polycythemia

Vitamin B$_{12}$
Cobalamin

Cobalamin is present in animal foods. Its resorption in the terminal ileum is possible in humans only if bound to the intrinsic factor secreted by the parietal mucosa cells of the stomach. In the blood cobalamin is tied to specific transport proteins (transcobalamins). The biologically active forms of vitamin B$_{12}$ catalyze reactions as coenzymes in protein and nuclein acid metabolism. The metabolism of vitamin B$_{12}$ is closely connected to the folic acid metabolism. Since the liver stores great amounts of cobalamin, a deficiency leads to clinical symptoms after 1–2 years. Vitamin B$_{12}$ deficiency causes distinctive dyserythropoietic abnormalities in the bone marrow - megaloblastic erythropoiesis - associated with abnormally large red cells in the peripheral blood i.e. macrocytosis. A serious avitaminosis leads to pernicious anemia and to the funicular myelosis.

Reference range

Vitamin B$_{12}$ deficiency	< 150 pg/ml
Adequate cobalamin supply	> 250 pg/ml
Elevated concentration	> 1000 pg/ml

Decreased
▶ Nutrition

- Strict vegetarian diet
▶ Intrinsic factor deficiency
- Genuine pernicious anemia
- Chronic atrophic gastritis
- Stomach (part) resection
- Caustic burn of the stomach mucosa
- Congenital defect of the binding of intrinsic factor
- Stomach polyposis
▶ Transcobalamin II deficiency
▶ Diseases of the terminal ileum
- Crohn's disease
- Ulcerative colitis
- Celiac sprue
- Lymphoma invasion
- Resection of the terminal ileum
- Enterocolic fistula
- Tropical sprue
- Amyloidosis
- Intestinal tuberculosis
- Exocrine pancreatic insufficiency
▶ Increased consumption, loss
- Pregnancy
- Fish tapeworm
- Bacterial colonization of the small intestine
- Chronic liver diseases
- Chronic kidney diseases

Increased
▶ Iatrogenic
- Vitamin B$_{12}$ supply
▶ Diseases of the liver
- Acute hepatitis
- Chronic hepatitis
- Hepatic tumor
  ○ Metastases
▶ Hematologic
- Leukemia
- Polycythemia

Vitamin C Deficiency
Scurvy
Risk factors
▶ Advanced age

- ▸ Alcoholism
- ▸ Mental illness
- ▸ Infant on processed milk without supplementation
- ▸ Unusual dietary habits

Vitamin D
Calciferol
Vitamin D is a fat-soluble steroid compound that is formed from provitamins in the skin under the stimulus of ultraviolet light. Hydroxylation in liver and kidney lead to the biologically active forms. The two most important calciferols are ergocalciferol (vitaminD2) and cholecalciferol (vitaminD3). They promote proper utilization of calcium and phosphorus, producing growth in children, with proper bone and tooth formation. The calciferols decrease the plasma-calcium level through increased intestinal calcium resorption and through mobilization of calcium from the bones.

Reference range

25(OH)D (calcifediol)	8-80 ng/ml
1,25(OH)$_2$D (calcitriol)	16-65 pg/ml
Children	approx. 20 % higher

Decreased
- ▸ Vitamin D deficiency
  - Lack of sun exposure (advanced age)
  - Malnutrition
  - Malabsorption
- ▸ Reduced hepatic production of 25(OH)D3
  - Severe chronic liver disease
  - Induction of hepatic P-450 enzymes (accelerating rate of degradation)
    - Carbamazepine
    - Phenytoin
- ▸ Reduced renal production of calcitriol - 1,25(OH)2 D3
  - Deficiency of 1-alpha-hydroxylase
  - Hereditary - vitamin-D dependent rickets type I

- • Chronic renal failure
- • Suppression of 1-alpha-hydroxylase action:
  - • Hypoparathyroidism
  - • Pseudohyperparathyroidism (end organ resistance)
- ▸ Resistance to calcitriol
  - • Vitamin D dependent rickets type II
- ▸ Increased vitamin D demand
  - • Children
  - • Pregnancy
  - • Lactation
- ▸ Increased metabolism
  - • Primary hyperparathyroidism
  - • Antiepileptics
- ▸ Nephrotic syndrome (excess excretion of vitamin D binding protein)
- ▸ Peritoneal dialysis

Increased
- ▸ Vitamin D hypervitaminosis
- ▸ Excessive UV light exposure
- ▸ High dose heparin-therapy

Vitamin M
See Folic Acid Deficiency → 148

Vitiligo, See Hypomelanosis → 203

VLDL Hyperlipidemia
Components: triglycerides, cholesterol and cholesterol esters. Calculation: VLDL cholesterol = (triglycerides / 5).

Reference range

10-31 mg/dl

Increased
- ▸ Idiopathic increased hepatic secretion of VLDL
- ▸ Diabetes mellitus
- ▸ Obesity

Vocal Cord Paralysis

Laryngeal nerve palsy, laryngeal paralysis, paralysis of the recurrent nerve

▶ Neoplasm
- Bronchial carcinoma with mediastinal metastases
- Mediastinal tumor
- Esophageal cancer
- Vagus neurinoma
- Tumors of the brain stem

▶ Trauma
- Intubation
- Post-surgical
  ○ Thyroid surgery
  ○ Carotid surgery
  ○ Neck dissection
  ○ Cardiac surgery
    – *Patent ductus arteriosus ligation (newborns)*
    – *Valve repair*
  ○ Tracheal surgery
  ○ Neurosurgery
- Head trauma

▶ Inflammation, infection
- Viral
  ○ Herpes simplex
  ○ Influenza viruses
- Lyme disease
- Collagen vascular disease
- Mononucleosis
- Sarcoidosis

▶ Drugs, toxins
- Alcoholism
- Arsenic
- Heavy metals
- Lead
- Mercury
- Phenytoin
- Vincristine

▶ Miscellaneous
- Diabetes mellitus
- Cerebrovascular accident

▶ DDx
- Larynx carcinoma
- Luxation or fixation (polyarthritis) of the arytenoid
- Complete vagal paresis (additional motoric and sensory dysfunctions)
- Paralysis of the four cranial nerves (glossopharyngeal nerve, vagal nerve, hypoglossal nerve, accessory nerve)
  ○ Lesions of the brain stem
  ○ Tumors of the base of the skull

Vocal Fremitus

Vibration in the chest wall, felt on palpation, produced by the spoken voice

Increased
▶ Pneumonia
▶ Atelectasis
▶ Bronchiectasia
▶ Congested lung

Decreased
▶ Obstructive atelectasis
▶ Pleural effusion
▶ Emphysema
▶ Pneumothorax

Vomiting, See Nausea, Vomiting → 252

Vulvar Pruritus

Vulvar itching. See Vulvitis → 381, See Vaginal Discharge → 372

Prepubertal girls
▶ Poor hygiene
▶ Contact dermatitis
▶ Atopic dermatitis
▶ Escherichia coli
▶ Beta-hemolytic streptococcus
▶ Scabies
▶ Pinworms
▶ Vaginal candidiasis

Young women
▶ Vaginitis, infection
- Vaginal candidiasis

- Trichomonas
- Bacterial vaginosis
- Herpes simplex virus
- Pediculosis pubis
- Scabies
- Human papillomavirus
- Molluscum contagiosum
- Tinea cruris
▶ Vulvar dermatitis
- Contact dermatitis
- Lichen simplex
- Lichen planus
- Hidradenitis suppurativa
- Psoriasis
- Seborrheic dermatitis
▶ Miscellaneous
- Vulvar intraepithelial neoplasia (papilloma virus)

Post-menopausal women
▶ Atrophic vaginitis
▶ Lichen sclerosis
▶ Paget's disease of the vulva
▶ Vulvar cancer
▶ Also causes seen in young women

Vulvitis

Inflammation of the female external genital organs, including the labia, clitoris, and the entrance to the vagina (vestibule).
See Vaginal Discharge → 372
Irritants
▶ Vaginal discharge
▶ Urine (incontinence)
▶ Other mechanical, chemical, thermal irritations
Allergies
▶ Soaps
▶ Fragrances
Infections
▶ Fungal (candida)
▶ Trichomoniasis
▶ Oxyuridae
▶ Bacterial
▶ Pediculosis

▶ Scabies
Vulvar dermatoses
▶ Chronic dermatitis
▶ Seborrhea
▶ Eczema
Systemic
▶ Low estrogen levels
- Prepubescent girls
- Postmenopausal women
▶ Diabetes mellitus
▶ Liver disease
▶ Hormone S deficiency

Warm Autoimmune Hemolytic Anemia

Autoimmune hemolytic anemia from IgG warm autoantibodies
In this form of hemolytic anemia antibodies are formed against red cell antigens resulting in premature destruction of cells.
See Anemia → 28
Causes
▶ Idiopathic (45%)
▶ AIHA associated with diseases (55%)
- Diseases of the lymphatic system
  ○ Chronic lymphatic leukemia
  ○ Other lymphomas
    - Non-Hodgkin-Lymphoma
  ○ Thymomas
- Infections
  ○ Bacterial infections
  ○ EBV
  ○ CMV
  ○ HIV
- Collagen vascular disease
  ○ Systemic lupus erythematosus
  ○ Scleroderma
  ○ Sjögren's syndrome (drying up of salivary, lacrimal and sebaceous glands)
  ○ Rheumatoid arthritis
  ○ Mixed connective tissue disease

U V

- Drug induced
- Miscellaneous diseases as a cause
  - Chronic inflammatory intestinal disease
  - Sarcoidosis
  - Pernicious anemia
  - Hashimoto thyroiditis
- Immune deficiency conditions
  - Wiskott-Aldrich syndrome
  - Hypogammaglobulinemias
  - Common variable immunodeficiency

Water diuresis
See Urine Osmolality → 369

Wax casts, See Cylindruria → 92

Weight Gain
See Obesity → 261
Causes
▶ Sedentary lifestyle
▶ Fluid overload
▶ Discontinuation of smoking
▶ Endocrine, metabolic
  - Hypothyroidism
  - Hyperinsulinism
  - Maturity-onset diabetes mellitus
  - Cushing's syndrome
  - Hypogonadism
  - Hyperprolactinemia
  - Insulinoma
  - Acromegaly
  - Hypothalamic disorder
▶ Drugs
  - Glucocorticoids
  - Nutritional supplements
  - Oral contraceptives
▶ Anxiety disorder with compulsive eating
▶ Congenital diseases
  - Prader-Willi syndrome
  - Laurence-Moon-Biedl syndrome

Weight Loss
Cachexia
See Malassimilation → 233
See Anorexia → 36
Insufficient nutrition
▶ Malnutrition
▶ Malassimilation (→ 233)
  - Maldigestion
  - Malabsorption
▶ Starvation
▶ Loss of appetite
  - Anorexia nervosa (→ 36)
  - Depression
  - Carcinoma
▶ Achalasia
▶ Stenosis in the gastrointestinal tract
▶ Chronic diseases
  - Hepatopathy
  - Renal failure
Reduced resorption
▶ Malabsorption
▶ Maldigestion
▶ Chronic diarrhea
▶ Gastrocolic fistula
▶ Celiac sprue
Losses
▶ Intestinal parasites
  - Worm infestation
▶ Intestinal fistula
▶ Hyperemesis gravidarum
▶ Diabetes mellitus
Increased demand
▶ Stress
▶ Drugs
▶ Hyperthyroidism
▶ Pheochromocytoma
▶ Leukemia
▶ Worm infestation
Psychic
▶ Psychosis
▶ Personality disorder
▶ Anorexia nervosa
▶ Depression

- Drugs/alcohol abuse

Infection
- Tuberculosis
- HIV

Gastrointestinal
- Hepatobiliar diseases
- Malassimilation
- Achalasia
- Pancreatitis
- Inflammatory bowel disease
- Cirrhosis
- After small intestine resection
- After gastrectomy
- Gastric outlet obstruction
- Carcinoid syndrome

Cardiovascular
- Heart failure
- Infectious endocarditis

Endocrine
- Hyperthyroidism
- Addison's disease
- Diabetes mellitus
- Hypopituitarism
- Carcinoid syndrome

Drugs
- Chemotherapeutics
- Drug abuse
- Hyperthyroidism factitia
- Amphetamines
- Digoxin

Systemic
- Cachexia
  - Malignant tumors
- Uremia
- Polyarteritis nodosa
- Autoimmune diseases
- Alcoholism
- Progredient muscular atrophy

Wheezing

Causes
- Asthma
  - Extrinsic
  - Intrinsic
  - Cold-induced
  - Drug-induced
    - Aspirin
    - Betablocker
    - Indomethacin
    - Tartrazine
- COPD
- Interstitial lung disease
- Infection
  - Pneumonia
  - Bronchitis
  - Bronchiolitis
  - Epiglottitis
- GERD (with aspiration)
- Aspiration
  - Foreign body
  - Gastric content
- Pulmonary embolism
- Cardiac asthma
- Anaphylaxis
- Airway obstruction
  - Neoplasm
  - Goiter
  - Edema of subcutaneous tissues
  - Hemorrhage
  - Aneurysm
  - Retropharyngeal erdema
  - Abscess
  - Congenital abnormalities
  - Strictures
  - Spasm
- Angioedema
- Carcinoid syndrome

Wound Healing, Impaired

Chronic disease
- Diabetes mellitus
- Peripheral vascular disease
- Chronic renal failure
- Leukopenia (leukopenia)
- Infection (leukopenia)
  - Hepatitis
  - Influenza

W
X

Malnutrition
- ► Weight loss
- ► Protein depletion
- ► Vitamin deficiencies
  - • Vitamin C deficiency (Scurvy)
  - • Vitamin A deficiency
  - • Vitamin B deficiency (leukopenia)
- ► Zinc deficiency

Protein deficiency
- ► Severe burns
- ► Tumor cachexia
- ► Chronic suppuration

Drugs
- ► Immunosuppressives
  - • Topical corticosteroids
  - • Systemic corticosteroids
  - • Chemotherapeutics
- ► Topical petrolatum (Vaseline)
- ► Topical antiseptics
  - • Alcohol
  - • Hexachlorophene
  - • Povidone-Iodine
  - • Hydrogen peroxide
  - • Chlorhexidine
- ► Topical hemostatic preparation
  - • Ferric subsulfate (Monsel's solution)
  - • Silver nitrate
  - • Aluminum chloride

Physiologic with advanced age

Xanthomas

Yellow nodules or plaques, especially on the skin, caused by storage of lipoproteins in macrophages.

Metabolic disorders
- ► Hypercholesterolemia
- ► Hypertriglyceridemia
- ► Glycogenosis
- ► Diabetes mellitus

Gastrointestinal disorders
- ► Chronic bile duct disease
- ► Biliary cirrhosis
- ► Chronic pancreatitis

Miscellaneous
- ► Nephrotic syndrome
- ► Myxedema (Hypothyroidism)
- ► Urticaria pigmentosa
- ► Amyloidosis
- ► Hand-Schüller-Christian disease
- ► Juvenile xanthogranuloma

Xerostomia

Dry mouth, dryness of the mouth.
With parotid gland swelling
- ► Sicca syndrome
- ► Sjögren's syndrome
- ► Heerfordt's disease

Without parotid gland swelling
- ► Drugs
  - • Alcoholism
  - • Antihistamines
  - • Antihypertensives
  - • Antiparkinsonian drugs
  - • Antispasmodics
  - • Atropine
  - • Bronchodilators
  - • Decongestants
  - • Diuretics
  - • Lithium
  - • MAO inhibitors
  - • Neuroleptics
  - • Tricyclic antidepressants
- ► Miscellaneous
  - • Alcoholism
  - • Radiation therapy
  - • Salivary gland surgery
  - • Diabetes mellitus
  - • Continuous vomiting
  - • Diarrhea
  - • Infections with high-fever
  - • Psychogenic
  - • Advanced age

Yellow-Nail syndrome
See Nail changes → 250

W
X

Zinc

Activator of various enzymes. Zinc deficiency can lead to: acrodermatitis, parakeratosis, wound healing impairment, hair loss, hypogonadism, microplasia, anemia. An intoxication leads to gastrointestinal impairment and hypochromic anemia.

Reference range

70–120 µg/dl

Decreased

▶ Nutrition
  - Parenteral nutrition
  - Alcoholism
▶ Decreased resorption
  - Acrodermatitis enteropathica
  - Ulcerative colitis
  - Crohn's disease
  - Celiac sprue
▶ Increased elimination
  - Nephrotic syndrome
▶ Faulty storage
  - Sickle cell anemia
▶ Changed zinc distribution
  - Stress
  - Infections
  - Cirrhosis
  - Myocardial infarction

Increased

▶ Iatrogenic
▶ Selfmedication

Y
Z

Medical Translator pocket

Better and easier communication with all your non-English-speaking patients!

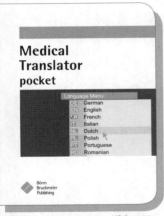

- Covers the 15 most commo languages in the US

- More than 580 ready-to-us phrases and questions used in history taking, physical examination, diagnosis, and therapy

- Easy phonetic pronunciatio for all non-English words and phrases

ISBN 978-1-59103-235-9   US $ 16.95

Drug pocket 2007

For students, residents and all other healthcare professionals

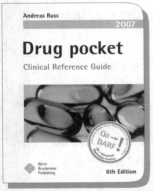

Andreas Russ
2007

Drug pocket
Clinical Reference Guide

Qo → DARF

Börm
Bruckmeier
Publishing

6th Edition

ISBN 978-1-59103-233-5   US $ 12.95

- The leading medical pocket guide, now in its sixth edition!

- Features information on more than 1,200 drugs

- Ideal for all physicians, nurses, and paramedics!

New in the 2007 edition:

- Prescription requirements and prescribing information for each individual drug

- Now includes the equation for precise calculation of dose adjustment in renal failure

- More detailed dosage information

Index

A

A2
- loud 171
Abdomen
- acute 7
Abdominal
- aortic aneurysm 32
- discomfort 5, 6
- discomfort, diffuse 5
- discomfort, epigastric and upper quadrants 5
- discomfort, left lower quadrant 6
- discomfort, left upper quadrant 5
- discomfort, lower quadrants 6
- discomfort, Mesogastrium 6
- discomfort, right lower quadrant 6
- discomfort, right upper quadrant 5
- enlargement 7
- enlargement, generalized 7
- enlargement, localized 7
- mass 7
- pain 7
- pain, extra-abdominal causes 9
- pain, in neonates, infants, and children 7
- pain, in surgical emergencies 7
- pain, in women 7
- pain, intra-abdominal causes 8
Acanthocytes 10, 132

Accident
- cerebrovascular 71
ACE 33
Achalasia 10
Aches 267
Acid phosphatase 10
Acidosis 34
- addition 11
- lactic 11
- metabolic 11
- respiratory 11, 12
- retention 12
Acneiform eruptions 105
Acrocyanosis 13
Acromegaly 13, 159
ACTH 14
Acute
- abdomen 7
- anemia 28
- coronary syndrome 86
- diarrhea 101
- glomerulonephritis 37
Acute-phase protein 72, 90
Addison
- disease 14
Addition
- acidosis 11
ADH 99
Adjustment disorder 98
ADNase 37
Adnexitis 15
Adrenal
- cortical insufficiency 14
- tumor 15
- tumor, bilateral 15
- tumor, unilateral 15
Adrenocorticotropic
- hormone 14
Adult
- respiratory distress syndrome 304
Adynamic
- ileus 207
Aerophagia 147

AFP 16
Ageusia 345
Agglutinin
- disease, cold 79
Agitation 95
Agranulocytosis 223
Agraphia 39
AIHA 47
Akinesia 277
Alanine
- aminotransferase 21
Albumin 16, 296, 297
Albuminuria 298
Alcohol
- abuse 78
- withdrawal 95
Aldosterone 17, 74
Aldosteronism 17, 186
Alexia 39
Alkaline phosphatase 17
- decreased 18
- increased 17
Alkalosis
- hypokalemic 18
- metabolic 11, 18
- respiratory 11, 19
Alopecia 19, 105
Alpha-1 Antitrypsin 20
Alpha-Fetoprotein 16
- decreased 16
- increased 16
ALT 21, 23
Alveolar
- ventilation, reduced 319
AMA 21, 36
Amaurosis 376
Amblyopia
- nocturnal 259
Amenorrhea 21
- ovarian 211
- physiologic 21
- primary 21
- secondary 21, 22
Aminotransferases 23

H

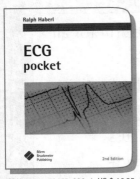
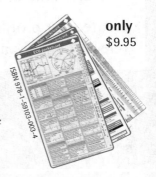

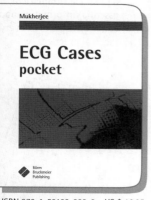

pocketcards

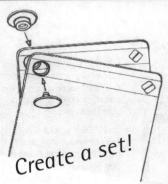

pocketcards cover vital medical information: pocket-sized, printed in color on white plastic.

Each **pocketcard** provides a practical summary of essential information about common aspects of everyday medical practice.

Create a set!

→ Alcohol Withdrawal pocketcard
→ Antibiotics pocketcard 2007
→ Antifungals pocketcard
→ ECG pocketcard
→ ECG Ruler pocketcard
→ ECG pocketcard Set (3)
→ Echocardiography pocketcard Set (2)
→ Epilepsy pocketcard Set (2)
→ Geriatrics pocketcard Set (3)
→ History & Physical Exam pocketcard
→ Medical Abbreviations pocketcard Set (2)
→ Medical Spanish pocketcard
→ Medical Spanish pocketcard Set (2)
→ Neurology pocketcard Set (2)
→ Normal Values pocketcard
→ Pediatrics pocketcard Set (3)
→ Periodic Table pocketcard
→ Psychiatry pocketcard Set (2)
→ Vision pocketcard

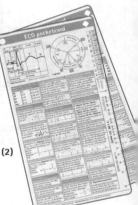

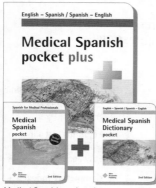

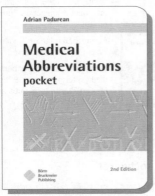

Börm Bruckmeier Publishing
PO Box 388
Ashland, OH 44805

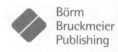

Börm
Bruckmeier
Publishing

Phone: 888-322-6657
Fax: 419-281-6883

Name		E-mail	
Address			
City		State	Zip

	Subtotal	
Sales Tax, add only for: CA 8%; OH 6.25%	+ Sales Tax	
Shipping & Handling for US address: UPS Standard: 10% of subtotal with a minimum of $5.00 UPS 2nd Day Air: 20% of subtotal with a minimum of $8.00	+ S&H	
	= Total	

Credit Card: ☐ Visa ☐ Mastercard ☐ Amex ☐ Discover
Card Number

Exp. Date   Signature

For foreign orders,
quantity rebate, optional
shipping and payment
please inquire:
service@media4u.com

Books and Pocketcards also available at ...   www.**media4u**.com

Börm Bruckmeier Products

	COPIES	PRICE/COPIES	PRICE
pockets			
Anatomy pocket		x US $ 16.95 =	
Canadian Drug pocket 2006–2007		x US $ 14.95 =	
Differential Diagnosis pocket		x US $ 14.95 =	
Drug pocket 2007		x US $ 12.95 =	
Drug pocket plus 2007		x US $ 19.95 =	
Drug Therapy pocket 2006–2007		x US $ 16.95 =	
ECG pocket		x US $ 16.95 =	
ECG Cases pocket		x US $ 16.95 =	
EMS pocket		x US $ 14.95 =	
Homeopathy pocket		x US $ 14.95 =	
Medical Abbreviations pocket		x US $ 16.95 =	
Medical Classifications pocket		x US $ 16.95 =	
Medical Spanish pocket		x US $ 16.95 =	
Medical Spanish Dictionary pocket		x US $ 16.95 =	
Medical Spanish pocket plus		x US $ 22.95 =	
Medical Translator pocket		x US $ 16.95 =	
Normal Values pocket		x US $ 12.95 =	
Respiratory pocket		x US $ 16.95 =	
pocketcards			
Alcohol Withdrawal pocketcard		x US $ 3.95 =	
Antibiotics pocketcard 2007		x US $ 3.95 =	
Antifungals pocketcard		x US $ 3.95 =	
ECG pocketcard		x US $ 3.95 =	
ECG Evaluation pocketcard		x US $ 3.95 =	
ECG Ruler pocketcard		x US $ 3.95 =	
ECG pocketcard Set (3)		x US $ 9.95 =	
Echocardiography pocketcard Set (2)		x US $ 6.95 =	
Epilepsy pocketcard Set (2)		x US $ 6.95 =	
Geriatrics pocketcard Set (3)		x US $ 9.95 =	
History & Physical Exam pocketcard		x US $ 3.95 =	
Medical Abbreviations pocketcard Set (2)		x US $ 6.95 =	
Medical Spanish pocketcard		x US $ 3.95 =	
Medical Spanish pocketcard Set (2)		x US $ 6.95 =	
Neurology pocketcard Set (2)		x US $ 6.95 =	
Normal Values pocketcard		x US $ 3.95 =	
Pediatrics pocketcard Set (3)		x US $ 9.95 =	
Periodic Table pocketcard		x US $ 3.95 =	
Psychiatry pocketcard Set (2)		x US $ 6.95 =	
Vision pocketcard		x US $ 3.95 =	